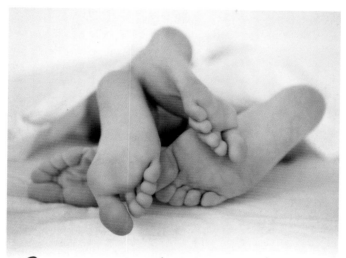

fertility & conception

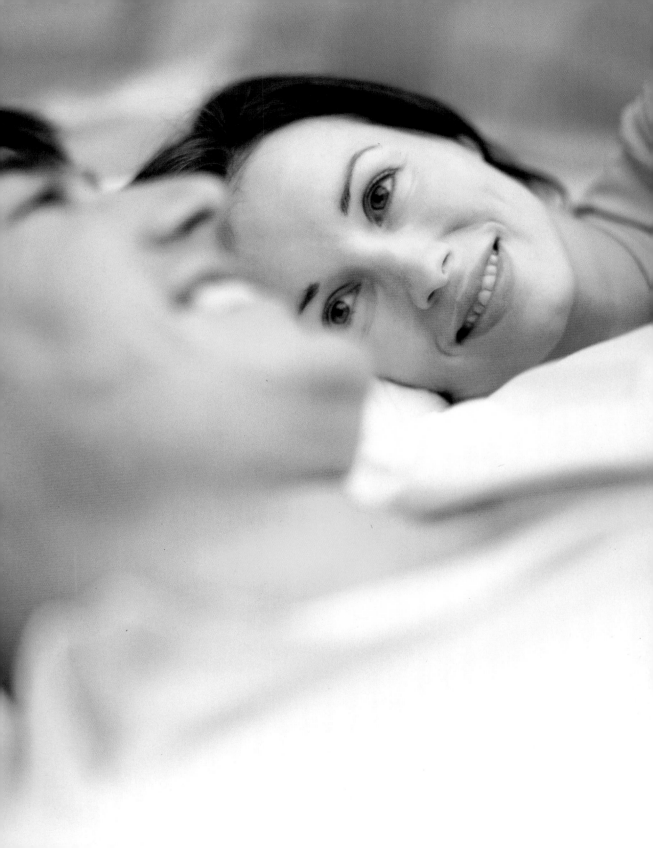

fertility & conception

conception

the complete guide to getting pregnant

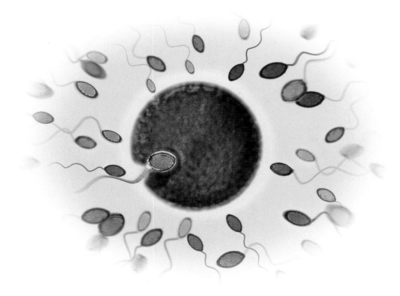

ZITA WEST

LONDON, NEW YORK, MUNICH,
MELBOURNE, DELHI

Zita West would like to dedicate this book to all the
clients she has helped over the years

Senior editors Salima Hirani, Jennifer Williams
Art editor Nicola Rodway
Project editor Jude Garlick
Editor Anne Esden
US Editor Christine Heilman
Designer Ann Burnham
DTP designer Karen Constanti
Production controller Mandy Inness
Managing editor Anna Davidson
Managing art editor Emma Forge
Picture researcher Franziska Marking
Jacket designer Chris Drew
Jacket editor Claire Tennant-Scull
Art director Carole Ash
Category publisher Corinne Roberts

First American Edition, 2004
10 9 8 7 6

Published in the United States by
DK Publishing, Inc.
375 Hudson Street
New York, New York 10014

A Cataloging-in-Publication record for this book
is available from the Library of Congress.

ISBN-13: 978-0-7894-9690-4

Reproduced by Colourscan, Singapore
Printed and bound in Singapore by Star Standard

Discover more at **www.dk.com**

contents

Sperm in a fallopian tube

foreword

Wanting a child is an instinctive desire that has deep cultural, social, and psychological implications. Over the last two and a half decades, I have dedicated most of my professional career to the treatment of patients who have trouble conceiving. The inability to conceive places an inordinate amount of stress on any relationship. This often leads to a delay in seeking much needed advice. In the process, valuable time is often wasted while the biological clock keeps on ticking. The first step towards resolution requires re-establishing control as rapidly as possible and this necessitates both knowledge and insight.

If I could make one general recommendation, it would be for every couple to have access to the information contained in this book. The author, Zita West, has succeeded in an unpretentious manner to unravel confusion and simplify otherwise complicated issues while constantly focusing on the ultimate objective of healthy parenthood. While maintaining an emphasis on providing valuable scientific information, the book also offers practical guidelines and tips on lifestyle, diet, and nutrition. For the millions of couples all over the world who want to achieve a healthy pregnancy as quickly as possible, or who are embarking on a journey from infertility to family, *Fertility and Conception* will provide an excellent road map and is a must-read.
—*Geoffrey Sher, M.D.*

Dr. Geoffrey Sher is the founder of the most far-reaching fertility practice in the United States and has been influential in the births of more than 10,000 IVF babies. Dr. Sher is the founder of The Sher Institute for Reproductive Medicine (SIRM), which is based in Las Vegas, with additional centers throughout the United States. SIRM offers the highest quality cutting edge breakthroughs in the field of assisted reproduction. Dr. Sher is the recipient of numerous awards and has published dozens of articles, abstracts, and books, including In Vitro Fertilization: The A.R.T. of Making Babies.

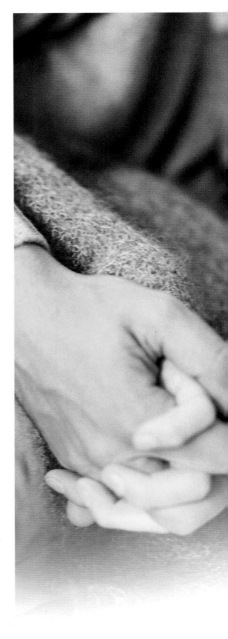

author's introduction

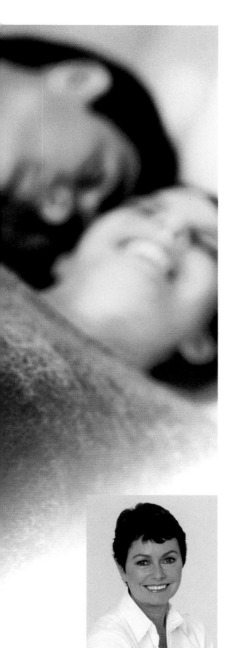

Do you see yourself with a baby? This is a question I ask all my clients when they come to the clinic.

Almost everyone can have a baby! Success depends on how far you are prepared to go to achieve it. Every couple is different in terms of what they are willing to consider, from natural conception to IVF, egg donation, surrogacy, and adoption.

My vocation is as a midwife; my deep commitment to fertility has come from that role. My passion is helping couples to focus on, plan for, and succeed in having a baby. It is a wonderful privilege to work with a couple prior to conception, get a positive pregnancy result, and look after them during pregnancy and birth.

My approach is rooted in long-held Chinese beliefs. These are based on knowledge of the human body that comes from listening, observing, and understanding natural laws and fertility cycles. In this book you will find many complementary techniques that enhance fertility and conception, combined with the very latest Western technology, making the most of ancient and modern.

If you've given all the natural methods your best shot and you're still not pregnant, I'll take you through all the options for assisted conception, with in-depth coverage of one of the most common fertility treatments: in vitro fertilization (IVF). Whatever you are faced with, remember: focus; don't give up everything; don't put your life on hold.

I do hope this book helps you to get closer to your goal of having a baby.

Zita West

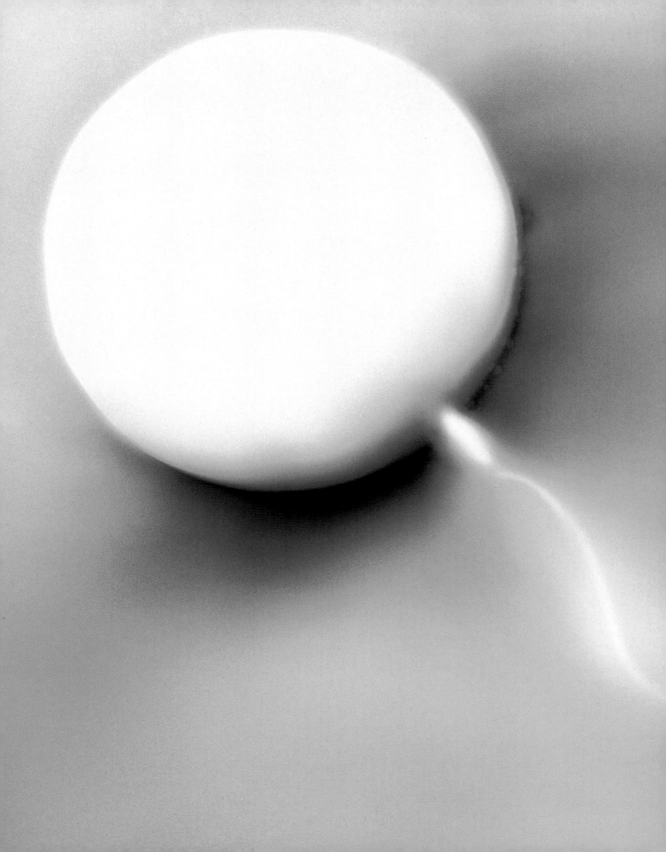

FERTILITY FACTS

MANY WOMEN AND MEN DON'T THINK MUCH ABOUT REPRODUCTION AND FERTILITY UNTIL THEY WANT A BABY. **YOU WOULD BE SURPRISED** JUST HOW MANY COUPLES I SEE WHO DO NOT FULLY APPRECIATE HOW THEIR SYSTEMS WORK. **IN KNOWLEDGE LIES THE ABILITY** TO IMPROVE YOUR OWN CHANCES OF CONCEPTION. **THE STARTING POINTS** ARE THE BASIC DETAILS OF THE FEMALE AND MALE REPRODUCTIVE SYSTEMS AND HOW THEY RELATE TO THE ALL-IMPORTANT ISSUE OF FERTILITY AND AGING.

reproduction in women

A woman's supply of eggs—several million initially—are created while she herself is in the womb. By puberty, between a quarter and half a million remain. During her life, only 400 or so of those will be released via ovulation.

HORMONES AND THE CYCLE

The ovaries are roughly the size of small plums, and they contain a lifetime's supply of immature eggs. Each month, an egg develops to maturity and is released from one ovary, ready for fertilization. The ovaries also produce estrogen and progesterone.

The average menstrual cycle is 28 days long and has two distinct phases. The first is the follicular phase, associated with the production of estrogen, which stimulates the egg to develop within the ovary until it is released (ovulation). The second is the luteal phase, associated with progesterone. During this phase the womb lining grows so that a fertilized egg can implant in it and be nourished.

THE FOLLICULAR PHASE

The first day of the menstrual cycle is the first day of bleeding (see page 12), which marks the start of the follicular phase. This is when the egg (ovum) grows and develops. Every female is born with some 2 million eggs, although only 300–400 will mature and be released during her lifetime. The nucleus of the ovum contains half the genetic material (chromosomes) needed to produce a new individual—the other half comes from the sperm.

At the start of the follicular phase, the hypothalamus in the brain (which regulates the pituitary gland) releases gonadotrophin-releasing hormone (GnRH). This signals to the pituitary gland to release follicle-stimulating hormone (FSH), which stimulates the eggs inside the ovary to grow. About 20 immature eggs respond and begin to develop within sacs known as follicles, which provide the nourishment the eggs need to grow.

As the eggs develop, the ovaries release estrogen. This hormone signals to the pituitary gland to reduce FSH production so that only enough is released to stimulate one egg to continue developing. The rest shrivel away. Estrogen also stimulates the lining of the uterus (endometrium) to begin to thicken, preparing it for implantation of the fertilized egg. The primary follicle contains the egg that has grown most rapidly. Once mature, it is about half the size of a grain of sand and is the largest cell in the human body.

The body's estrogen level continues to rise until it triggers a surge of luteinizing hormone (LH) from the pituitary gland. This stimulates ovulation, in which the follicle ruptures and the egg is gently released along with its follicular fluid onto the surface of the ovary.

THE LUTEAL PHASE

Having released the egg, the ruptured follicle continues to receive pulses of LH. This enables it to turn into a small cyst known as the corpus

Crystals of estradiol, a naturally occurring estrogen.

A mature human egg just before ovulation.

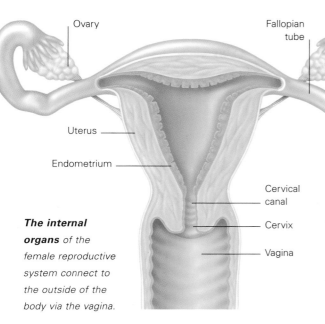

The internal organs of the female reproductive system connect to the outside of the body via the vagina.

Labels: Ovary · Fallopian tube · Uterus · Endometrium · Cervical canal · Cervix · Vagina

luteum, whose job is to produce progesterone. Progesterone has three important functions: it builds and thickens the endometrium, developing glandular structures and blood vessels that supply nutrients to the developing embryo; and it switches off production of FSH and LH. It also raises the basal body temperature (BBT) by half a degree, warming the uterus for a fertilized egg.

THE JOURNEY OF THE EGG

The egg is surrounded by a protective shell known as the zona pellucida. This in turn is surrounded by a mass of sticky cells known as the cumulus oophorous. These cells allow the fimbriae, fingerlike projections at the end of each fallopian tube, to pick up the egg and sweep it into the tube.

A fallopian tube is roughly the diameter of a pencil, with a narrow channel within it leading from the fimbriae to the uterus. The channel is lined with microscopic hairs called cilia, which,

together with muscular contractions, help to move the ovum along the tube to the uterus. The journey from the ovary to the uterus takes about six days. The egg will never complete this journey if it is not fertilized: instead, it disintegrates and is absorbed. Fertilization needs to occur within 24 hours of ovulation, making the window of opportunity quite short.

FERTILIZATION

Most healthy sperm can live in the female reproductive tract for several days, which means that intercourse can take place up to three days before ovulation and fertilization will still be possible. Cervical mucus acts as a barrier to abnormal sperm, which are unable to swim up the channels in the mucus. This ensures that only strong, well-formed sperm make it through the cervix and uterus to the fallopian tube. The journey from ejaculation to the fallopian tube takes 30–60 minutes, with many barriers along the way. It is a distance of only 4 in (10 cm).

An egg is about 550 times wider than the tiny sperm head, so it presents a large target. The sperm's first task when it reaches the egg is to get through the cumulus oophorous. Only good-quality, motile sperm are able do this, and many of them die in the process. The sperm then has to attach to the egg and penetrate the zona pellucida. This is a major barrier, four times thicker than the head of the sperm. The release of solubilizing enzymes and a change in the sperm's swimming technique—lashing its tail 800 times a second to generate sufficient force—allow it to penetrate this barrier within about four hours. Most sperm fail to attach and simply bounce off. The zona pellucida thus encourages the strongest and healthiest sperm to penetrate the egg successfully.

The lining of the fallopian tube.

The lining of the uterus (endometrium) at mid-cycle.

Once the shell is breached, the sperm sheds its tail so that only the head, the part containing the genetic information, fuses with the nucleus of the egg. The fertilized egg now contains a full complement of 46 chromosomes, which it needs to develop into a fully functioning, complete human body. A chemical reaction in the egg immediately hardens the zona pellucida so that no more sperm can get in. Cell division begins.

The fertilized egg, which is known as a zygote at this stage of development, divides into two after 36 hours (on average). It generally has four cells within 46 hours and eight cells within 54–56 hours of fertilization. The rapidly developing embryo travels along the fallopian tube for the next few days until it reaches the uterus, nourished by mucus secreted by cells in the lining of the tube.

If fertilization does not occur, the egg is absorbed by the body. Without production of the pregnancy hormone human chorionic gonadotrophin (HCG—see below), progesterone levels will fall. The endometrium begins to disintegrate, the uterus sheds the broken blood tissue through the vagina (menstruation), and the cycle begins again.

IMPLANTATION

After ovulation, as a result of a signal from luteinizing hormone (LH), a number of changes have been taking place in the lining of the uterus in preparation for implantation. Specialized structures called pinopodes develop in cells within the endometrium, creating the ideal conditions for implantation. They remove fluid from the uterine cavity to ensure good contact between the embryo and the maternal surface. The endometrium also secretes proteins that aid attachment.

By the time it reaches the uterus, the embryo has about 30 cells and is known as a blastocyst. It now starts to break out of the zona pellucida. As women age, the zona becomes tougher, making it more difficult for the embryo to hatch out. IVF (in vitro fertilization) procedures may include assisted hatching, whereby the shell is broken slightly to help the embryo to emerge.

The embryo arrives in the uterus about 4–5 days after fertilization. By this stage the endometrium is about ½ in (10 mm) thick. The more developed the blastocyst before it implants, the greater the chance of a successful pregnancy.

Implantation is aided by the uterus, which presses its back and front walls together over the embryo rather like a closed fist, holding it firmly in place until it is safely embedded in the endometrium. Part of the growing embryo soon makes contact with the mother's blood supply.

The attachment of the embryo to the endometrium stimulates the production of the pregnancy hormone HCG. This is the hormone that is detected by tests to confirm pregnancy. It stimulates the corpus luteum to continue to produce progesterone to maintain the pregnancy until the placenta produces sufficient progesterone to take over (by the 12th week of pregnancy). This then takes over the role of producing progesterone.

Sperm try to penetrate the thick surface of an egg in order to fuse with the egg nucleus.

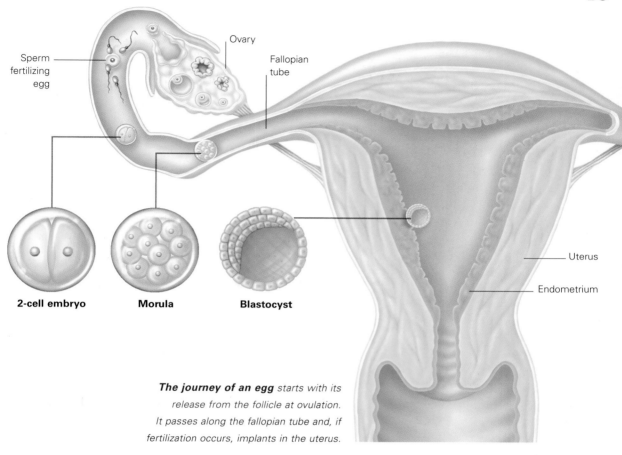

Sperm fertilizing egg

Ovary

Fallopian tube

Uterus

Endometrium

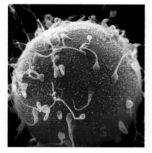

2-cell embryo

Morula

Blastocyst

The journey of an egg starts with its release from the follicle at ovulation. It passes along the fallopian tube and, if fertilization occurs, implants in the uterus.

During fertilization, the sperm—seen here as hairlike structures—attempt to penetrate the thick surface of the egg in order to fuse with its nucleus. Only one sperm will be successful in doing this.

A zygote is a fertilized egg— this is what it looks like one day after fertilization. This primitive embryo contains all the genetic material inherited from the father's sperm and the mother's ovum. It is about to start cell division.

A morula is an embryo about four days after fertilization. There has been a series of cell divisions by this time and there are about 12–16 cells present. The cells are enclosed by a very thin protein layer.

The blastocyst stage occurs at about five days after fertilization. The embryo can be seen "hatching" from a hole in the zona pellucida. At this stage an embryo consists of at least 30 cells and may have many more.

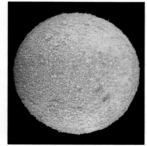

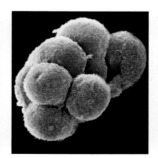

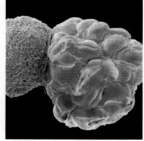

reproduction in men

Unlike women, men are fertile all the time. From puberty, they manufacture sperm constantly: an adult male produces many millions of them every day.

HORMONES AND SPERM PRODUCTION

Hormonal processes are similar in men and women. In both, the hypothalamus releases gonadotrophin-releasing hormone (GnRH). This occurs every 60 to 90 minutes in men, triggering the pituitary gland to release follicle-stimulating hormone (FSH) and luteinizing hormone (LH). A man produces FSH and LH at an even rate throughout the month, allowing sperm cells to be produced and matured constantly. So in theory, he is always fertile. This fertility does, however, depend upon a perfect balance between FSH and LH being maintained at all times.

Luteinizing hormone stimulates the leydig cells in the testes to produce testosterone. This hormone plays a very important part in several reproductive (among other) functions, including sexual arousal, the production of seminal fluid and the maturation of sperm.

The testes are roughly the same size as the ovaries and are located in the scrotal sac outside the body. They are made up of thousands of tiny coiled tubes known as seminiferous tubules. FSH stimulates spermatocytes—primary sperm cells within the tubules—to divide and develop into spermatids—young, tailless sperm. The spermatids develop here over a 72-day period, nourished by the sertoli cells lining the tubules.

During this period, each spermatid grows a head containing genetic material (chromosomes), a middle piece containing materials that generate energy for the sperm's movement, and a tail.

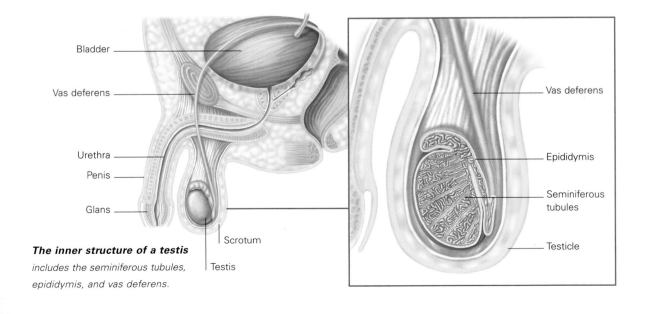

Bladder

Vas deferens

Urethra

Penis

Glans

Scrotum

Testis

Vas deferens

Epididymis

Seminiferous tubules

Testicle

The inner structure of a testis *includes the seminiferous tubules, epididymis, and vas deferens.*

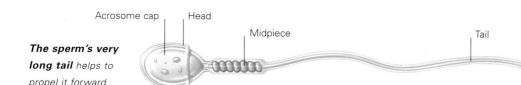

Acrosome cap   Head   Midpiece   Tail

The sperm's very long tail helps to propel it forward.

When the sperm is almost fully mature, it leaves the tubules and enters the epididymis, a long, coiled tube attached to the back of a testicle. This tube is an astonishing 18 ft (6 m) in length, but only one three-hundredth of an inch in diameter.

SPERM AND SEMEN

It takes several days for sperm to move along the length of the epididymis and develop full motility, the ability to beat their tails to propel them forward and swim in a straight line rather than around in circles. The sperm then move into the vas deferens to await ejaculation. This tube has a huge capacity—it may take about 30 ejaculations to empty the vas deferens of its full load.

The first contractions of orgasm come from the epididymis and the vas deferens, and these move sperm up into the urethra. En route, the seminal vesicles and other male accessory glands contract violently, expelling fluid. Muscular contractions of the penis then move the ejaculate (semen), which consists of the sperm plus the fluids, forcefully out through the end of the penis.

Sperm form less than 20 percent of the volume of ejaculate. The composition of semen includes more than 22 different chemicals, including fructose (sugar), vitamins B12, C, and E, the minerals potassium, sulfur, and zinc, prostaglandins and other (essential) fatty acids.

EJACULATION

Seminal fluid is ejaculated as a viscous, coagulated mass (coagulum) that usually liquefies after about 10 minutes. This protects the sperm in the hostile, acidic environment of the vagina and provides them with energy (after liquefaction) so that they have the power to swim through the cervical

FACTS ABOUT SPERM

- 380 cell divisions are needed to make one sperm, compared with only 23 cell divisions required to produce one egg.
- Up to 1,500 sperm per second are produced within each testicle.
- Sperm swim at a rate of ⅛ in (3 mm) per hour.
- Even if a man ejaculates up to 300 million sperm at a time, only about one million of them will make it as far as the cervix. Two hundred at most will make it as far as a fallopian tube and therefore have a chance of fertilizing an egg.

mucus to find an egg and then to cling to it. About 250 million sperm are ejaculated at one time. Why so many? Because they face the prospect of an incredible journey that has very many obstacles along the way. The chances are that relatively few sperm, even out of millions, will have the strength or level of fitness to complete the journey to the egg successfully.

These sperm are passing along a tube in the rete testis. This tube links the seminiferous tubules with the vas deferens.

age and fertility

Female age is a very important consideration in the probability of conception. Male age is less important, although age does have some impact on male fertility.

THINGS TO CONSIDER

There are several crucially important factors to consider when you are assessing your fertility and whether or not your age will make a difference.

Ovarian reserve The so-called biological clock has a significant impact on a woman's fertility. A woman is born with all the eggs she will ever have.

STATISTICS

The older the couple, the more difficult it becomes for them to conceive. A study in the US in 1957 found that:

- **by age 30**, 7% of couples had problems conceiving
- **by age 35**, 11% of couples had problems conceiving
- **by age 40**, 33% of couples had problems conceiving
- **by age 45**, 87% of couples had problems conceiving. Recent studies would suggest that, for a number of reasons, infertility rates are higher among couples in the US today than among those studied in the late 1950s.

O AGING AND FEMALE FERTILITY

Declining fertility is more of an issue for women than men. Assuming that ovulation occurs normally, that sexual intercourse takes place at the right time, and there are no medical or health problems, statistics show that:

- **at the age of 15**, a woman has a 40 to 50% chance of conceiving per cycle
- **at 25**, she has a 30 to 35% chance
- **at 35**, she has a 15 to 20% chance
- **at 45**, she has a 3 to 5% chance.

Her store of eggs (ovarian reserve) slowly declines with increasing age, particularly after the age of 35. The number of fertilizable eggs has run out long before a woman's last menstrual period.

Egg quality A "good egg" is defined by normal chromosomes and, once those chromosomes have combined with those from a sperm cell, the egg's ability to divide efficiently. Older women have older eggs, which may carry chromosome abnormalities, so it may take them longer to get pregnant than younger women. When they do, they are more likely to miscarry and there is a greater risk of chromosome abnormalities (such as Down's syndrome)—1 in 476 for 25 year olds, 1 in 192 for 35 year olds and 1 in 21 for 45 year olds.

Egg quality declines as a woman gets older, but you can't assess it accurately just by age. Two women of the same age can have different chances of conceiving in any given month. Furthermore, a woman of 45 may have good-quality eggs and still be fertile, while a 25-year-old woman may have poor-quality eggs and be infertile. These are extreme examples, but the point is that, although egg quality declines significantly in the late 30s and even faster in the early 40s, individuals do not always conform to statistics. Your egg quality may be average for your age, or better or worse.

There are screening tests for egg quality, but they are far from perfect. Blood tests on days 2–3 of your cycle to check levels of follicle-stimulating hormone (FSH) and the number of antral follicles (small follicles) are used by infertility specialists to assess your ovarian reserve and your eggs.

Ovulation Ovulation occurs less frequently during the perimenopause—the years leading up to the menopause. As ovulation starts to decrease, a developing follicle does not send a hormonal message to the pituitary gland, which continues to produce FSH and luteinizing hormone (LH) and levels remain high. A pregnancy is therefore less likely as estrogen levels decline and progesterone production, which only occurs after ovulation, drops off. If you suspect you are perimenopausal, ask your doctor to test your levels of estrogen, progesterone, FSH, and LH.

What can you do? If you have reached the point when you cannot get pregnant because of reduced egg quality and quantity, you might consider egg donation (see page 183). This would allow you to experience a pregnancy and give birth to your own child. There are many social, psychological, and emotional issues to consider with this route, however. Whether you try to conceive naturally or by means of assisted reproductive technology, make sure you are as healthy as possible (see chapters 2 and 3).

Vitamins and minerals may improve your chances of achieving a pregnancy. A study by doctors at Leeds University in England indicated that women can produce better eggs and boost their fertility simply by taking a daily dose of multivitamins and minerals. Researchers studied 215 women undergoing in vitro fertilization and found that women who took a daily multivitamin pill increased their chances of becoming pregnant by as much as 40 percent. It is impossible to say how many women might be helped by this, but improving your health in this way is well worth doing if you are trying to get pregnant.

AGE AND MALE FERTILITY

There is continual replenishment of sperm throughout a man's adult life, so age is not considered to pose such a threat to his fertility. The quality and quantity of sperm, however, do change with advancing age. This is partly due to a

> ### SIGNS OF REPRODUCTIVE CHANGES IN WOMEN
>
> Do not hesitate to ask your doctor for advice on potential fertility problems if:
>
> - **you notice changes in the length of your menstrual cycle:** it is either shorter or longer than usual
> - **you notice changes in your periods,** such as lighter or heavier bleeding, a different color or type of bleeding, or spotting between periods or after intercourse
> - **you have recently been breast-feeding** and you are still getting leakage from your breasts (and you are concerned about the conception of a second or subsequent baby)
> - **you are generally concerned** if you are in your mid-30s or beyond about your natural reproductive potential and/or your chances of success using assisted reproductive techniques should they be necessary.

decrease in the number of testosterone-producing cells (leydig cells). As in women, levels of FSH and LH increase, suggesting that men are subject to reproductive failure in old age. There is an increased incidence of chromosomal abnormalities in the sperm of older men, leading to an increased risk of birth defects. Sperm development (spermatogenesis) is affected in older men. Sperm count and motility also decrease, and there is an increase in the numbers of abnormal sperm.

Conditions that become more prevalent in men as they get older may contribute to a decline in sperm production and quality, either as a result of the disease itself (such as diabetes) or of the medications prescribed for it (such as drugs for hypertension). "Male menopause," or andropause, including a decline in fertility, was recently revealed in a study demonstrating that men of 35 and older are 50 percent less likely, during a 12-month period, to conceive a baby with a similarly fertile female partner than men who are younger than 25.

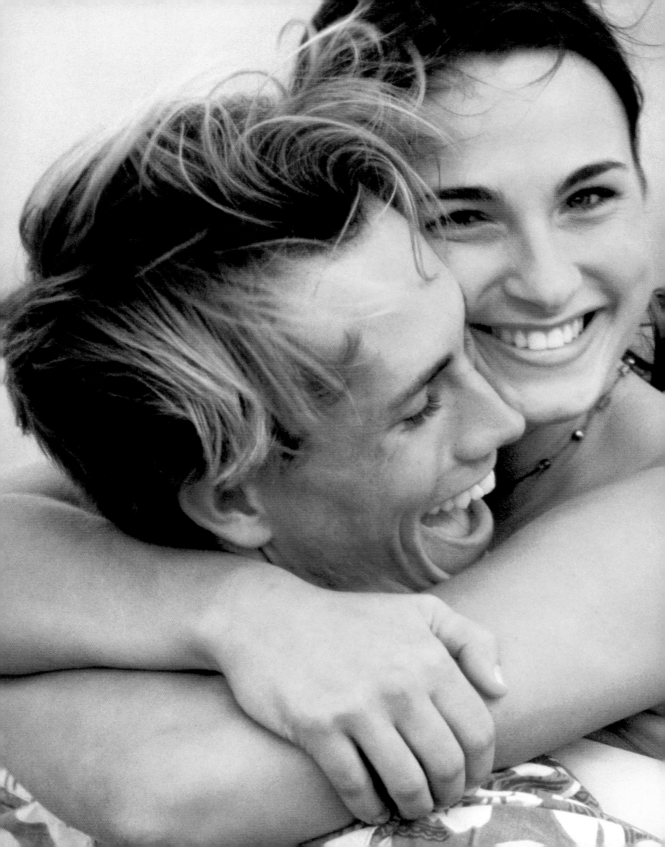

LIFESTYLE & FERTILITY

WHEN PLANNING A PREGNANCY, THE FIRST THING YOU NEED TO DO IS TO **EVALUATE YOUR PHYSICAL CONDITION** AND THAT OF YOUR PARTNER AS THESE HAVE A BIG IMPACT ON YOUR FERTILITY. BY TAKING STOCK IN THIS WAY, YOU CAN IDENTIFY THE AREAS OF YOUR LIFE IN WHICH YOU NEED TO MAKE SOME ADJUSTMENTS IN ORDER TO IMPROVE YOUR CHANCES OF **NATURAL CONCEPTION**. UNDERSTANDING THE IMPORTANCE OF THE INTERPLAY OF REPRODUCTIVE HORMONES AND BEING AWARE OF THE **FACTORS AFFECTING FERTILITY** ARE FUNDAMENTAL. ARMED WITH THIS INFORMATION, YOU CAN **IMPROVE YOUR CHANCES** OF GETTING PREGNANT.

planning for a baby

It's important to prepare yourself when you plan for a baby. You and your partner need to be in the best possible health, but you also need to be mentally prepared for what is a 15-month commitment, if you include preconception and postnatal care.

STARTING A FAMILY

So you've decided that you want a baby. Now's the time for both you and your partner to start taking a good look at your overall health and well-being. This is not only to ensure that your body is ready to nurture an unborn child, but also to give you the best chance of conceiving successfully.

But being ready physically isn't everything. You also have to prepare yourself psychologically. When you begin to plan your family, take some time to consider the following questions that I always ask my clients.

Can you see yourself with a baby in your life? As a practitioner, I feel very pleased when couples reply to this question positively, and describe how they can see themselves with a baby. I believe that it is very important to be able to visualize yourselves as part of a family unit.

ZITA'S TIPS

If you've already been trying to conceive for some time, I know that the picture of you and your partner with your own baby may have started to recede as you become more anxious. Don't give up on the dream. Make a plan to review your situation after another six months, and in the meantime, try to relax and not to put yourselves under pressure.

Have you made space and time in your life for a baby? Many women's lives are filled with work, socializing and a hundred other interests, to the extent that they simply don't have any space left over for a baby. If you and your partner have a grueling schedule, the chances are that you won't have time for sex; it will also be harder to follow a balanced diet and ensure a healthy lifestyle—all of which is vital to allow yourself a good chance of becoming pregnant. You need to create that space and time in your lives.

Have you made space in your home for a baby? Look around your home and imagine how your baby will fit in and what the baby's room will look like. If the room is cluttered, roll up your sleeves and clear a space in your home for your baby.

TRYING WHEN YOU ARE OLDER

Increasingly, women are so busy with relationships and developing their careers that the decision to have a baby is left on the back burner until they are well into their 30s. We often wait for that magical point (which hardly ever happens) when everything will be "just right."

Then the biological clock starts ticking. We find the right partner. Work is no longer our sole priority. Suddenly we want a baby—and we want it *now*. We've all grown used to getting the material things in life as and when we want them. We're accustomed to having control over most areas of our lives—and this includes our fertility.

Indeed, up until now we have spent years making sure that we don't get pregnant. We take for granted that having a baby is part of the natural order of things, so it never occurs to us that it may not happen according to plan.

NATURAL CONCEPTION

But having a baby is not absolutely in your control, and this fact can be very frustrating, especially if you've been trying to get pregnant for a while.

To help maximize your chances of a natural conception, you first need to understand how human fertility works. Many women fail to take into account the possibility that a pregnancy may not necessarily come about just because they have stopped using contraception (see page 47).

Compared with other animals, reproduction in even the most fertile humans is inefficient. Most species ovulate multiple eggs and conceive every time ovulation coincides with sexual activity. Humans have on average a 25 percent chance of conceiving each month, with most fertile couples achieving a pregnancy within one year. So, with 100 fertile couples, 20 will be pregnant after one month, 16 (20 percent of 80) after two months, and so on (see chart, below).

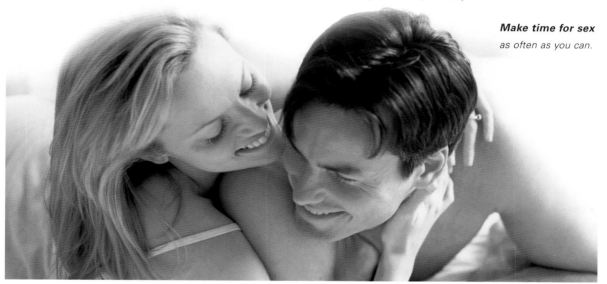

Make time for sex as often as you can.

AVERAGE CONCEPTION RATES IN FERTILE COUPLES

After a year of trying, 72–73 out of 100 couples achieve a pregnancy, at the rates set out below.

MONTH	1	2	3	4	5	6	7	8	9	10	11	12
NUMBER OF COUPLES	100	90	81	73	66	60	54	49	44	39	35	31
NUMBER PREGNANT	10	9	8	7	6	6	5	5	5	4	4	4 or 3
NUMBER NOT PREGNANT	90	81	73	66	60	54	49	44	39	35	31	27–28

self-assessment

The first step in planning a pregnancy is for you and your partner to get in shape and cut out things that undermine fertility. You need to prepare mentally and emotionally, improve your well-being, and optimize your chances of a natural conception. If you have already been trying to conceive for some time, I hope the plan in this book will help you find new encouragement.

TAKING STOCK

There are many factors that have an effect on fertility in both men and women, so evaluating your fertility status is a good place to start preparing for conception. The checks here will help you and your partner make that evaluation and decide which factors can be improved. They comprise a list of points to consider that a fertility specialist would raise, and are designed to help you pinpoint any possible problems. On consideration, if you feel you may have a fertility problem, visit your doctor or a specialist for advice and tests (see Chapter 4), so you don't waste time. For most people, these checks will help you move toward Plan A (see page 46), making the changes necessary to give you the best chance to get pregnant naturally.

YOUR FERTILITY CHECK

● **Your age** The older you become, the less fertile you are, so if you are over 35, try to conceive for no longer than six months before having fertility tests (see pages 99–103).

● **Your weight** If you are more than 10 percent under the weight recommended for your height (see page 29), hormone production may be affected. If you are overweight and find it hard to lose weight, you may have a thyroid problem (see pages 106–107). Ask your doctor for advice and have tests to check for underlying medical conditions.

● **Your contraceptive history** Contraceptive methods you have used in the past may have affected your fertility (see page 47). Intrauterine devices, for example, have been linked with pelvic inflammatory disease (see page 108). Ask for tests if you suspect any damage.

● **Your menstrual history** If your periods are irregular or absent, or if your cycle is shorter than 25 days or longer than 31 days, visit a gynecologist to have your hormone levels checked. Severe menstrual cramps may be caused by endometriosis (see pages 114–16), which will affect your fertility. Excessive bleeding may indicate fibroids (see pages 117–19). Bleeding or spotting between cycles should be checked because it may indicate a serious medical problem. You may need a smear test: talk to your doctor.

● **Your sexual history** You and your partner need to have regular sex—less than twice a week and you may not be doing it enough to get pregnant. Painful intercourse may be a symptom of endometriosis. If you have been using a lubricant, this may be blocking the movement of sperm to the cervix. If you have had previous sexual partners, you may have been exposed to sexually transmitted infections (STDs—see pages 108–112). Have a swab and blood test taken at a clinic to rule out STDs.

● **Your general physical condition** Do you have regular smear tests? If not, have one immediately. If you smoke, drink alcohol, take recreational drugs, exercise strenuously

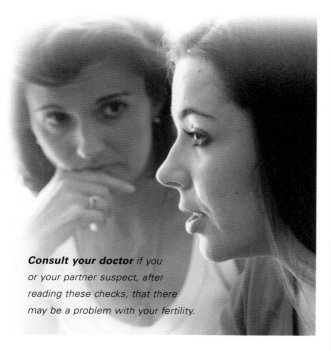

Consult your doctor if you or your partner suspect, after reading these checks, that there may be a problem with your fertility.

more than 3–4 times a week, or don't get regular exercise or adequate sleep, your fertility may be compromised.

- **Your family history** Ask your parents about their medical histories to find out if you might have inherited a tendency to low hormone production or genetic problems.

- **Previous operations, illnesses, and medical conditions** Operations on the thyroid or pituitary glands can affect fertility, as could anemia (see page 105), gynecological surgery, cancer, or ongoing medication. You need to know if you have immunity to rubella: check with your doctor.

- **Your pregnancy history** A previous pregnancy shows you can conceive, and it's likely you can repeat it. If you've had two or more miscarriages (see pages 122–23), talk to your doctor. Have tests to rule out damage to reproductive organs or infection if you've had a miscarriage, an ectopic pregnancy, or a termination with complications, or if you experience excessive, prolonged bleeding.

YOUR PARTNER'S CHECK

- **His age** Male fertility doesn't usually decline until over 50 (see page 17) but reduced sperm counts are more common today. No man should try for a baby for more than six months without a sperm test (see pages 132–37).

- **His weight** If your partner is more than 20 percent under his recommended weight, his hormone production may be affected. Obesity may be linked to other health problems, such as diabetes, which can affect fertility.

- **His general physical condition** Ideally, your partner should have a thorough physical examination. If he drinks, smokes, or takes drugs, encourage him to stop, and to get adequate sleep, relaxation, and exercise to promote healthy sperm production. He should avoid extreme diets and getting too much exercise. Wearing tight pants made of synthetic fibers during a physical workout, or the heat in steam rooms or saunas may impair sperm production.

- **History of pregnancies with previous partners** If your partner has previously fathered a child, there is every chance he can do so again if he has had no physical changes due to illness or injury. If a previous partner suffered early miscarriages, he should have his sperm checked for chromosomal defects (see page 137).

- **His sexual history** If your partner has had previous sexual partners, he should have tests to rule out STIs.

- **His family history** Your partner should ask his parents about their medical histories to see if he is likely to have abnormal hormone production or genetic problems.

- **Previous operations, illnesses, and medical conditions** Varicoceles, undescended testicles, mumps, hernia, accidental damage, serious illness, or surgery may have affected your partner's fertility (see pages 138–41). He should talk to his doctor if he is worried.

your state of mind

This is an exciting time in your life, and naturally you're eager to do all the "right" things. You may embark on lots of research and make many healthy changes, only to find that you both feel under unnecessary pressure. Always try to relax, be sensitive to each other's feelings, and enjoy plenty of sex!

MAKING CHANGES

There are many positive changes you can make to improve your fertility, as this book will show. The woman (I find it usually is the woman in a couple) starts the research, reading any literature she can find on the subject (buying books like this one, for example), investing in every vitamin supplement under the sun, and embarking on a radical regimen that involves changing her lifestyle to incorporate healthy influences and giving up many things she enjoys in life but that reduce her fertility. And she expects her partner to do the same, although many men are much more reluctant to do so.

It is important to find out as much as you can about the options open to you and the best ways to get yourself in peak condition for conception and pregnancy. Making sure you and your partner eat a well-balanced diet is, of course, vitally important for all parents-to-be. But I advise moderation. Remember that "a little of what you fancy does you good" sometimes.

COPING WITH OTHERS

Don't be self-conscious about the changes you make. Couples often worry that friends will notice they have stopped smoking or drinking and draw the obvious conclusions. But these are all things that many people do in the cause of general fitness, so don't worry that they will draw attention to a decision you'd rather remained private for now.

Because you're trying to get pregnant, it follows that you will become acutely aware of other people's bumps and babies. Suddenly they seem to be everywhere. Try not to get fixated on them. You may find yourself having to navigate through a sea of myths, rumors, advice, and tips from family and friends, or being hurt by thoughtless remarks and comments. These can be particularly difficult to cope with if you seem to be taking awhile to conceive. You know the kind of thing: "He only has to look at me and I get pregnant," or "You're lucky having all that disposable income and no kids to tie you down."

It may help to have a prepared response for the even worse direct inquiries about when you're going to have a baby or why you don't have one already. However you decide to deal with tactless inquiries, try not to lose your sense of perspective—or humor. If social events become daunting, don't isolate yourself by avoiding them.

MAINTAINING A HEALTHY RELATIONSHIP

Driving your partner crazy by nagging him to make all sorts of changes to lifestyle and eating habits is likely to put a strain on your relationship. Take things one step at a time. At the risk of making generalizations, in my experience, men are less than brilliant at taking supplements. I suggest you resist presenting him with a whole health-food store of pills and capsules, but instead find one good, all-around mineral and multivitamin so that he only has to take one pill each day.

The imperative to start a family is not always the same for the man as for his partner. However ready, willing, and supportive your partner may be, the need to conceive rarely assumes the same

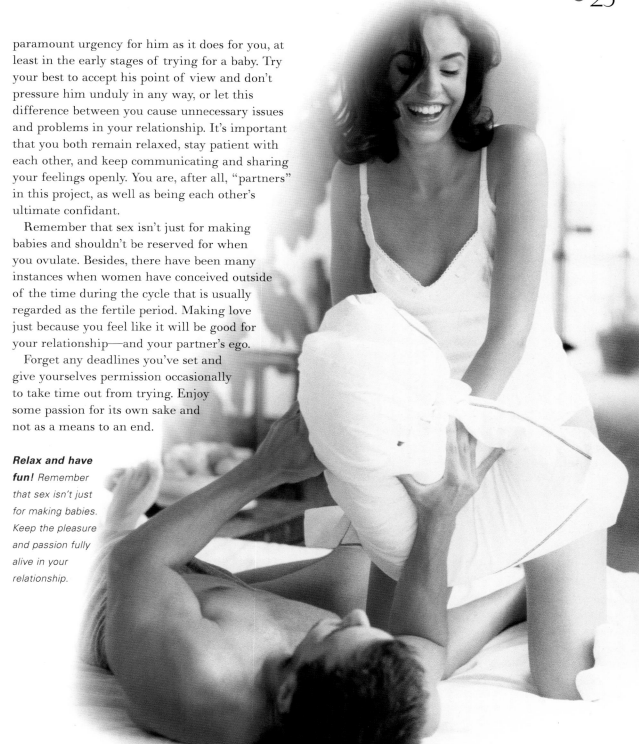

paramount urgency for him as it does for you, at least in the early stages of trying for a baby. Try your best to accept his point of view and don't pressure him unduly in any way, or let this difference between you cause unnecessary issues and problems in your relationship. It's important that you both remain relaxed, stay patient with each other, and keep communicating and sharing your feelings openly. You are, after all, "partners" in this project, as well as being each other's ultimate confidant.

Remember that sex isn't just for making babies and shouldn't be reserved for when you ovulate. Besides, there have been many instances when women have conceived outside of the time during the cycle that is usually regarded as the fertile period. Making love just because you feel like it will be good for your relationship—and your partner's ego.

Forget any deadlines you've set and give yourselves permission occasionally to take time out from trying. Enjoy some passion for its own sake and not as a means to an end.

Relax and have fun! *Remember that sex isn't just for making babies. Keep the pleasure and passion fully alive in your relationship.*

your hormones

The proper interactions between hormones are vitally important for the general health of women and men, and for their fertility in particular. Many factors can interfere with and impede these interactions, but you can also influence them for the better.

A DELICATE BALANCE

Hormones are chemical messengers, made in special glands or in the brain, that are carried around in the bloodstream to various parts of the body, where they have an effect on the functioning of organs and body processes. In the case of the female and male reproductive systems, this means the uterus, ovaries, and breasts, and the testes, respectively. Each hormone depends on the presence of correct levels of counterpart hormones at a given time in order to carry out its own special role. If the delicate interaction between hormones is adversely affected in any way, then your health may be compromised. If the hormones involved in the reproductive cycle (see pages 10–15) are similarly compromised, your fertility will be affected.

Hormonal imbalance may be triggered by many different causes. An underlying medical condition may affect your hormones, especially if it is a glandular condition such as an underactive thyroid (see pages 106–107). Reproductive dysfunction may, on the other hand, prevent hormones from functioning properly (see pages 113–123).

Dietary and lifestyle factors are common causes of hormonal imbalance. We are increasingly exposed to environmental pollutants that may seriously upset the harmony between and within our body systems. A poor diet may bring about deficiencies in the vitamins, minerals, and trace elements that have a vitally important role in the production of hormones. Smoking, drinking alcohol excessively, and taking recreational drugs further deplete our resources of these precious substances.

TESTING HORMONES

Your doctor can arrange for your hormone levels to be checked with simple tests, usually on the blood.

- **Blood tests** A blood test on days one to three of your menstrual cycle can measure levels of most of the reproductive hormones (see page 99–100). A second blood test after ovulation (on day 21 of a 28-day cycle, for example) can check progesterone levels.

- **Saliva testing** is an alternative method of checking levels of important hormones for reproduction, but it isn't used as frequently. You can take samples yourself at home and then send them to a laboratory for testing. This method needs to be done in conjunction with a doctor, who will then be able to prescribe any medication necessary once you have the test results.

DETECTING IMBALANCE

You can, however, encourage hormonal balance in the body by following dietary and lifestyle guidelines. First, you have to detect imbalance by recognizing signs and symptoms. If you have suspicions, ask your doctor for a blood test (see box, left) so he or she can help you to determine the cause of any problem. If you have a significant imbalance, dietary and lifestyle guidelines will help you only so far. You will need medical help.

diet and hormones

There are many dietary factors that influence hormonal balance. If you are overweight or eat unhealthily, your fertility may well be compromised. A healthy diet and weight will support all your body's functions, including hormone production and interaction.

YOU ARE WHAT YOU EAT

Your hormonal balance and fertility are profoundly affected by what you eat, your nutrient levels, and how well your digestion works. Hormone production may be blocked, for example, if you're short of EFAs (essential fatty acids), vitamin A, vitamin B6, zinc, magnesium, and antioxidants, resulting in an imbalance that makes conception less likely.

THE EFFECTS OF A POOR DIET

A well-balanced diet can optimize your fertility status (see pages 54–58). We'd never put second-rate fuel into our cars, because we know it would damage them and they wouldn't perform well. Junk food is second-rate fuel for our bodies. It's low in nutrients and contains pollutants and preservatives. The body has to expend valuable energy to detoxify itself when subjected to such pollutants. This added stress on the liver results in energy being diverted away from body functions not necessary for survival (such as fertility) and into the detoxification process.

Allergies that cause disruption to your digestive function will also allow your body to absorb excess pollutants (see page 28), so it is important to detect allergens and stop consuming them.

Adequate fiber and good liver function (see page 50) are vital as well because once hormones have carried out their tasks, they're taken in the blood to the liver and passed to the digestive tract for elimination. This process cannot be successful if you don't consume enough fiber, or if your liver is overburdened with a poor diet.

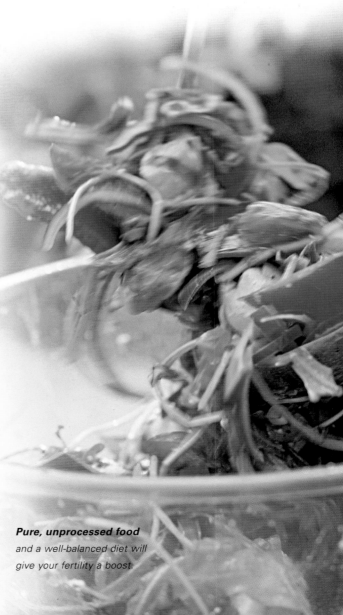

Pure, unprocessed food and a well-balanced diet will give your fertility a boost.

TESTING FOR ALLERGIES

Wheat and dairy are the most common allergens, perhaps because they form a major part of many people's daily diet. If you suspect that you might be suffering from a food allergy, consider consulting a nutritionist for advice and a comprehensive allergy screening.

○ SELF-HELP PLAN

The following plan is designed to help you identify which food or foods you might be allergic to. Cut out all wheat and dairy products from your diet.

Wheat can be replaced with:

- corn pasta, brown rice, rice cakes, oat cakes, rye biscuits, rolled oats, rice flour, millet flakes, and whole-grain cornflakes. (Beware of wheat that is hidden as an ingredient in many processed foods.)

Dairy products can be replaced with:

- rice milk, oat milk, and tofu. Eat plenty of nuts, seeds, and green leafy vegetables.

After two weeks, introduce a lot of wheat at one meal and monitor how you feel over the next few days. Try the same thing with dairy foods.

If you think you have a reaction, cut them out again for three months. If you have no reaction, reintroduce them into your diet slowly, but try not to allow levels to creep too high.

ALLERGIES

It is worth investigating whether or not you have an allergy that may be adversely affecting your digestive functions. If you find you do have an allergy and work out how to avoid the substance that triggers it, everything else will start to fall into balance, including your hormone production.

Well-known allergens such as peanuts or shellfish produce an easily identified reaction. But there are other intolerances that can seriously affect your nutritional status, undermine your general health, and provoke less specific but debilitating symptoms. Because these symptoms often don't appear for a day or two, their cause can be difficult to detect.

HEALTHY DIGESTION

A healthy gut wall is permeable, which means that it allows for the transfer of nutrients. Digested fats, proteins, carbohydrates, vitamins, minerals, phytonutrients, and water are transported into the bloodstream. A healthy gut won't allow toxins through, but they can get across into the bloodstream if there is a low intake of beneficial minerals, such as calcium, magnesium, and zinc, or if alcohol consumption is high.

LEAKY GUT SYNDROME

A weak digestive system and a leaky gut wall can be the result of repeated exposure to allergens. Certain substances (such as allergens or antibiotics) act as a local irritant to the gut wall and make it more porous and "leaky" than it should be. The leakier the gut, the more toxins enter the bloodstream. These pollutants trigger an immune system response, resulting in symptoms such as headaches, joint pain, indigestion, flatulence, heartburn, bloating, water retention, mood swings, irritability, food cravings, diarrhea, and constipation.

In a healthy gut, minerals are transported across the gut wall by protein carriers, but these can be damaged easily if the gut wall is leaky. The more permeable the gut becomes, the less the body is able to absorb minerals.

So, if you have leaky gut syndrome, no matter how many vitamins and minerals you take, you will not be able to absorb the nutrients you need unless you eliminate allergens from your diet.

DECREASED ABSORPTION

Other substances that affect the level of minerals your body absorbs include:

- high consumption of alcohol, which destroys B vitamins
- caffeine, which also robs the body of these minerals.

Wheat and dairy are major sources of phytates that bind to calcium, iron, and zinc and prevent their absorption. Even if you are not allergic to them, limit your consumption of them.

WEIGHT AND HORMONAL BALANCE

Too many women have an issue with their weight. It's important to be "the right weight," and BMI charts (see below) can be useful, but don't get fixated on them! You'll probably know if you are the wrong weight. If you have issues with food, see a counselor.

You do need to know the implications of weight for fertility. These may make you rethink your target weight, and encourage you to aim for a sensible weight at which you can stay fit and healthy. They may also make you rethink your ideal body shape: research has shown that pear-shaped women are often more fertile.

BEING OVERWEIGHT

Excess weight can lead to raised estrogen levels and prevent ovulation. Fat cells continually release estrogen, which suppresses the pituitary gland, affecting the release of FSH (follicle-stimulating hormone). Losing a small amount of weight might restore hormonal balance and stimulate ovulation.

BEING UNDERWEIGHT

Being underweight (by more than 15 percent) can also stop you from ovulating. Too little body fat may cause estrogen levels to fall and menstruation to be intermittent or even stop altogether. It may also affect the quality of cervical mucus.

FINDING THE BALANCE

If you are underweight, you should gain weight, and if you are overweight, you should lose some. Avoid crash diets at all costs. Follow the dietary and lifestyle guidelines in Chapter 3. The detox program (see pages 50–53) will clear out your liver, helping to redress any hormonal imbalance. I would advise against a radical detox program if you are trying to conceive, however.

The body mass index (BMI) is used by doctors and nutritionists to gauge your total body fat content. It is calculated by dividing your weight in kilograms by the square of your height in meters. Read the figure for one off against the other on the chart. A BMI of less than 18.5 means you are underweight, while more than 25 suggests that you are overweight.

BODY MASS INDEX

Weight (stone)	(lb)	(kg)	58	60	62	64	66	68	70	72	74	76	78
24st 4lbs	340	154	71	66	62	58	55	52	49	46	44	41	39
22st 12lbs	320	145	67	62	59	55	52	49	46	43	41	39	37
21st 6lbs	300	136	63	59	55	51	48	46	43	41	39	37	35
20st	280	127	59	55	51	48	45	43	40	38	36	34	32
18st 8lbs	260	118	54	51	48	45	42	40	37	35	33	32	30
17st 2lbs	240	109	50	47	44	41	39	36	34	33	31	29	28
15st 10lbs	220	100	46	43	40	38	36	33	32	30	28	27	25
14st 4lbs	200	90	42	39	37	34	32	30	29	27	26	24	23
12st	180	82	38	35	33	31	29	27	26	24	23	22	21
11st 6lbs	160	73	33	31	29	27	26	24	23	22	21	19	18
10st	140	63	29	27	26	24	23	21	20	19	18	17	16
8st 8lbs	120	54	25	23	22	21	19	18	17	16	15	15	14
7st 2lbs	100	45	21	20	18	17	16	15	14	14	13	12	12
5st 10lbs	80	36	17	16	15	14	13	12	11	11	10	10	9
Height (in)			58	60	62	64	66	68	70	72	74	76	78
(feet)			4'10	5'	5'2	5'4	5'6	5'8	5'10	6'	6'2	6'4	6'6
(cm)			147	152	157	163	168	173	178	183	188	193	198

KEY
- 19 or under, underweight
- 20–24, desirable weight
- 25–29, overweight
- 30–40, obese
- More than 40, severely obese

hormonal imbalance

It is imbalances between levels of estrogen and levels of progesterone that are responsible for many of today's hormonal problems. Estrogen is dominant in the first part of your cycle and progesterone in the second part (see pages 10–11).

TOO LITTLE ESTROGEN

This condition is most common in older women. The perimenopause, the years leading up to menopause, can begin at any time after your mid-30s, and sees a decline in estrogen and hence ovulation. But estrogen deficiency, particularly in the first half of the cycle, may occur if too much estrogen is removed from the body as a result of too much wheat fiber in the diet, or if too little estrogen is recycled via the bowels and liver.

Other causes of deficiency include low body weight—more than 15 percent below normal—which may cause menstruation to stop and levels of estrogen to fall; deficiency in vitamin A; excessive amounts of exercise, causing menstruation to cease and estrogen levels to fall; smoking, which alters the metabolism of estrogen so that women who smoke are likely to be estrogen deficient; taking antibiotics, which destroy the healthy bacteria that are present in the gut; and years of taking the contraceptive pill.

Symptoms of estrogen deficiency include irregular periods, vaginal dryness, painful intercourse, hot flashes and night sweats, bladder infections, dry skin, lethargy and depression, and signs of premature aging, such as memory problems.

Solutions include eating phyto-estrogens (see box, opposite) or taking low-dose natural estrogen, available from a qualified herbalist, who may also suggest herbal remedies. Para-aminobenzoic acid (PABA) is a component of vitamin B-complex and is involved in the stimulation of the pituitary gland to produce estrogen. (See page 64 for good food sources of PABA.)

TOO LITTLE PROGESTERONE

Progesterone plays a pivotal role in synchronizing the activity of other hormones. The body uses it to produce three major estrogens, testosterone, and the stress hormones cortisol and aldosterone. It helps to control water balance, it assists in the use of fat for energy, it aids proper thyroid function, and it is a natural antidepressant.

Progesterone deficiency is the most common example of hormone imbalance in women of all ages.

As with estrogen, progesterone production drops off during perimenopause, when ovulation declines. When ovulation fails, no progesterone is produced in the luteal phase (see pages 10–11), or production doesn't keep going long enough. This may happen after using the Pill, miscarriage or breast-feeding. It is known as a luteal phase defect (LPD). Pregnancy is unlikely unless the luteal phase is longer than 10 days.

Progesterone maintains a pregnancy in the beginning, so a deficiency may cause miscarriage. You are also more likely to be deficient in progesterone if you have polycystic ovary syndrome (PCOS, see pages 119–21). Progesterone deficiency may also be associated with the faulty secretion of other reproductive hormones such as FSH (follicle-stimulating hormone), LH (luteinizing hormone), or prolactin, and is linked to endometriosis (see pages 114–16) and menstrual cycle irregularities (see pages 126–28).

Symptoms include painful or lumpy breasts, headaches that are linked to your menstrual cycle, anxiety and irritability, sleeping problems, unexplained weight gain, PMS (premenstrual syndrome—see pages 126–28), bleeding between periods, and reduced libido.

Solutions might include progesterone therapy (taken orally or in a pessary), which has caused controversy among healthcare professionals. Natural progesterone cream can also be used, but only under supervision. Vitamin and mineral supplements that might help include vitamins B6 and E, magnesium, and evening primrose oil. Herbs such as *Vitex agnus-castus*, obtainable from a qualified herbalist, can help to regulate progesterone production. Useful lifestyle changes include reducing stress (see pages 40–43), not exercising excessively, and increasing low body weight.

TOO MUCH ESTROGEN

Excessive amounts of estrogen circulating in the blood are increasingly common, not because women's ovaries are making more hormones, but because of greater exposure to environmental estrogens, found in pesticides, plastics, and PCBs—chemical pollutants in water, air, and soil. These estrogens are structurally similar to the body's estrogen and, although the implications for health are not fully understood, they are believed to mimic its actions, upsetting the balance of estrogen and progesterone in men and women alike.

Poor diet, with too much refined carbohydrate and saturated animal fat and too little fiber, is also responsible. Saturated fats may stimulate the reabsorption of "old" estrogens from the bowel. A high-fiber diet helps to prevent this. Eat plenty of fresh fruit, particularly apples and pears, and vegetables, whole grains, oats, and oat bran (not wheat bran, which can irritate the intestinal lining). Buy organic produce whenever you can to minimize exposure to hormone-disrupting pesticides, antibiotics, and growth promoters. The methods the body uses to expel estrogens need optimum digestive (especially liver) function, which is compromised by poor diet and a stressful lifestyle.

A high-fat diet is, of course, linked to an increase in obesity, which has a disruptive effect on the menstrual cycle. Having too much fatty tissue in the body gives it a greater ability to convert male hormones into estrogen. Moderate exercise is beneficial to hormone balance as well as weight control.

Symptoms in women include puffiness and bloating, water retention, rapid weight gain,

PHYTOESTROGENS

Phytoestrogens are natural plant compounds that closely resemble our own estrogen, but are much weaker. They attach themselves to estrogen receptors on body cells, blocking the effects of both estrogen and environmental estrogens, while causing estrogen-like effects, but weaker ones than those of estrogen.

A diet rich in phytoestrogens can help reduce the heaviness and length of menstrual flow, correct estrogen/progesterone ratios, lengthen the luteal phase of the cycle, and inhibit an estrogen-dependent carcinogen that causes breast cancer. Phytoestrogenic foods are also rich in immunity-enhancing flavonoids, vitamins and minerals, amino acids, essential fats, and fiber.

● GOOD FOOD SOURCES

Most fruits, vegetables, grains, beans, and seeds have a degree of phytoestrogenic activity. Particularly good sources include:

- all legumes
- alfalfa sprouts and flax seeds
- oats and hops
- fennel
- parsley, cabbage, Brussels sprouts, broccoli, and radicchio
- cherries

Soy is a rich source of natural phytoestrogens, but it may also have mild contraceptive properties. It is not recommended, therefore, for women who are trying to become pregnant.

breast tenderness, heavy bleeding, mood swings—causing anxiety, depression, and weepiness—sleep problems, migraine, a flushed face, reduced libido, foggy thinking, and high levels of copper in the bloodstream. In the longer term, women may develop conditions such as endometriosis or fibroids—associated with the stimulatory effects of estrogen—gall bladder problems, poor blood-sugar control, and an underactive thyroid.

Symptoms in men include hair loss, headaches, bloating, weight gain, prostate enlargement, irritability, and breast enlargement.

Solutions include changing to a low-fat, high-fiber, nutrient-rich diet that will improve hormonal balance, reduce symptoms, and optimize conditions generally for becoming pregnant. Other dietary measures include eating live yogurt containing *Lactobacillus acidophilus* to encourage estrogen metabolism and the excretion of estrogen in particular; eating phyto-estrogens (see box, page 31) to slow down the conversion of androgens into estrogen and to prevent excess estrogens from binding to receptor sites; eating vegetables of the cabbage family, which increases the rate at which the liver converts estrogen into a water-soluble form that can be excreted; increasing protein intake to improve estrogen metabolism in the liver; and taking vitamin B6 to reduce the effects of estrogen excess. Getting more exercise will aid the excretion of estrogens, alleviate stress, and help you to lose weight if you need to.

TOO MANY MALE HORMONES

Both men and women may suffer from excess androgens, which are the male hormones, in the blood. In women, this condition is usually the result of polycystic ovary syndrome, or PCOS (see pages 119–21). Other causes are poor diet, especially one containing excessive amounts of sugar, refined foods, and simple carbohydrates; disorders of the adrenal system; the use of anabolic steroids or corticosteroids; or obesity.

Symptoms include acne, ovarian cysts—which are associated with PCOS—excess body hair, unstable blood-sugar levels, thinning hair on the head, mid-cycle pain, and erratic menstruation.

Solutions include a high-fiber vegetarian diet that's low in saturated fats and high in phyto-estrogens (see box, page 31), but you should seek medical help.

THE EFFECTS OF CORTISOL

Cortisol deficiency in both men and women is the result of the adrenal glands becoming fatigued because of long-term, low-level stress and/or poor nutrition. Whenever you react to stress, your body responds by producing the adrenal hormone cortisol. This competes for receptor sites with progesterone, making the progesterone less "active" and leading, after a long period of stress, to estrogen dominance. (Cortisol also increases estrogen production.) Too much stress will also result in the exhaustion of the adrenal glands and a deficiency of cortisol, which causes hormonal imbalance.

Symptoms of cortisol deficiency include unstable blood-sugar levels and debilitating tiredness. The tiredness is exacerbated by stress or poor diet and manifests itself in two stages. The symptoms of stage one include allergies, candidiasis, fatigue and insomnia, premenstrual syndrome (PMS), a loss of libido, susceptibility to viral infections, and low blood pressure. Stage two symptoms include alcohol intolerance, chronic fatigue and weak muscles, depression, headaches, and unstable blood-sugar levels.

Solutions include reducing your intake of stimulants such as sugar, tobacco, caffeine, and alcohol, and making sure that your diet is as healthy as possible (see pages 54–64). Use relaxation techniques to reduce stress levels (see pages 40–43) and then to keep them under control.

negative influences

Some things are good for you, while others are bad. The good things can help to protect you from the bad, but only so far. In general, avoiding the negative influences that cause damage to living cells will improve your health and fertility.

MAKING SACRIFICES

I know that many of you have probably willingly given up things that you enjoy for the sake of conceiving a healthy baby, and that you may feel as though you've been "going without" forever. There is a danger in becoming too obsessive and rigid, and "a little of what you fancy"—the occasional glass of wine, for example—will almost certainly do you no harm. But there are some things you should reduce your exposure to as much as you possibly can.

MUTAGENS

There are substances and pollutants that you may be exposed to every day, so you should understand the effect they have on your fertility. The substances to avoid are known as mutagens, so called because they can cause genetic damage. They are most damaging during the development of the egg, sperm, and embryo. The main culprits are caffeine, tobacco, alcohol, recreational and medical drugs, dietary mutagens, and environmental hazards.

CAFFEINE

Caffeine is one of the first things I ask clients to give up. The way decaffeinated coffee is processed makes that just as bad as normal coffee. Caffeine robs the body of water and valuable minerals and stimulates the body to produce cortisol (see opposite), which competes for the receptor sites of progesterone, causing deficiency. A moderate to high caffeine intake (more than 2–3 cups of coffee

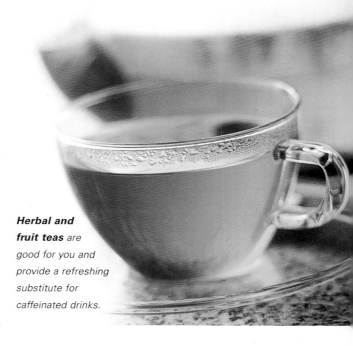

Herbal and fruit teas are *good for you and provide a refreshing substitute for caffeinated drinks.*

a day) can increase the time it takes to conceive by up to 50 percent. Caffeine is excreted more slowly during the luteal phase (see pages 10–11), which means there will be more circulating in your system during implantation and cell division.

Caffeine increases the risk of miscarriage, low birth weight, and preeclampsia. There's evidence that if the father has a high coffee intake before conception, the risk of premature birth is increased. So avoid coffee and any soft drink containing caffeine. Tea is not as bad.

SMOKING

Smoking robs the body of zinc, selenium, and vitamin C, and increases levels of cadmium and lead in the blood. Tobacco smoke contains at least 30 chemicals that can adversely affect fertility. Smoking reduces the rate of cell replication in all organs, so it may do the most damage during the first days and weeks of pregnancy.

Women who smoke are more likely to:
• be infertile
• have lower estrogen and progesterone levels
• have an inadequate LH (luteinizing hormone) surge, causing irregular or no ovulation
• take longer to conceive
• have an increased risk of miscarriage
• bleed during pregnancy
• deliver babies with low birth weight
• have an earlier menopause.

Men who smoke are likely to have:
• decreased sperm density and count
• less motile sperm (see page 136)
• an increase in abnormal sperm
• reduced testosterone
• offspring with congenital abnormalities (because of higher lead concentrations) or a higher risk of developing health problems such as asthma.

These risks increase with the number of cigarettes smoked. Also, I've found that a lot of women going through IVF (in vitro fertilization) who smoke have thinner womb linings because of reduced supplies of oxygen in the bloodstream.

ALCOHOL

Many people today think of alcohol as a great de-stresser, and it's easy to get into the habit of a glass or two of something at the end of a hard day. The benefits to your general well-being of not drinking any alcohol are considerable, however: you'll sleep better, be more focused, have more energy, and feel better all around. If you're trying to conceive, a very occasional glass of wine or the odd beer is unlikely to have a damaging effect, especially if you have it during the first half of

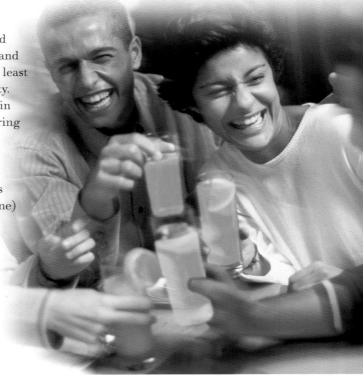

Socializing with friends is a great way to relax—even without alcohol.

your cycle. But give up alcohol completely if you can. Studies have shown that women who drink less than five units (five small glasses of wine) of alcohol a week are twice as likely to conceive within six months than women who drink a larger amount. Even as little as two units per week can increase your levels of the sex hormone prolactin, which will adversely affect hormonal balance.

Alcohol affects fertility in women by:
• reducing the body's absorption of zinc and vitamin B6 and so indirectly increasing the absorption of lead and cadmium. Zinc and B6 are both vital for the proper production of male and female sex hormones, and low levels of zinc have been overwhelmingly linked to fertility problems
• increasing the excretion of folic acid in the urine—deficiency of folic acid can lead to neural tube defects.

Alcohol is one of the most common causes of male impotence, and 80 percent of male alcoholics are sterile. It affects male fertility by:

- exposing sperm to the toxic effects of acetaldehyde, a breakdown product of alcohol metabolism
- causing chromosomal abnormalities if consumed around the time that sperm are forming (approximately three months before conception)
- causing atrophy of the tubes that carry semen
- causing a deterioration in sperm concentration and a decrease in sperm output and motility
- adversely affecting the formation of sperm tails
- increasing the production of abnormal sperm cells
- adversely affecting the body's testosterone output, damaging the liver's ability to clear used hormones, allowing female hormones to build up and depress sperm production.

However, these effects are reversible. If your partner gives up alcohol until you have conceived, there will be an improvement in his sperm profile.

RECREATIONAL DRUGS

Cocaine affects the brain chemistry responsible for releasing reproductive hormones. Many couples don't think they have a problem because they do, perhaps, only a couple of lines of coke on weekends. But *cocaine and babies don't mix.*

Cocaine has a negative influence on fertility by:

- adversely affecting the fallopian tubes and even causing birth defects
- binding to the sperm, affecting motility and causing problems at fertilization when the sperm tries to penetrate the egg.

Marijuana has an active ingredient called tetrahydrocannabinol that is chemically related to testosterone. It accumulates in the ovaries and testes. Even if used in moderate amounts, marijuana can:

- have a toxic effect on the developing egg and disrupt ovulation
- cause a low sperm count, poor sperm motility, and an increase in the number of abnormal sperm.

Smoking just one joint lowers testosterone levels and libido for up to 36 hours.

PRESCRIPTION AND NONPRESCRIPTION DRUGS AND HERBAL REMEDIES

I am always amazed at the number of people who try for a baby while taking over-the-counter or prescribed drugs without realizing the effects they have on fertility. Some are toxic to eggs and sperm. You should be aware of the effects of some commonly prescribed drugs for everyday problems:

- **painkillers** nonsteroidal anti-inflammatory drugs (NSAIDs) such as ibuprofen, with heavy use, may interfere with ovulation. Acetaminophen is safe.
- **acne relief agents** you should not take Accutane if you are considering a pregnancy; it has been linked to miscarriage and serious birth defects.
- **antibiotics** make sure you tell your doctor you are trying for a baby if you need antibiotics. Some affect sperm production or motility.
- **antidepressants** all antidepressants can interfere with the hormones involved in the reproductive cycle. Consult your doctor if you are taking these drugs while trying to conceive.
- **antihistamines** these drugs are used in cough and cold preparations to dry up nasal mucus secretions, but can have the same effect on cervical mucus. They are also used in sleep-aid products.
- **diuretics** if you experience a dry mouth as a side effect of taking these drugs, then they will probably have a drying effect on cervical mucus.
- **expectorants** these are designed to thin bronchial mucus, so making cervical mucus more stretchy, but beware of guaifenesin, which may be toxic.

DRUGS TO AVOID

The following drugs may have an adverse effect on fertility, either on cervical mucus, ovulation, or sperm count:

- antibiotics
- antihistamines
- inhalers
- sleeping pills
- Prozac
- antiviral drugs
- decongestants
- antihypertensives
- antimalarial pills
- painkillers

- **steroids** drugs such as cortisone and prednisone, used to treat conditions such as asthma and lupus, can, if taken in high doses, prevent the pituitary gland from producing enough of the hormones needed for normal ovulation.
- **anti-vertigo agents (motion-sickness pills)** like diuretics, these drugs tend to dry the mouth and therefore are likely to affect cervical mucus also.
- **antimalarial pills** these have been linked to abnormalities in embryos.

Drugs affecting male fertility include those used to treat ulcers or gout, which interfere with sperm production; some antidepressants, which may cause erection difficulties; high doses of steroids, which reduce sperm counts; and beta-blockers, used to control blood pressure, which may cause impotence and decreased sperm counts and motility.

Finally, many drugs affect the way in which the body absorbs nutrients, often causing vitamins and minerals to be excreted. If you or your partner are taking any prescribed drugs, discuss the possibility of drug–nutrient interactions with your doctor.

Herbs to avoid because of their negative effects on fertility include burdock, catnip, celery seed, chamomile, cohosh, fennel, juniper, pennyroyal, and sage. A recent study showed that St.-John's-wort, echinacea, and ginkgo biloba may reduce sperm quality and the ability of sperm to penetrate an egg.

DIETARY DANGERS

Dietary mutagens can be caused by "pyrolysis," a process that occurs when foods (especially proteins) are cooked at high temperatures. Pyrolysis adversely affects eggs and the genetic material they contain.

This damaging effect increases if food is cooked in unsaturated fats heated to over 212°F (100°C), as in grilling, barbecuing, frying, and roasting. Stick to poaching and braising using olive oil.

Many of the harmful substances produced by this pyrolysis of protein can be destroyed in the digestive tract, especially in the presence of dietary antimutagens (see Zita's Tips, page 38). But some mutagens are absorbed and penetrate all the body's

systems. Limit your intake of fish, meat, eggs, and cheese cooked at temperatures above that of boiling water, but do not eat undercooked meat or poultry.

Other factors can increase the damage caused by mutagens, including having low nutrient levels of vitamins A, B1, B2, B5, B6, B12, E, folate, vitamin C, the minerals zinc, magnesium, and selenium, and essential fatty acids. (See Zita's Tips, page 38.)

Low protein levels You may be at risk of reduced egg production if your protein levels are low and if you're deficient in individual amino acids. Low protein levels also lead to slow synthesis of DNA and result in a high percentage of embryonic deaths.

In 1989, a study of 200 women representative of all "social classes" found there was a better pregnancy outcome for those women who ate 2.6 oz (75 g) of protein daily compared with those who

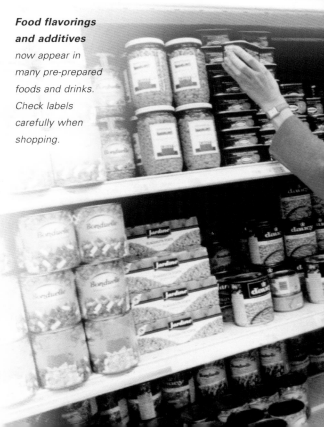

Food flavorings and additives now appear in many pre-prepared foods and drinks. Check labels carefully when shopping.

ate 2.2 oz (63 g) daily. Protein intake level was found to be most critical around the time of ovulation. The women consuming 2.6 oz (75 g) of protein daily from this time to the end of the first trimester produced babies weighing between 7.5 and 9.5 lb (3.5 and 4.5 kg) and those eating the lower-protein diet produced babies weighing less than 5.5 lb (2.5 kg).

Flavorings and additives appear in many pre-prepared foods and drinks. While 30 or 40 years ago foods came from obvious sources, many foods today are created from a vast range of chemicals.

Several thousand additives are used in food processing, but only a small percentage of these ever appear on food labels. Sulfur dioxide is a preservative that enhances the color of dried apricots, for example. Even approved additives

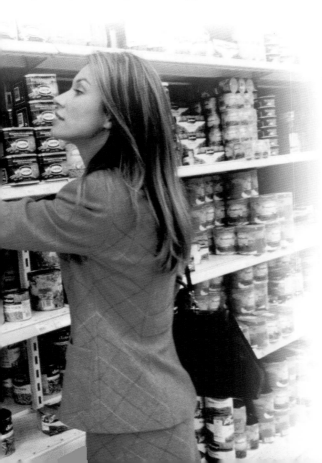

have not all been fully tested, and their effects in combination are unknown. Avoid them if you can.

Salt is necessary, but the amounts added to foods today are very high. I have noticed a direct link between salt intakes and hormonal imbalance.

Aspartame is likely to be found in any sweetener you put in your drink, and it's an ingredient in most foods that are labeled "diet" or "sugar free." When the temperature of aspartame exceeds 86°F (30°C), which it does once it is ingested, the wood alcohol in it converts to formaldehyde (a poison used to preserve body parts) and then to formic acid, which is highly toxic.

Aspartame can have an adverse effect on every stage of the reproductive process and can cause miscarriage by triggering an immune response that could destroy the fetus. Check all labels carefully and especially avoid "diet" drinks.

Monosodium glutamate (MSG) is found in a lot of food in Chinese or Mexican restaurants and prepared foods. It has been shown to cause infertility in animals. Look out for it also in flavored chips, meat seasonings, and soups.

ENVIRONMENTAL HAZARDS

Nitrous compounds, pesticides, herbicides, fertilizers, and environmental estrogens have all entered the food chain and water supply through industrial farming and as pollutants from factories. Environmental estrogens may also leach out of plastics such as plastic wrap, plastic water bottles, and food wrappers, particularly if they come into contact with fatty foods.

Every year we each eat approximately 11 lb (5 kg) of preservatives and additives, and consume one gallon of pesticides and herbicides that have been sprayed on our fruit and vegetables.

Some of this exposure is unavoidable, but eating organic food and drinking filtered or bottled water (from glass bottles) will vastly reduce your intake.

Lead is introduced into our environment through car exhaust fumes, industrial pollution, old water pipes, vegetables exposed to pollution,

ZITA'S TIPS

There are vitamins, minerals, and other nutrients you can eat to help combat the damaging effects caused by pollutants. Most are naturally occurring constituents of plants, including fruits and vegetables. Particularly effective are:

- **vitamins A, C, and E,** which are potent in the digestive tract and continue their action in the blood and around cell membranes. They are antioxidants and help to limit damage by pollutants. An excess of Vitamin A, however, can cause birth defects, so the RDA for pregnant women is under 3,000 IU

- **calcium, magnesium, selenium, and zinc,** which are powerful antimutagens (see page 33) and reduce uptake of aluminum, cadmium, lead, and mercury

- **green tea,** which contains substances known as catechins that are powerful antimutagens

- **chlorella,** which is considered to be an exceptionally broad-spectrum antimutagen supplement. A freshwater algae that is a rich source of nutrients, chlorella binds to heavy metals and chemicals that have accumulated in the body

- **cilantro,** which is a powerful heavy metal detoxifier, as well as pectin-rich foods such as apples, pears, and bananas

- **dietary fiber,** from fruit, vegetables, whole grains, oats, oat bran, and legumes, which helps in the excretion of toxins from the body. (Wheat bran can block mineral absorption.) Soak half a cup of flax-seed in juice overnight and add to food the next day.

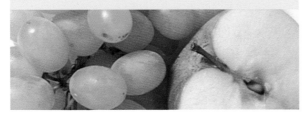

and even shampoos. High levels build up in your body if your intakes of calcium, zinc, iron, and manganese are low. Cigarette smoking is believed to increase lead uptake by as much as 25 percent.

Recent studies have revealed high percentages lead in some sperm samples. Lead is thought to be responsible for malformed sperm, low sperm counts, poor sperm motility, and altered spermatogenesis (sperm production).

In women, lead is believed to affect the quality of eggs, leading to an increased risk of infertility, miscarriage, congenital abnormality, and stillbirth.

Vitamin C may assist with the removal of lead from the body, along with pectin, which is found in apples, pears, and bananas. You would also be well advised to eat foods containing sulfur- and nitrogen-rich amino acids. These include garlic, onions, cooked beans, and eggs. Drink two quarts (liters) of bottled water a day.

Cadmium is linked to increased rates of miscarriage and embryo defects. It accumulates in the body from cigarette smoke, processed foods, and some drinking water, as well as from exposure to sewage sludge and high-phosphate fertilizer. It also builds up if you're deficient in vitamins B6, C, and D, or zinc, manganese, copper, selenium, and calcium. Taking zinc in food or supplements (see page 63) can reduce the adverse effects of cadmium.

Mercury is an extremely toxic substance that has been linked to neurological problems and slow cognitive development. It is absorbed by the body from pesticides, fungicides, industrial processes, and dental fillings, and from certain kinds of fish. The FDA warns that swordfish, king mackerel, shark, and tile fish should be avoided before and during pregnancy. The FDA also urges women to eat no more than 6 oz (170 g) of tuna per week, before and during pregnancy.

Aluminum is easily absorbed by the body and binds with other substances, destroying vitamins and causing long-term mineral loss. High levels of aluminum can lower fertility in both men and women. Major sources of aluminum in the environment are saucepans, indigestion tablets, deodorants and antiperspirants, food additives, tea, and also foods that come wrapped in foil.

Copper in high levels in the body is toxic and can reduce male and female fertility. Sources are water pipes, saucepans, jewelry, the contraceptive pill, and the copper IUD. Taking zinc with vitamin C can help to detoxify the body of copper.

Phthalates are chemicals that were used in the manufacture of soft plastics and children's toys. They are now banned, but are still found in some makeup products, toiletries, and perfumes. They can adversely affect reproduction (as hormone disrupters), so check labels on products carefully.

ADDITIONAL RISKS

There are many items used in everyday life that may, perhaps surprisingly, present a degree of risk to your fertility and general health.

Electromagnetic fields caused by cellular phones may have an affect on fertility, but this has yet to be established. So to be safe, limit your use. Don't use electric blankets: some research suggests that exposure to the current may cause miscarriage.

Tampons interrupt the free flow of blood out of the body, according to Chinese beliefs. If you need to use them on a particular occasion, buy unbleached 100 percent cotton ones (available from health stores) and, as with all tampons, change them regularly.

Botox is being used by more and more women to delay the evidence of aging on the face, but we do not know the long-term effects of this on fertility or any other aspect of health.

Flying is a tricky one. I'm often asked about the safety of flying when trying for a baby. I don't like my clients to fly once pregnant because the risk of miscarriage is greater, especially on long-haul flights. But if you're trying for a baby, the issue is whether you are pregnant but are unaware of it. Weigh up the odds and don't put your life on hold or miss out unnecessarily on getting away for a break. Avoid taking antimalarial pills.

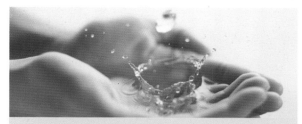

POLLUTION CONTROL

Pollution occurs in so many forms in modern life that it is impossible to avoid it altogether. But there are steps you can take to protect yourself by minimizing exposure and limiting any potential damage to your fertility. **Try taking as many of the precautions listed below as you can.** This list may be daunting, but taking any steps you can may improve your chances of conception.

○ DIETARY

Eat a balanced diet supplemented by essential vitamins and minerals (see pages 59–64). Whenever possible, buy organic, natural, and unprocessed foods. Wash, and peel if necessary, all fruits and vegetables. Avoid processed ham, bacon, preserved meats, and smoked foods because they contain nitrous compounds. Avoid canned food, unless the can has a white lining, as with cans of organic foods. The aluminum in unlined cans leaches into the product. Go on the liver detox program (see pages 50–53). Avoid copper and aluminum cookware and aluminum foil. Drink filtered or glass-bottled water: never drink water from the hot faucet.

○ ENVIRONMENTAL

Wash your hands before touching food. Avoid passive smoking. Avoid heavy traffic, and close car windows in tunnels. Refuse dental fillings containing mercury. Go outside—natural sunlight helps to eliminate toxic metals from the body and metabolizes desirable minerals. Avoid using any deodorants and antiperspirants that contain aluminum. Avoid air fresheners, hairsprays, perfumes, and shower gels that contain artificial musks or phthalates because the chemicals they carry affect hormone levels. Avoid chemical cleaning agents and garden pesticides. Do not stand near the microwave oven when it's in use.

avoiding stress

We're well equipped to deal efficiently with stressful situations, but long-term stress, too often part of 21st-century life, has an adverse effect on health—and therefore fertility.

STRESS AND THE BODY

Stress is our body's response to a "stressor." It puts us into "defense mode" by sending a message to the pituitary gland, via the hypothalamus, to start the fight-or-flight response. This response:

• activates the adrenal glands to produce adrenaline, cortisol, and DHEA (see page 42), which interferes with hormone production
• increases heart rate and blood pressure
• constricts blood vessels (restricting the blood flow necessary for making sperm)
• releases blood sugar to give us the extra energy we need to fight the saber-toothed tiger or get away fast, which interferes with hormone production.

All this happens in a split second, allowing us to deal with the situation instantly and then return to a state of balance.

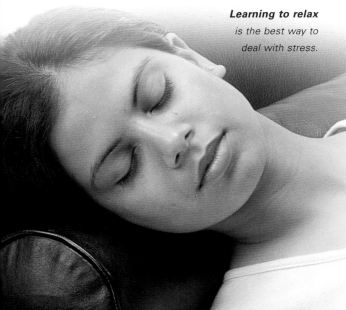

Learning to relax is the best way to deal with stress.

MODERN STRESS

Many of the stresses that people have to deal with today do not involve life-threatening situations. Most of the clients I see, both men and women, are locked into a permanent stress response that they're unable to switch off.

Many are working long hours—12- to 14-hour days—and coping with stressful situations on a daily basis. They don't have enough time to exercise, eat properly, or get sufficient sleep regularly. They drink too much alcohol and rely on nicotine and caffeine to keep them going. They barely have enough time and energy to maintain a relationship and have a regular sex life.

Complex stressors (such as job difficulties, power struggles, rush-hour traffic, or money worries) do not have a simple beginning, middle, and end, so the stress response remains switched on and we start to interpret more and more things as being stressful. Over an extended period of time, this leads to exhaustion.

It's hardly surprising that under such relentless pressure, something has to give, and very often that something is reproduction. Most of the body's energy is devoted to survival, maintenance, and essential repairs. In such extreme circumstances, reproduction falls further down the priority list.

THE ANATOMY OF STRESS

Once the body is locked into a prolonged stress response, nonessential functions start to slow down or switch off altogether, as does nonessential chemical production (metabolism). Most of the body's organs and systems are affected:

- excessive cortisol is released, upsetting the body's hormonal balance
- digestion is inhibited
- excess stomach acid is produced
- sex drive decreases
- white blood cells decrease, impairing the immune system, slowing down healing, and increasing susceptibility to infection
- blood pressure goes up
- weight is gained
- memory and concentration suffer
- excess adrenaline production leads to dopamine deficiency and depression
- vital nutrients—vitamins B and C, calcium, and magnesium—become depleted
- you feel permanently tired

Blood sugar When you're stressed, the hormones adrenaline and cortisol cause your blood-sugar (glucose) levels to rise so that you have more energy ready for the fight-or-flight response. But then the body produces more insulin to get the sugar out of the blood and into the body's cells, so the blood-sugar level falls abruptly. This is known as hypoglycemia, and a vicious cycle of sugar cravings and tiredness begins.

Twenty percent of the body's entire intake of glucose fuels the brain—which includes the pituitary gland, responsible for reproductive hormones—so this is one of the first bodily functions to be affected when glucose levels drop.

THE IMPLICATIONS FOR FERTILITY

Stress can have a profound effect on fertility. Stress hormones affect the hypothalamus and pituitary glands and reproductive organs. In women, the reproductive hormone prolactin is overproduced, and this can interfere with ovulation. The hypothalamus stops secreting GnRH (gonadotrophin-releasing hormone), which in turn will affect the release of LH (luteinizing hormone) and FSH (follicle-stimulating hormone). Because these hormones stimulate ovulation, fertility is affected.

CONTROLLING BLOOD SUGAR

There are many ways to control hypoglycemia.

○ EATING SENSIBLY

Avoid stimulants such as tea, coffee, cigarettes, alcohol, and sugar. Always eat breakfast. Eat less and more often and try to include some protein with every meal. Take a multivitamin and mineral supplement. Snack between meals, but only the right snacks! Nuts, sunflower and pumpkin seeds, rice crackers, crispbreads and oat biscuits with hummus, cottage cheese or guacamole, fresh fruits, bananas with live yogurt are ideal. Often just a little will be enough to satisfy any cravings you may have.

○ THINGS TO TRY

Mix protein and carbohydrates in the same meal as this gives a gradual release of glucose into the bloodstream. You will feel fuller for longer and consequently have more energy. Eat complex carbohydrates—brown, dense, and grainy with all the vitamins, minerals, and fiber retained. Eat fresh fruit and vegetables, either raw in salads or as snacks between meals, or steamed, baked, or stir-fried. Add a little unsaturated fat to meals—such as avocado, olives, almonds, peanuts, sunflower seeds, pine nuts, and cold-pressed organic olive oil. Dress vegetables and salads in olive oil, lemon juice, black pepper, and fresh herbs and seeds. Eat peas and beans—such as kidney, flageolet, cannellini, and butter beans. They are a ready-made mixture of protein and carbohydrates. Add them to casseroles, soups, and salads.

○ THINGS TO AVOID

Avoid processed or refined foods—such as sugary cakes, biscuits and sweets, soft drinks, "juice drinks," white bread, rice, and pasta. These are quickly digested, causing your blood sugar to rise rapidly, prompting an increase in insulin production. This will cause your blood sugar to then fall quickly, leaving you tired and low in energy, soon craving another sweet "fix." A steady release of energy is needed to maintain your energy levels throughout the day. Always read the labels. Avoid eating fruit after meals as this can sometimes cause bloating in sensitive digestive systems.

Menstruation may become irregular and the luteal phase of the cycle may be disrupted. In men, the sperm count goes down. Semen samples from men under stress show a decrease in volume and greater numbers of sperm with abnormalities.

Stress can also cause a drop in levels of DHEA (dehydroepiandrosterone), which is converted into other hormones. This, together with the cortisol (see page 32) released when you are stressed, may bring about hormonal imbalance such as too high an estrogen level (see page 31), affecting fertility.

DEALING WITH STRESS

If your body is locked into a stress state, you need to address the causes before trying to get rid of the symptoms. Think of it as a paper jam in a printer: even when the paper is removed, the machine won't work because it is still registering a jam. It has to be switched off and on, or reset.

Similarly, you need to develop a strategy to help identify and deal with the causes of stress in your life. Write them down, then decide how best to manage them *realistically*. Remember that stress is caused by a reaction to a situation, not the situation itself. Everything depends on how you interpret it and respond to it.

The most common stress factors are:

- work—don't give it up, but do try to cut back your hours and perhaps your level of responsibility, or learn to delegate
- your relationship—it's vital to talk to your partner if you are to give and receive mutual support
- failure to conceive—this produces a vicious circle of alternating hope and anxiety. Limit the time you spend thinking about having a baby each day

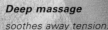

Deep massage
soothes away tension.

- coping with fertility treatment—deciding what the next steps should be, how long to continue with it and worrying about the cost. Carry out research and try to remain philosophical, for the sake of your own health and fertility

SELF-HELP STRESS RELIEF

There are a number of ways in which you can help yourself feel some release from the stresses and strains of daily life.

Exercise Regular exercise is the best way to relieve stress and improve your general health and sense of well-being.

Massage This is a wonderful way of easing tension from the body. Deep massage releases long-held levels of stress and promotes a profound feeling of relaxation.

Deep-breathing techniques Breathing is involuntary, but how we breathe reflects our state of mind and emotion. Very few of us breathe deeply enough, especially when we are stressed. When relaxed, we breathe deeply, the lungs fill easily and more oxygen is exchanged. Consciously breathe slowly, deeply, and smoothly.

Dao yin is a Chinese system of breathing (and exercise) that helps you to relax, thereby reducing tension and stress, as well as allowing your *qi* (life energy) to circulate more freely, unblocking meridians, balancing yin and yang (see page 72), and charging the kidneys—believed by the Chinese to have an important association with reproduction—with vital energy.

Lie comfortably on the floor and make your breathing soft, slow, and continuous. Breathe in through your nose for a count of eight, then out (also through the nose) for a count of eight. Practice this for one week until it becomes natural. Once you've mastered the breathing, focus your mind on the palm of your hand and slowly move your focus along the meridians, finally coming to rest on the conception vessel (see diagram, page 73). Do this exercise for ten minutes every day.

Visualization Some people believe that what you think will happen to you has a powerful effect on what eventually does happen to you. Remind yourself that the body heals and repairs itself, and put positive thoughts about health, fertility, and conception into your brain. Send thoughts of health and strength to every cell of your body. Refuse to allow negative thoughts into your mind. Positive thoughts will encourage you to do what you have to do, so be an optimist. You will feel better for it.

Transcendental meditation (TM) The physiological effects of TM include a drop in the metabolic rate, which stress revs up. Taking a short course to learn TM can be an investment for life.

Aromatherapy Add drops of an essential oil such as chamomile, lavender, neroli, mandarin, rose, ylang-ylang, or sandalwood to a base oil used for massage. Diffuse calming vapors around the room with a few drops of essential oil on a lightbulb ring or a tissue placed on a hot radiator. A couple of drops in the bath will give you a relaxing soak.

Bach Flower Remedies These are available from drugstores or health-food stores and may help stress and emotional problems (see page 147). Add a few drops of an appropriate remedy to water.

ZITA'S TIPS

It may sound obvious, but adequate, regular sleep is essential if the body is to rest, renew, and repair itself. If you have trouble sleeping, try any of the tips below to help you set up positive sleeping habits.

- **Get up at the same time every day,** regardless of how much sleep you have had or what time you went to bed.

- **Try to go to bed at the same time** every evening to get your body into a regular rhythm.

- **Try going to bed half an hour earlier** for a week to see if this makes you feel better.

- **Keep the bedroom quiet and cool,** with an open window, if possible.

- **Keep the bedroom as dark as possible** so the brain registers that it's time to sleep.

- **Keep the bedroom for resting,** sleeping, and lovemaking—no phones, computers, or piles of papers should distract or disturb you.

- **If you don't fall asleep** within 30 minutes of trying, get up again for a little while. Take a walk around the house, make yourself a warm drink, and maybe listen to some soothing music.

- **Limit a daytime nap** to 30 minutes.

- **Take a hot bath with lavender oil** 90 minutes before you go to bed.

- **Try to eat dinner before 7 PM** so that your meal is digested by the time you go to bed.

- **Avoid caffeine and alcohol** for at least 5 hours before bedtime.

- **Get some fresh air and exercise** every day.

- **Talk through any problems or fertility issues** with your partner before you go to bed.

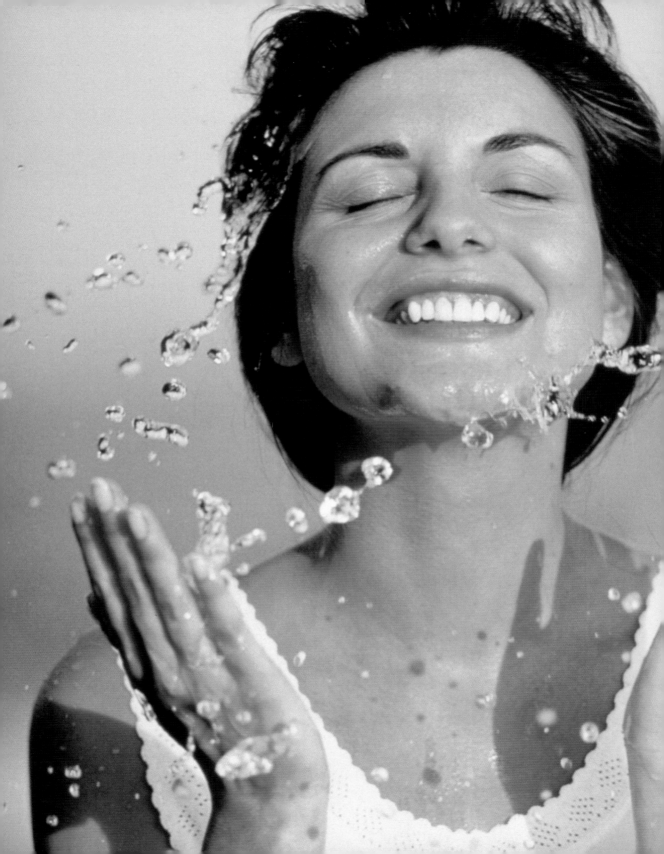

NATURAL CONCEPTION

INVESTING TIME AND ENERGY IN **PRECONCEPTION CARE** IS A GOOD PLAN IF YOU WANT TO GET PREGNANT. **SPEND AT LEAST THREE MONTHS** IMPROVING YOUR FERTILITY STATUS BY ADJUSTING YOUR DIET SO THAT IT SUPPLIES **ESSENTIAL NUTRIENTS TO BOOST FERTILITY,** GETTING ADEQUATE AMOUNTS OF EXERCISE, MANAGING STRESS, AND REDUCING YOUR EXPOSURE TO ALL THE THINGS THAT COMPROMISE FERTILITY. YOU ALSO NEED TO GET TO KNOW YOUR CYCLE SO THAT YOU CAN IDENTIFY YOUR FERTILE TIME AND, DURING THE **COUNTDOWN TO CONCEPTION,** DO EVERYTHING YOU CAN TO MAXIMIZE YOUR CHANCES OF CONCEIVING.

plan A

Now that you know how fertility can be compromised, you will appreciate how lifestyle changes you and your partner make over the coming months will make a difference as you put Plan A—natural conception—into practice.

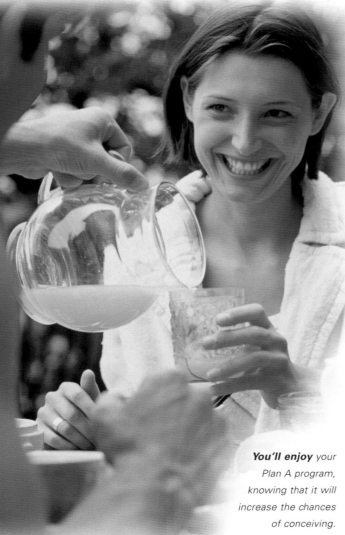

You'll enjoy your Plan A program, knowing that it will increase the chances of conceiving.

TAKING THE FIRST STEPS

You need to consider making lifestyle changes to enhance your fertility status. These will include getting regular exercise (but not too much); following a healthy eating plan, which may include taking nutritional supplements to balance your hormones and get all your body systems functioning as well as possible; and losing or gaining weight, if necessary.

Work to reduce your stress levels and use complementary therapies to increase your general health and sense of well-being. Acupuncture may be of great benefit in this respect, and it may also enhance your fertility (see pages 72–73). You might like to consider seeing an acupuncturist regularly while you are trying to conceive.

Research indicates that, if you have been taking the contraceptive pill, you may be very fertile for a while immediately after you stop taking it (see opposite), so don't miss this opportunity to conceive.

Meanwhile, your partner should also get himself in shape. He, too, can start with a healthy eating plan and use the guidelines for physical fitness and a balanced diet that will enhance his general health as well as his sperm production.

It is very exciting to start trying for a baby by looking at and then improving significant areas of your life—physically, nutritionally, and emotionally. Understanding your fertility and having frequent sex—and I cannot stress enough the importance of the latter—is a good foundation for successful conception and pregnancy.

contraception

You may think this is the last thing you need to think about when you're trying for a baby, but it is possible that any invasive methods of contraception you've used in the past may have had an impact on your fertility, so you need to plan accordingly.

THE PILL

The contraceptive pill works by preventing ovulation, altering the natural balance of estrogen and progesterone and inhibiting production of LH (luteinizing hormone). Cervical mucus becomes hostile to sperm, and the endometrium becomes too thin for implantation.

The Pill contains progestogens (synthetic progesterone) and estrogens whose molecules are similar to natural hormones, but are present in greater amounts.

One in 200 women finds her periods stop when she comes off the Pill: others, used to having scant 2–3-day bleeds while taking the Pill, may find their periods are now heavier. The Pill depletes zinc and magnesium, upsets the balance of zinc and copper, and depletes vitamin A (see pages 59–63). Long-term use may weaken the immune system and exacerbate allergies. Young women are advised to think carefully about the Pill as a long-term contraceptive method.

Recent research now suggests that, with modern contraceptive pills, conception rates are often higher immediately after women stop taking them. Then the rates dip considerably and do not return to pre-Pill levels for as long as 18 months.

Careful vitamin and mineral supplementation will help to correct nutritional imbalances. Follow Plan A for three months while you are still taking the Pill, in case you become pregnant quickly after stopping it.

CONTRACEPTIVE INJECTION

This is a hormonal injection given every three months, and is much like the progesterone that a woman produces during the last two weeks of every cycle. Women using contraceptive injections tend to bleed less and suffer less cramping, and, after three or so injections, may stop having periods altogether. It can take from a few months to well over a year—and commonly takes about 12 months—for your periods to return to normal once you have stopped having the injections. Side effects of this form of contraception include irregular periods, weight gain, depression, and PMS.

IMPLANTS

This involves match-size rods inserted under the skin that time-release progesterone to prevent ovulation and make mucus more hostile to sperm. Side effects include headaches, weight change, unscheduled bleeding, lighter or no periods, breast tenderness, and depression.

INTRAUTERINE DEVICES

The IUD (intrauterine device), or coil, is a mechanical device inserted into the uterus. The main action of copper-containing IUDs is to kill sperm (the copper immobilizes them). This should not be considered a first-line choice of contraception for women at risk of sexually transmitted infections (STDs), although new IUDs with short, single-filament tails have minimal risk of infection ascending into the uterine cavity. There is also a mild risk of cervicitis. If you have used an IUD in the past, it's a good idea to check your nutritional status: look out for mineral imbalances, especially raised copper and lower zinc levels.

physical fitness

We're well aware of the wide-ranging benefits of physical exercise and yet, with our busy lives, it's all too easy to forget, to let it slip, to put it off until we've finished the other 101 things we need to do. But staying in shape and keeping active is known to be beneficial for fertility, so it's time to get moving!

THE BENEFITS OF REGULAR EXERCISE

Incorporating a regular exercise routine into your daily life is vital, but not just for losing weight or shaping the body (although these can be welcome side effects). Regular exercise increases fitness and strength, enabling us to cope with the physical demands of the day and unexpected emergencies. For couples trying to conceive, it oxygenates the body and increases blood flow to supply the reproductive organs with essential oxygen.

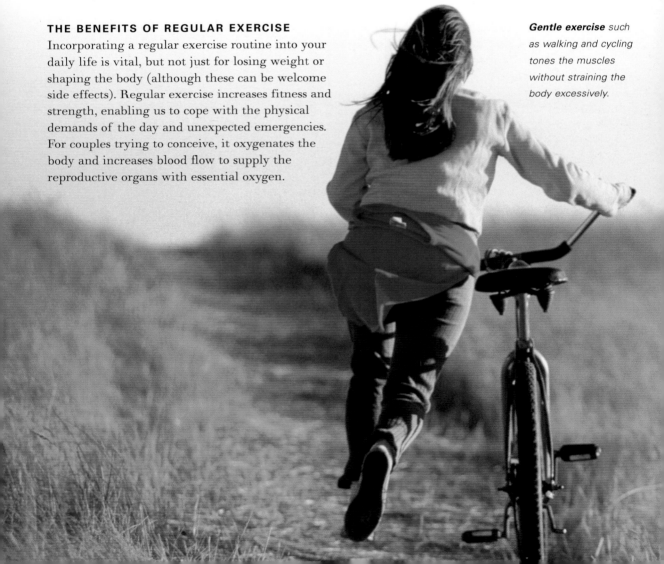

Gentle exercise such as walking and cycling tones the muscles without straining the body excessively.

Moderate physical exercise that fits comfortably into your regular schedule, and which you *enjoy*, improves your well-being at every level, by:

- boosting the immune system (by raising levels of immunoglobins and white blood cells)
- releasing endorphins (the body's natural painkillers) so that you are less likely to feel depressed and more likely to feel good
- increasing mental speed, efficiency, and concentration
- relieving stress
- reducing anxiety
- raising energy levels
- improving self-image and self-esteem
- promoting relaxation and restful sleep
- increasing bone density and mass, helping bones to resist mechanical stress and fracture, and reducing the risk of developing osteoporosis
- increasing muscle and reducing excess fat
- stretching and stimulating the muscles and internal organs, keeping the spine and joints supple, and maintaining the body's correct alignment to gravity
- increasing insulin sensitivity (so helping to prevent non–insulin-dependent diabetes)
- alleviating the symptoms of PMS (premenstrual syndrome)
- preparing the body for pregnancy: pregnant women who exercise moderately and sensibly suffer far less from constipation, hemorrhoids, or morning sickness.

If you're not used to exercising regularly, avoid launching yourself into a grueling fitness regimen. Strenuous exercise more than three times a week can have the opposite effect of what you have in mind and inhibit your chances of conceiving. Instead, find an activity that builds up your fitness levels gradually and, most important, one that you'll enjoy and look forward to doing. You'll start to feel the benefits of exercise by doing just 20 minutes three times a week. Swimming, brisk walking, and cycling are all perfect.

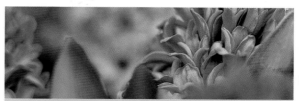

SEASONAL EXERCISE

The Chinese adjust exercise to match the season. Spring, summer, and late summer are times of **yang energy** (of warmth, activity, growth, and upward, outward motion). Fall and winter are times of **yin energy** (of cold, rest, reflection, recuperation, and downward, inward motion).

O SPRING
Spring corresponds to the element of wood and is associated with the tissues and ligaments of the human body. Evenings lengthen, the air is fresh, and people emerge from indoors. Gear exercise to stretching, walking, and weight training, gently building up muscles.

O SUMMER
Summer corresponds to fire and is associated with the heart and circulation. The days are long and the sun is strong. Get as much outdoor and aerobic exercise as possible: swimming, cycling, dancing, and jogging.

O LATE SUMMER
Late summer corresponds to earth and is associated with digestion and metabolism. It is harvest time; the sun is hot. Exercise outdoors: try power walking, cycling, and swimming.

O FALL
Fall corresponds to metal and is associated with the lungs and colon. Evenings draw in and the frosts arrive. Build up winter strength with qigong, Pilates, stretching, and walks.

O WINTER
Winter corresponds to water and is associated with the kidneys and bladder. The weather is cold and the days dark. Conserve energy and exercise gently and meditatively with deep breathing, yoga, tai chi, and qigong.

detoxifying the liver

The liver processes most of the chemicals that enter the body, as well as waste produced by the body itself. If this major detoxification organ doesn't function properly, harmful toxins can build up and compromise your health.

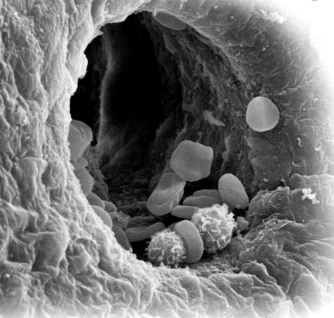

GOOD LIVER FUNCTION

The hormonal balance needed for fertility depends on good liver function. Your liver detoxifies many substances—caffeine, alcohol, drugs, pesticides, herbicides, food additives and preservatives, environmental toxins (from tobacco smoke and gasoline fumes, for instance), and toxins produced by bowel bacteria. It chemically alters excess or used hormones for recirculation or excretion.

To give your liver health and function a boost, I recommend a liver detoxification program (see box below). Many of my clients have found it beneficial. It gives your liver a well-deserved rest, since, for either seven or ten days, you don't eat

This cross section of liver tissue shows a healthy liver capillary (with red and white blood cells). Capillaries supply liver cells with nutrients and oxygen for proper functioning.

THE LIVER DETOX PROGRAM

The liver detox program can be undertaken over a seven- or ten-day period. It is based on two lists of foods (see pages 52–53). "Foods to eat liberally" lists foods that are good for the liver, and "Foods to eat moderately" lists foods that are easy on the liver. On most days you can eat foods from both lists, but for two days of the diet, base your meals solely on the "Foods to eat liberally" list. During this time, eliminate all foods in "Foods to avoid." Eat three meals per day, snack as necessary, and drink plenty of water.

⊙ 10-DAY DETOX
- Days 1–4 and days 7–10: consume foods from either "Foods to eat liberally" or "Foods to eat moderately" lists.
- Days 5–6: consume foods from "Foods to eat liberally" list.

⊙ 7-DAY DETOX
- Days 1–3, and days 6–7: consume foods from either "Foods to eat liberally" or "Foods to eat moderately" lists.
- Days 4–5: consume foods from "Foods to eat liberally" list.

any foods that make your liver work hard. Instead, you eat foods that are good for the liver, or those that it doesn't have to work too hard to process.

WHY DETOX?

If your liver is constantly burdened, the process of detoxification becomes less efficient. This leads to an increased level of toxins in the bloodstream, which can have a negative effect on your metabolic processes. Toxins that your body cannot eliminate build up in the tissues, typically in your fat stores.

HOW TO DETOX

The liver detox program excludes direct sources of toxins such as alcohol and caffeine and also common allergenic foods, such as wheat and dairy, since these can irritate the lining of the gastrointestinal tract, making it more porous and allowing any circulating toxins to pass across into the blood (see leaky gut syndrome, page 28).

Meat intake is reduced, and fruit and vegetable intake are increased significantly in order to help cleanse the bowel of toxins. This is important because these bowel toxins can be reabsorbed back into the blood, after which they will pass into the liver for detoxification. The high fiber intake also encourages the body to eliminate toxins that are already present in the body.

Once you start the detox program, you might experience withdrawal headaches in the first few days, but these usually pass as your body adapts.

SUPPLEMENTS THAT SUPPORT THE LIVER

An herb and supplement program taken during detoxification will give the liver an added boost. These substances are known to help liver function.

Silymarin is a potent liver protective agent. Clinical trials have documented the efficacy of silymarin (an extract of the antioxidant herb milk thistle) for a variety of liver disorders. It helps to protect the liver in people undertaking long-term drug programs, without interfering with the clinical effects of the drugs.

DETOX GUIDELINES

While you are following the liver detoxification program, bear in mind a few general guidelines in order to maximize its effects and minimize any side effects:

- don't detox if you are on any medication until you've checked with your doctor
- stop the program if you feel pain or discomfort
- get plenty of fresh air and, if possible, sunshine
- keep warm and get plenty of rest and sleep
- don't do any exercise
- start the program on a weekend
- consider lymphatic drainage as well (see page 149)
- if you have been taking medication, or you smoke, drink alcohol, or have a high caffeine intake, drink grapefruit juice with warm water to lessen side effects.

Choline can be bought from health-food stores in lecithin granules and sprinkled over foods. It is needed to make methionine, which has a significant role in liver detoxification. It is a sulfur-containing amino acid, as are cystine and lysine, all of which are key to liver detoxification.

Lactobacillus acidophilus are beneficial bacteria. They complement this supplement program by improving the health of the gastrointestinal tract and reducing toxicity. They are found in live natural yogurt, but are best taken as a supplement.

Other useful supplements include vitamins C, E, and B-complex, beta-carotene, the minerals magnesium, selenium, manganese, zinc, copper, and molybdenum, and glutathione.

MAINTAINING LIVER HEALTH

After you complete the liver detox program, reintroduce allergens (such as wheat and dairy products) one by one. If you don't react adversely, reintroduce them completely, but excluding as many of the items on the "Foods to avoid" list as possible during the preconception period in order to maintain the benefits of the detox program.

FOODS TO EAT

FOODS TO EAT LIBERALLY

Vegetables—*eat a large variety of vegetables, especially:*

- broccoli, cabbage, and cauliflower (all members of the cabbage or Brassica family with detoxifying properties)
- garlic and onions (with detoxifying, sulfur-containing compounds)
- asparagus, avocado (containing detoxifying glutathione)
- green leafy vegetables, such as kale and cabbage (containing detoxifying B vitamins)
- artichoke (a natural detoxifier)
- beets (another natural detoxifier)
- carrots, sweet potatoes, pumpkin, beets, spinach, celery, watercress, peas (all of which contain antioxidants)
- herbs such as parsley and cilantro

Fruit—*again, eat as much variety as possible, especially:*

- apples, pears (core fruits, which contain pectin)
- apricots, peaches, mangos, melons, papayas, pineapples, bananas, kiwi fruits, all berries (containing valuable antioxidants to support the liver)
- lemons—use the juice for salad dressings
- legumes—peas, beans, and lentils (for soluble fiber and protein)
- whole grains/cereals—whole-grain rice and millet
- olive oil—for cooking and salad dressings

Drinks

- fruit (except orange) and vegetable juices—try beet, celery, apple, and carrot or apple, pear, carrot, and ginger
- dandelion "coffee"—three cups daily (a liver cleanser)
- fruit and herbal teas
- juice of half a lemon in warm water 20 minutes before breakfast or on waking.
- water—filtered or bottled only.

FOODS TO EAT MODERATELY

- white meat—chicken, game
- white fish—sole, cod, haddock, plaice, skate, herring, sardines, pilchards, tilapia
- eggs
- nuts—almonds, Brazil nuts, walnuts
- seeds—sunflower, pumpkin, sesame, flaxseed (ground)
- dried fruit—dates, figs, apricots, raisins
- grains—barley, rye, oats
- cow's milk substitutes—oat, almond, or rice milk
- potatoes
- tomatoes
- live natural organic yogurt

FOODS TO AVOID

- nonorganic foods
- alcohol
- caffeinated drinks—e.g., coffee, tea, colas (also avoid the decaffeinated alternatives, which still contain substances requiring detoxification by the liver)
- orange juice
- sugar and foods containing lots of sugar—candies, chocolate (these stress the immune system)
- refined carbohydrates—white versions of foods such as bread, pasta, rice, and also cakes and cookies
- red meats (these are pro-inflammatory)
- dairy products (these are pro-inflammatory)
- wheat—found in bread, pasta, pastry, cakes, biscuits
- foods containing additives and preservatives
- packaged and processed foods, including processed meats
- salt

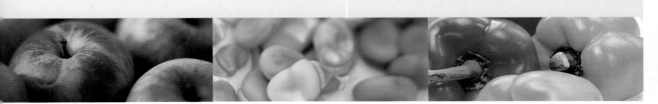

EXAMPLE MENUS

DAYS WHEN USING BOTH LISTS

Breakfast

- homemade granola, e.g., combinations of rolled oats, barley, millet, and rye, with extra oat germ and coconut flakes if desired. Add seeds, such as sunflower, whole or ground pumpkin, ground flaxseed, and ground sesame seeds. Top with a selection of fresh fruit and cinnamon for flavoring, if desired, and serve with oat milk or fruit juice
- oatmeal made with almond milk or oat milk

Lunch

- grilled organic chicken or poached fish with salad or steamed vegetables, served with whole-grain rice
- vegetable soup with rye bread (make sure no wheat flour has been added)
- baked potato with hummus
- dessert—fresh fruit salad

Evening meal

- vegetable stir-fry, e.g., onions, vegetables from the Brassica family, red cabbage, yellow/red peppers and carrots, cooked in olive oil and flavored with garlic and ginger. Serve with whole-grain rice or millet
- chili topped with live yogurt
- poached egg on a bed of spinach

Drinks

- 2 quarts (liters) of water throughout the day, fruit and herb teas, dandelion coffee, vegetable juices, fruit juices

Snacks

- seasonal fruits, nuts, seeds, dried fruits

"FOODS TO EAT LIBERALLY" DAYS

Breakfast

- slice of melon, banana, apple, pear
- poached fruit, such as apples, peaches, or plums, topped with sunflower seeds

Lunch

- salads, e.g., bean salad (kidney beans, chickpeas [garbanzos], green peas), carrot salad (grated carrots, grated apple, thinly sliced red cabbage) and mixed green salad (arugula, lettuce, and watercress) with millet. Serve with a dressing of olive oil and lemon juice
- guacamole with raw carrot and cucumber slices
- fresh vegetable soup with beans, lentils, and chickpeas
- dessert—a drink of sweet freshly squeezed fruit juices, or fresh fruit salad

Evening meal

- steamed vegetables or vegetable stir-fry, e.g., snow peas, baby corn, broccoli, kale, onions, garlic, or winter vegetables, e.g., leeks, parsnips, rutabaga, turnip, with garlic. Serve with whole-grain basmati rice
- mixed roasted Mediterranean vegetables served with whole-grain basmati rice
- dessert—a drink of sweet freshly squeezed fruit juices, or fresh fruit salad

Drinks

- 2 quarts (liters) of water throughout the day, fruit and herb teas, dandelion coffee, vegetable and fruit juices

Snacks

- seasonal fruits, vegetables, e.g., avocado, celery, carrot

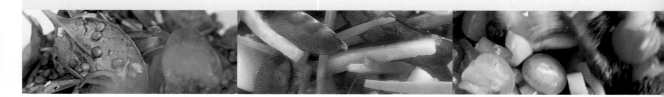

healthy eating

Once you've followed the detox program, keep up the good work by adopting sensible eating habits to maintain your long-term health and hormonal balance.

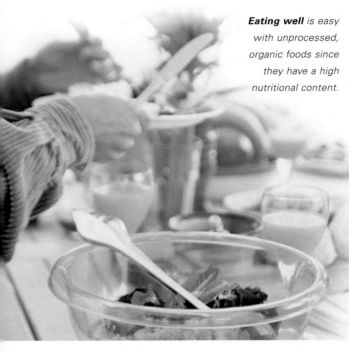

Eating well is easy with unprocessed, organic foods since they have a high nutritional content.

Most of the nutrients, vitamins, and minerals we need should come from the food we eat. But food production has changed. Although there is a huge range of foods available now, most are grown miles away in soil robbed of nutrients by intensive farming, artificial fertilizers, and pesticides. Food storage and preservation methods are now so good that we cannot tell how fresh our food really is. Processing, refining, and cooking strips away more value. The result is that we no longer receive the correct amount of vitamins and minerals.

REDRESSING THE BALANCE

I want to explain how you can balance your whole system through food. But it's no good telling you exactly what to eat and what to avoid, especially if you feel you have already given up too many of the things you enjoy. It's easier to change old habits if we understand *why* we should.

Food is not just fuel to give you energy. The quality of the food you eat makes a difference in the functioning of the cells in your body, including the hormones and cells in your reproductive system.

Try writing down everything you eat and drink over the next few days—you may be surprised at what it reveals. Avoid going on a "diet," because it has such negative connotations. Just think nutrients instead of calories, and eat the best, freshest, and most wholesome foods you can afford.

Nutritious foods are those that are closer to their natural form—fruits, vegetables, nuts, and seeds. Nutritionally inferior foods are generally highly processed and packaged—fast foods, store-bought cakes, cookies, pies, chips, and prepared meals.

NUTRITIONAL REQUIREMENTS

I don't believe that the "balanced diet" we hear so much about actually exists. For a start, the level of nutrients absorbed from food varies from person to person. Each of us goes through periods of eating well or badly at different times, and we each have specific nutritional requirements, depending on lifestyle, metabolism, and genetic makeup. Smokers, drinkers, dieters, excessive exercisers, or anorexics will all be depleted of certain nutrients, while people who have been on the contraceptive pill or are on medication or daily aspirin will have different requirements again.

EATING WELL THROUGHOUT THE DAY

All food is made up of:

- macronutrients (proteins, fats, and carbohydrates)
- micronutrients (vitamins and minerals) and phytochemicals (such as flavonoids, antioxidants, and carotenes).

Which of these foods we need to eat, and when, is governed by our internal body clock:

- To start the day, we need to eat protein-rich energy foods. According to traditional Chinese medicine, 7 AM to 9 AM is the peak time for the stomach, when digestion is at its best, so it's important to eat breakfast.
- Lunch should be a small, high-protein meal to trigger a rise in dopamine, a chemical found in the brain associated with energy. Eating too many carbohydrates will release serotonin and make you feel sleepy.
- By dinnertime, the body is anticipating sleep, so eating carbohydrates will aid relaxation. This is why cravings for sweet foods are more common in the evening. During the night, the stomach empties 50 percent more slowly than during the day, so it is best to eat your evening meal four hours before bedtime. That way, your digestion will be better, you will burn more calories, and your sleep will be undisturbed. According to the Chinese, 7 PM to 9 PM is the stomach's rest period.

PROTEINS

Proteins provide the building blocks of the body. They are needed to:

- repair and renew cells
- transport oxygen and nutrients
- produce hormones
- make antibodies to fight infection
- grow new tissues for muscles, bones, and general repairs

Proteins are made of amino acids, and a full supply is essential for egg production (animal studies have shown that inadequate protein intake results in poor-quality eggs) and to produce the hormones FSH (follicle-stimulating hormone) and LH (luteinizing hormone). Cysteine, found in white meat, lentils, beans, nuts, and seeds, is a particularly important amino acid.

Both men and women need approximately 2.2–2.5 oz (60–70 g) of protein a day, making up roughly 20 percent of our diet. Protein is found in animal products such as meat, fish, eggs, and dairy produce, and in vegetable sources such as lentils, peas and beans, nuts, brown rice, sunflower and pumpkin seeds, and quinoa.

The best sources of vegetable protein come from combining legumes and grains—such as lentils and rice, for example.

Vegetarians and even "raw food" vegans can have sufficient protein in their diet, but they must eat much larger quantities of food. The more amino acids there are in

PROTEIN VALUES

- **Egg** 6 g per egg
- **Lean meat, fish, poultry** 25–30 g per 100 g (4 oz)
- **Tempeh** 30 g per 200 g (8 oz)
- **Milk** 8–9 g per cup (250 ml)
- **Yogurt** 8–10 g per cup (250 ml)
- **Cream cheese** 2 g per 25 g (1 oz)
- **Cheddar cheese** 7 g per 25 g (1 oz)
- **Parmesan cheese** 10 g per 25 g (1 oz)
- **Cottage cheese** 28 g per 200 g (8 oz)
- **Nuts and seeds** 2–3 g per tablespoon
- **Rice, cooked** 5 g per 200 g (8 oz)
- **Cornmeal, cooked** 2 g per 200 g (8 oz)
- **Bulgur wheat, cooked** 8 g per 200 g (8 oz)
- **Oatmeal, cooked** 5 g per 200 g (8 oz)
- **Wheat germ, toasted** 8 g per 50 g (2 oz)
- **Bread** 2–11 g per slice (check the label)
- **Adzuki beans, cooked** 17 g per 200 g (8 oz)
- **Kidney beans, cooked** 15 g per 200 g (8 oz)
- **Potato, medium-size, baked with skin,** 5 g
- **Nutritional yeast, flakes** 4 g per heaping tablespoon
- **Most fruits** 1 g per fruit
- **Vegetables** 1–3 g per 100 g (4 oz)

a protein food, the more value it has as a protein source. Beans and rice are good sources of protein, as long as you eat them in large enough quantities.

In some early research, there was concern about needing to combine proteins so that all essential proteins were available at each meal. Later research has determined that this is not necessary. While all essential amino acids are needed, they do not have to be eaten together.

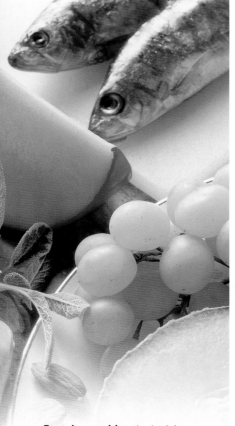

Protein provides the body's building blocks, while slow-releasing carbohydrates give sustained energy.

A "real food" diet with variable protein sources will usually cover all essential amino acids.

Protein in food is slowly released into the bloodstream, allowing for maximum utilization of amino acids. When nutrients are "loaded" into the system, your body must work hard to remove the overload. So eating protein early in the day and at more than one meal will feed your body best.

Certain kinds of diet seem to come in and out of fashion. There has been a craze to reduce fat and protein (of any kind) and eat mainly carbohydrates, but I do not believe this will lead to long-term health. The body needs wholesome, natural protein and high-quality fats in order to function properly. Contrary to "media nutrition," we do not eat too much wholesome protein. We do, however, eat too many processed fats; processed, preserved, and salted proteins; refined carbohydrates; and nonnutritive calories.

If you do not eat fish and red meat, you may need to supplement zinc, a component of proteolytic enzymes found in fish, seafood, and red meat. Zinc is not only important to protein digestion, it is also key to a healthy immune system, fertility, mood, and energy.

High-protein diets (such as the Atkins diet) are currently in vogue. Too much protein in the diet, however, may be as problematic as too little. It can lead to excessive levels of ammonia in the body as well as calcium depletion.

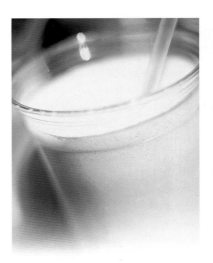

If you enjoy drinking milk, try almond or rice milk instead of cow's milk.

FATS

Fats are vitally important for health and fertility. They are called essential fatty acids because they are just that—essential. They:

• make hormones
• transport cholesterol
• help reduce inflammation

Deficiency may be manifested as dry skin, cracked lips, PMS, and tender breasts.

Sources of fats include butter and margarine, vegetable oils, whole milk and milk products, meats, nuts, and seeds.

There are two basic types of fat: saturated and unsaturated.

• Saturated fats are found in meat and dairy products. They turn solid at room temperature and are best kept to a minimum, since they contribute to heart disease, obesity, high cholesterol levels, and an increased risk of some cancers.

- Unsaturated fats are found in olive oil, nuts, seeds, and fish. Certain unsaturated fats, known as omega-6 and omega-3 oils, are essential for the brain, nervous system, immune system, cardiovascular system, and skin. Some key compounds that are essential for proper hormonal balance are manufactured by the body from omega-6 and omega-3 oils. Unsaturated fats should make up about 20–25 percent of the diet. Good sources include flaxseed oil (made from ground flaxseed), pumpkin seeds, evening primrose oil, and oily fish.

CARBOHYDRATES

As the body's basic fuel source, carbohydrates should account for about 55 percent of the food you eat. They are vitally important as far as fertility is concerned because sufficient amounts of energy are needed for reproduction to be able to take place and to maintain balanced hormones and balanced blood-sugar levels.

Food sources of carbohydrates include whole grains, sugar, syrup, honey, fruits, and vegetables.

There are two kinds of carbohydrate:

- "fast-releasing" or simple carbohydrates, such as sugar, refined white flour, and processed foods, which tend to give you lots of calories but not many nutrients. You should reduce intakes of these

- "slow-releasing" or complex carbohydrates, such as fruit, vegetables, legumes, and whole grains. These are the best carbohydrates because they contain plenty of fiber, give you sustained energy, and may contain phytoestrogens (see page 31). They can lower blood cholesterol, stabilize blood sugar, regulate bowel movements, and give you more stamina. These are the carbohydrates you should focus on.

MICRONUTRIENTS AND PHYTOCHEMICALS

Micronutrients include essential vitamins and minerals (see pages 59–64) and also plant-based phytochemicals, which include vitally important nutrients such as bioflavonoids, carotenoids, antioxidants, and phytoestrogens. These are found in unprocessed foods. Eating a minimum of five portions of fruit and vegetables a day should ensure that you get a good supply of these precious

An ideal daily fiber intake of around 1.2 oz (35 g) has many vital health benefits.

substances, which play an important role in the functioning of all body systems. You cannot have too much of them.

Fiber has great health benefits, including fewer constipation and bowel problems, a reduced risk of breast and colon cancer, and a reduction in the incidence or severity of gallstones, diabetes, and cardiovascular disease. Eating a minimum of five portions of fruit and vegetables a day should provide you with adequate amounts of fiber. The ideal intake is no less than 1.2 oz (35 g) a day, although most of us only get about 0.8 oz (22 g). The best sources are whole grains, vegetables, fruits, nuts, seeds, and legumes. Too much wheat fiber in your diet can rob the body of estrogen. You don't need to sprinkle wheat bran all over your cereal, for example: too much may block the uptake of vital nutrients. Use flaxseed instead (see Zita's Tips, page 38) to improve bowel movements, which are important for getting rid of old hormones.

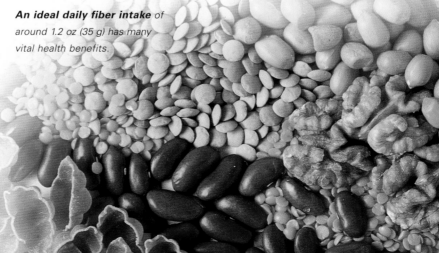

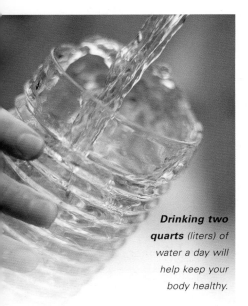

Drinking two quarts (liters) of water a day will help keep your body healthy.

Water is the most important nutrient to the body after oxygen. It makes up 70 percent of the adult body, 83 percent of blood, 73 percent of muscle, 25 percent of fat, and 22 percent of bone. It is needed for the functioning of every body system, including the elimination of toxins, production of energy, transportation of hormones, and development of follicles, and to make sperm, semen, cell membranes, and cervical mucus.

Every day, the body loses approximately 1.5 quarts (liters) of water in perspiration, breath, and urine. Alcohol, tea, and coffee cause us to lose more water and rob us of valuable minerals.

Most of us are dehydrated and don't even realize it, and the consequences can be serious.
• If there is only low-level dehydration, the brain doesn't switch on the thirst mechanism.

• Dehydration increases the production of cholesterol, which surrounds cells to seal in and conserve water, preventing nutrients from entering and toxins from escaping. Taking supplements is a waste of time if you are dehydrated.
• With long-term dehydration, the body rations the available water, diverting it to the essential organs (the brain and heart) and away from the ovaries and the testicles.

To replace lost water, we need to drink at least two quarts (liters) a day. But it takes time to rehydrate. If you pour water onto a plant that has dried out, it will sit on the soil surface or run down the sides without being absorbed. Our bodies react the same way, so for a week or two it will feel as though the water is running straight through you. Increase your water consumption gradually. Drink filtered or glass-bottled water. Keep a pitcher of water at hand at all times to remind you to drink regularly. Also, drink juiced raw fruits and vegetables or fruit and herb teas.

ZITA'S TIPS

● **Ensure tap water is filtered,** because chlorinated tap water contains trihalomethanes (THMs), chemical compounds that occur when chlorine, used to kill bacteria in drinking water, reacts with organic matter. THMs have been linked to colon, bladder, and kidney cancer as well as spina bifida, infant heart problems, and miscarriage.

● **When drinking bottled water,** make sure the bottles are made from glass, not plastic. "Out-gassing" from plastic can pollute your body.

As you begin to rehydrate, the toxins stored in the cells will start to escape into the lymph system. To aid this gentle process of detoxification, go for a deep body massage, have a sauna, and take up regular skin brushing.

BALANCED EATING SUMMARY

● Consume fresh food that is in season, and buy organic whenever possible.
● Eat protein regularly.
● Choose "good" unsaturated fats and avoid "bad" saturated fats.
● Rely on complex carbohydrates for your main source of energy.

● Eat a broad range of different fruits and vegetables.
● Eat sufficient fiber.
● Limit the amount of wheat and dairy in your diet.
● Cut out tea, coffee, alcohol, and sugar.
● Drink two quarts (liters) of water daily.

essential nutrients for conception

Whether it's the many B vitamins, which are vital for hormonal balance, folic acid for developing eggs, or the antioxidant properties of vitamin C, our intake of a range of important nutrients are essential for good health and especially fertility.

NUTRIENTS FOR FERTILITY

Although there are many key nutrients for maintaining a healthy body, some play a specific role in enhancing fertility in women. (For key nutrients for male fertility, see pages 76–79.) Your main source should always be food, but modern farming methods have robbed the soil of many vital minerals. Your lifestyle may mean you need extra nutrients, making supplementation advisable.

HOW SUPPLEMENTS HELP

Taking supplements guarantees that you get the nutrients you need. Research has shown that couples who took nutritional supplements over a 14-month period conceived earlier than those taking no supplements. I do not recommend taking vitamins or minerals ad hoc, however. They need to be taken in balance with each other: high doses of one can lead to depletion in another (see page 62). If possible, consult a nutritionist for an analysis of your individual needs and a personal program to start at least three months before conception.

If you don't consult a nutritionist, take supplements according to the recommended dosages, and ensure that you take them in a way that will maximize absorption and hence their benefits.

KEY NUTRIENTS FOR FERTILITY

AMINO ACIDS

These perform a vital role in the body and are necessary for egg production. They are found in protein foods (see page 55). There are no RNIs (see page 62).

VITAMIN A

This vitamin is essential for producing female sex hormones. Food sources include eggs, yellow fruits and vegetables, whole milk and milk products, dark green leafy vegetables, and oily fish.

Vitamin A has antioxidant properties, protects cells against damage, and is very important for a developing embryo. There are, however, many concerns about women who are either trying to conceive or who are pregnant taking vitamin A. This is because, in the past, pregnant women have been encouraged to eat liver, which contains vitamin A in the form of retinol. High doses of retinol have been linked to fetal abnormalities. The National Institutes of Health (NIH) Recommended Dietary Allowance (RDA) for Vitamin A is 2,565 IU for pregnant women.

Beta-carotene is a plant pigment that is converted to vitamin A in the body. In studies, cows fed diets deficient in beta-carotene had delayed ovulation and developed more ovarian cysts. The corpus luteum (see page 10) has the highest concentration of this nutrient in the body. It produces progesterone, so beta-carotene may be important for cycle regularity and in early pregnancy. Supplementation is known to reduce the incidence of ovarian cysts. Food sources include peas, broccoli, carrots, spinach, and sweet potatoes. There is no RNI for beta-carotene.

B VITAMINS

B vitamins are very important for fertility, especially B6, folate (folic acid is the supplement), and B12.

B vitamins are water-soluble and many are lost in urine. Lifestyle factors such as stress and alcohol, tobacco, and antibiotic use inhibit absorption. B vitamins are very important for the production and balance of sex hormones. The hypothalamus, which releases sex hormones, is sensitive to severe B-vitamin deficiency.

Vitamin B1 (thiamin) In studies of animals, deficiency in B1 prior to mating has been linked to failed ovulation or implantation.

Important food sources of B1 include molasses, brewer's yeast, whole grains, nuts, brown rice, organ and other meats, egg yolks, fish, poultry, legumes, and seeds.
▶ **DOSAGE** RNI women 0.8 mg/day.

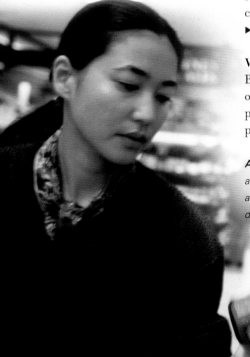

Vitamin B2 (riboflavin)
Deficiencies in B2 have been linked to sterility, miscarriage, and low birth weight. The liver uses vitamin B2 to clear away used-up hormones, including estrogen and progesterone. If these are allowed to accumulate, messages to the hypothalamus and pituitary glands about hormone production may be inhibited and levels fall.

Food sources of B2 are much the same as for B1. The presence of other B vitamins aids absorption.
▶ **DOSAGE** RNI women 1.1 mg/day.

Vitamin B5 (pantothenic acid)
B5 is particularly important at and around the time of conception for fetal development.

Food sources include those for B1 plus wheat germ, salmon, sweet potatoes, broccoli, oranges, cashews, pecans, and strawberries.
▶ **DOSAGE** RNI adults 3–7 mg/day.

Vitamin B6 Together with zinc, B6 is essential for the formation of female sex hormones and the proper functioning of estrogen and progesterone. The ovaries respond

A huge range of vitamin, mineral, and other nutrient supplements are available from health-food stores or drugstores.

to deficiency in vitamin B6 by shutting down progesterone production, leading to estrogen dominance (see page 32). Studies show that supplementation helps to prevent luteal phase defects (LPDs) and encourages the production of progesterone. Research has also shown that if women who have problems conceiving take B6, their fertility improves during a six-month period.

Food sources of B6 include those for B1 plus green leafy vegetables. Zinc aids absorption.
▶ **DOSAGE** RNI women 1.2 mg/day, but I suggest you can take up to 50 mg/day.

Vitamin B12 Together with folate, B12 is needed for the synthesis of DNA and RNA. These are important compounds that are part of our genetic blueprint and are involved in the makeup of every cell in the body. Adequate levels of B12 maximize the uptake of folate or folic acid.

The only reliable sources of B12 are animal products, in particular lamb, sardines, and salmon. Vegans need to eat fermented foods that contain bacteria, but they are advised to take supplements to ensure adequate intakes of B12. Calcium aids absorption.
▶ **DOSAGE** RNI women 1.5 mcg/day, but I suggest you can take up to 50 mcg/day.

Folate Every woman should take a multivitamin that contains a minimum of 400 mcg of folic acid daily for at least three months before she starts trying to conceive, and for at least two months after conception, in order to reduce the risk of neural-tube (brain and spinal cord) defects in the developing embryo.

Good food sources of folate are dark-green leafy vegetables, broccoli, organ meats, brewer's yeast, root vegetables, whole grains, oysters, salmon, milk, legumes, asparagus, oatmeal, dried figs, and avocados.

Vitamin C aids absorption. It is worth noting that it takes about three months to reestablish adequate folate levels after taking the contraceptive pill.

▶ **DOSAGE** RNI women 200 mcg/day.

VITAMIN C
Vitamin C is an antioxidant that blocks the damaging action of free radicals. Too high a dosage (in excess of 1,000 mg/day) might, however, act as an antihistamine and dry up the cervical mucus.

Good food sources of vitamin C include citrus fruits, rosehips, cherries, sprouted alfalfa seeds, cantaloupe, strawberries, broccoli, tomatoes, sweet peppers, black currants, mangos, grapes, kiwi fruit, pineapples, asparagus, peas, potatoes, parsley, watercress, and spinach.

▶ **DOSAGE** RNI women 40 mg/day, but I would advise women to increase this to 500 mg/day.

VITAMIN E
Research on animals has indicated that taking vitamin E along with vitamin C in the treatment of unexplained infertility may improve ovulation. Also, deficiency in vitamin E has been linked to miscarriage in some studies.

Food sources of vitamin E include cold-pressed oils, wheat germ, organ meats, molasses, eggs, sweet potatoes, leafy vegetables, nuts, seeds, whole grains, and avocados. A natural (d-alpha-tocopherol), as opposed to synthetic (dl-alpha-tocopherol), supplement of vitamin E is more easily utilized by the body and retained for longer in the body tissues. Check the packaging when you buy a supplement to see which it is. Take with selenium and vitamin C for a healthy endometrium.

Vitamin E has anticoagulant properties, so be careful if you are taking aspirin or heparin.

▶ **DOSAGE** RNI women >3 mg/day, but I would recommend 400 IUs.

IRON
Low levels of iron can affect fertility (see page 105), and iron deficiency is very common. Adequate amounts of iron help to guard against miscarriage.

Food sources include organ meats, lean meat, eggs, fish, poultry, molasses, cherries, dried fruits, prunes, green leafy vegetables, kelp, spinach, parsley, pumpkin and sunflower seeds, broccoli, oatmeal, sardines, and nuts.

Tea, coffee, and tobacco all inhibit the absorption of iron.

▶ **DOSAGE** RNI women 14.8 mg/day, but I recommend 20 mg/day. Only take iron supplements if you are certain that you have a deficiency.

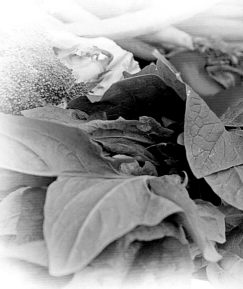

Green leafy vegetables are packed with nutrients, particularly folic acid, vitamin C, B vitamins, and iron.

MAGNESIUM
A deficiency in magnesium is associated with female infertility and possibly an increased risk of miscarriage. Animal studies that show magnesium deficiency inhibits the use and excretion of vitamin B1. We need magnesium and B1 for energy production; deficiency causes a decrease in the rate of cell metabolism.

The average Western diet tends to be low in magnesium because its common dietary staples—such as fish, meat, milk, and most fruits—do not contain the mineral.

Food sources of magnesium are kelp, green leafy vegetables, tofu, legumes, rye, buckwheat, millet,

combining supplements

Most people benefit from taking a good multivitamin and mineral supplement. If you are trying to conceive a baby, specific additional nutrients may be recommended. You may need advice about how to combine supplements to fulfill all your needs.

IDENTIFYING NEEDS

Nutrients should ideally come from the food you eat. Ensure that you eat a wide range of nutrient-rich foods. Do not use supplements to compensate for poor nutrition. It is important, however, to take a good vitamin-and-mineral supplement and an essential fatty acid (see opposite) supplement.

Depending on the kind of life you lead, you may be deficient in some nutrients. For example, there is evidence that micronutrient intakes in Europe are falling. Those nutrients giving cause for concern include vitamins B2, B6 and C, folate, copper, magnesium, iron, iodine, zinc, and selenium. If your lifestyle is stressful, you have been taking the contraceptive pill,

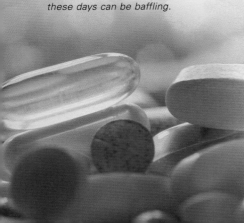

The choice of supplements these days can be baffling.

or you drink a lot of alcohol, it is advisable to supplement vitamin B-complex with some additional zinc and extra vitamins C and E. If you have certain gynecological conditions, specific nutrients might be recommended in higher amounts (see pages 109–130). In addition, greater amounts of some nutrients are believed to be good for sperm health (see pages 76–79).

Remember that too much of one vitamin or mineral may deplete levels of another, and taking certain medications may deplete your body of vital nutrients.

OFFICIAL GUIDELINES

Nutrient intakes are recommended in many countries by health departments. In the UK, the Reference Nutrient Intake (RNI) has replaced the Recommended Daily Amount (RDA), although the two are largely interchangeable. The two benchmarks are of little practical use, in fact, and many health experts believe that it would be better to consider the amounts of nutrients necessary to prevent chronic disease rather than aiming merely to prevent overt deficiency.

DO'S & DON'TS

Follow specific instructions on the packet and also consider:

- **fat-soluble vitamins**, such as D and E, should be taken with fats; and water-soluble vitamins, such as B and C, with water

- **certain medications** can rob the body of vital nutrients: antibiotics may reduce vitamin and mineral levels; aspirin may deplete vitamin C levels; vitamin B levels may be reduced by taking antidepressants; and folate can be depleted by contraceptives

- **large intakes of zinc** may interfere with iron and copper absorption (vitamin C enhances iron absorption)

- **iron supplements** may deplete zinc levels

- **taking any B vitamin** will enhance the absorption of other B vitamins, but too much of one may deplete the others

- **coffee and tea** affect absorption of some nutrients

molasses, brown rice, bananas, dried figs and apricots, nuts, barley, seafood, and whole grains. It is a good idea to supplement magnesium and selenium (see below) together, along with calcium and vitamins B6 and D to aid absorption. Take with protein foods. Alcohol, tea, coffee, and smoking inhibit absorption.

▶ **DOSAGE** RNI women 270 mg/day. I would recommend up to 400 mg/day.

SELENIUM

As with magnesium, a deficiency in selenium is associated with female infertility and even an increased risk of miscarriage.

Good food sources of selenium include tuna, herring, brewer's yeast, wheat germ and bran, whole grains, and sesame seeds.

▶ **DOSAGE** RNI women 60 mcg/day, but I would recommend 200 mcg/day.

MANGANESE

Studies on animals have shown that manganese deficiency can lead to defective ovulation. It is also believed to inhibit the synthesis of sex hormones.

Manganese competes with iron for absorption, so food sources of iron should ideally not be eaten with manganese-rich foods, which include whole grains, green leafy vegetables, carrots, broccoli, ginger, legumes, nuts, pineapples, eggs, oats, and rye. It is advisable to take manganese supplements with protein foods or vitamin C. High intakes of zinc may inhibit the absorption of manganese.

▶ **DOSAGE** RNI women 1.4 mg/day, but the upper limit for manganese is 15 mg/day.

ZINC

Zinc deficiency is one of the most common nutritional problems that I come across. It is vitally important for growth and proper cell division in a fetus. Zinc is needed for many enzymes to work. Low levels of zinc slow down the metabolizing of protein, which is needed for the production of good-quality eggs. Zinc also maintains the menstrual cycle.

Folic acid and iron inhibit the absorption of zinc. In addition, if you drink a lot of alcohol or you have been taking the contraceptive pill, you are more likely to have low zinc levels.

Good food sources include lean meat, fish, seafood, chicken, eggs, pumpkin and sunflower seeds, rye, oats, whole grains, legumes, ginger, parsley, mushrooms, brewer's yeast, and wheat germ.

Vitamins B6 and C may aid absorption: tea, coffee, alcohol, and high fiber intake may inhibit it.

▶ **DOSAGE** RNI women 7 mg/day, but I believe you can take up to 30 mg/day, depending on your lifestyle.

COENZYME Q10 (CO-Q10)

Coenzyme Q10 is a fat-soluble substance that is present in every cell in the body, and is important for energy production. Research has indicated that co-Q10 levels tend to be lower in women who have had a recent miscarriage.

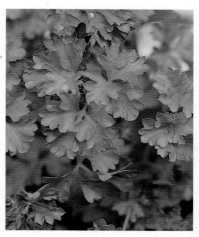

Parsley *is a good source of zinc and can be added to many dishes.*

Supplementing coenzyme Q10 may improve fertilization rates in women who are undergoing ICSI treatment (see page 174).

Most of the research into co-Q10 has been in connection with heart disease and improving blood flow. I therefore encourage women with fertility problems to take it to improve blood flow generally and especially prior to commencing fertility treatment.

It is difficult to obtain sufficient amounts of this nutrient from food sources (although it has been found that vegetarians have higher levels in their bodies). So, supplementation is the only reliable way of increasing your intakes of co-Q10. There is no RNI.

ESSENTIAL FATTY ACIDS

EFAs act as hormone regulators. I cannot stress enough the importance of taking these nutrients as a supplement.

Omega-3 EFAs have a derivative called DHA (docosahexaenoic acid). Eight out of ten women are deficient in DHA. This and the omega-6 derivative, arachidonic acid, are important structural elements of cell membranes. They form body tissue and are essential for brain development in a fetus. DHA is needed for the production of cell membranes in the ovaries.

Women should be supplementing EFAs at least three months before they want to become pregnant, since it takes time for DHA to be incorporated into human tissue. Arachidonic acid must also be present for DHA to be properly synthesized in a baby's system.

Food sources of omega-3 EFAs are flaxseed and oily fish, walnuts, and green leafy vegetables. Tuna oil is the richest source, but women planning a pregnancy are advised not to eat more than 6 oz (170 g) of tuna a week because of the risk of mercury contamination. Supplements are screened for toxins and purified. Fish oils also have anticoagulant properties and may be beneficial if you have had recurrent miscarriages. Be careful, however, if you are taking aspirin or heparin. Food sources of omega-6 EFAs are seeds and their oils. There is no RNI, but 700–1,000 mg/day is beneficial.

OTHER KEY NUTRIENTS

There are other important nutrients that are necessary for the maintenance of general good health and well-being.

Vitamin B3 (niacin) This is important for energy production and for sex hormones. Good food sources include poultry, fish, lean meats, peanuts, brewer's yeast, milk products, and rice bran. B-complex aids absorption: stress, alcohol, and antibiotics hinder it.

PABA Based on studies done as long ago as the 1940s, para-aminobenzoic acid (PABA) has been linked to male fertility. This B-complex component may also be of benefit for folate production by intestinal bacteria, production of red blood cells, and processing of proteins. Food sources of PABA include organ meats, whole grains, brewer's yeast, molasses, spinach, and mushrooms. Folic acid and B-complex vitamins aid absorption of PABA, while high stress levels and antibiotics hinder it.

Vitamin K This is essential for blood clotting. Good food sources of vitamin K include green leafy vegetables, egg yolks, safflower oil, molasses, and cauliflower.

Calcium This mineral is needed for blood clotting and hormonal balance. Good food sources are milk and its products (but these should be eaten in moderation), green leafy vegetables, shellfish and bony fish, parsley, watercress, spinach, broccoli, cottage cheese, hard cheese, kelp, sesame seeds, flaxseed, and tofu. Tea, coffee, and tobacco all inhibit the absorption of calcium.

Chromium This is needed for the regulation of blood sugar and hormonal balance. Food sources are honey, grapes, raisins, corn oil, clams, whole-grain cereals, and brewer's yeast. Supplements should be taken with protein. Vitamin B3 maximizes absorption: tea, coffee, and tobacco inhibit it.

Copper This is essential for the production of DNA and RNA (see page 60). Copper deficiency is rare, but excess copper can be toxic. Food sources are organ meats, nuts, legumes, molasses, and raisins.

Iodine This trace element is needed for the manufacture of thyroid hormones. Food sources are seafood, kelp, and iodized salt.

Phosphorus This is the most abundant mineral in the body. It functions alongside calcium. Sources are fish, poultry, meat, eggs, legumes, milk and milk products, nuts, and whole-grain cereals.

Potassium This regulates blood pH levels. Together with sodium, it maintains fluid balance in the body and transportation of nutrients to all cells. Good food sources of potassium include bananas, avocados, carrots, apples, tomatoes, pineapples, leafy green vegetables, potatoes, dried apricots, peaches, melons, lean meats, whole grains, legumes, and sunflower seeds.

Sodium, sulfur, and molybdenum These minerals are also needed.

identifying nutritional deficiencies

As well as maintaining a balanced diet, it's important to pinpoint whether or not you are suffering from any vitamin or mineral deficiencies and to identify toxins that may be stored in your body. You can then take steps to restore the healthy nutritional balance that will improve your well-being and fertility.

TESTING FOR NUTRITIONAL DEFICIENCIES

Before you rush out to buy a pile of vitamin, mineral, and other nutritional supplements, you need to remember three important things.

- Vitamins and minerals work together in synthesis—they depend on each other to work efficiently.
- Everyone's individual needs are different.
- A good, well-balanced diet that is rich in vitamins, minerals, and other essential nutrients will protect and support the workings of your body in the best possible way.

To determine whether, for whatever reason, you are deficient in particular vitamins or minerals, I recommend that you start by visiting a nutritional expert for a full consultation. They will ask you to fill out a very detailed questionnaire about your dietary habits and general lifestyle that will help them to determine where deficiencies might lie. There are a number of alternative methods of detecting either deficiencies or the presence of toxic substances that you might like to consider.

Hair analysis There is debate among health professionals about the use of hair analysis. Many laboratories have produced inconsistent results and reference ranges vary enormously, leaving couples concerned and confused. It is used in forensic science, however, to reveal metal poisoning that does not show up in blood or urine tests.

Hair cells are among the fastest-growing cells in the body: as they grow, they record all the nutrients and toxins you have been exposed to. Levels of essential nutrients such as magnesium, selenium, manganese, or zinc, as well as toxins such as lead, mercury, and aluminum, can be assessed. A supplementation program can then be devised. Permed, tinted, or highlighted hair does not give accurate readings and, if you swim regularly, algicides in pool water may distort copper readings.

Iridology The iris is the colored part of the eye and the only visible part of the nervous system. It serves as an indicator of what is going on in your body, providing a noninvasive diagnostic tool.

An iridologist studies color, lines, markings, and rings. Dark patches indicate specific problems or weaknesses, so are an early warning of potential trouble spots. Iridology may reveal allergy, vitamin or mineral deficiency, or hormonal imbalance.

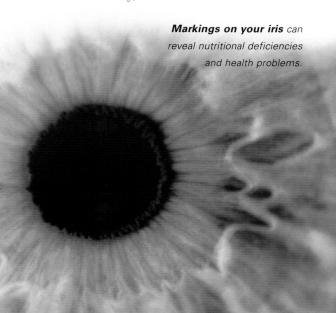

Markings on your iris can *reveal nutritional deficiencies and health problems.*

you and your cycle

Getting to know your cycle is the key to understanding your fertility. You need to appreciate what is happening to your body at every stage of the month so that you can interpret signs and work with your natural rhythms to enhance your fertility.

GETTING TO KNOW YOUR CYCLE

In my experience, most women take their menstrual cycle completely for granted until they want to conceive. Then they tend to focus solely on ovulation. Ovulation is important, of course, but so is every aspect of the cycle to achieve a pregnancy.

I work very closely with clients to help them understand exactly what is happening at each stage of the month and to recognize physical, hormonal, and emotional changes. I'm often astonished at how little women know about the processes of their bodies.

Many women have spent most of their adult lives trying to avoid getting pregnant. They have viewed their monthly bleeds as an inconvenience and barely noticed the parts of the cycle in between. Menstrual flow is a good indicator of general health as well as fertility, but women tend not to discuss the details of their cycle, even with close friends, so they have no idea of "normal" (see below) even though they may complain of feeling "out of sync" if their cycle is irregular. Only when they want to conceive do they become interested in what is happening inside their bodies.

WHAT IS NORMAL

What constitutes a normal cycle is in fact very hard to describe. Different women have different lengths of cycle and volumes of bleed. What is normal for some women—with regard to amount of blood loss, for example—will for others be an indication of hormonal imbalance (see pages 30–32 and 126–30). You should always consult your doctor about any changes in bleeding patterns that you experience.

Western medicine pays little attention to the details of a woman's cycle, but in traditional Chinese medicine, every detail is considered to be important for diagnostic purposes—the duration, color, volume, and consistency of menstrual flow, as well as physical changes and your emotional feelings throughout the month.

Any cycle lasting between 25 and 35 days is regarded as within the normal range by Western medicine, provided there are no underlying problems. In Chinese medicine, the ideal cycle for conception is thought to be 28 to 32 days, which is closer to the lunar cycle (see page 69). Acupuncture throughout the month can help to promote ovulation (see pages 72–73).

All the charts in this book, such as the one opposite, are based on a 28-day cycle, which is the average. Yours, of course, may be shorter or longer (see page 81), and this will affect your fertile time.

THE PERFECT BALANCE

Your menstrual cycle is the result of a complex interaction of hormones produced by the ovaries, the hypothalamus, and the pituitary gland, which all work together as a unit, sending messages to each other via hormones (see page 10). This interaction affects you in many different ways, from the degree to which you feel sexually attractive to energy levels to mental processing.

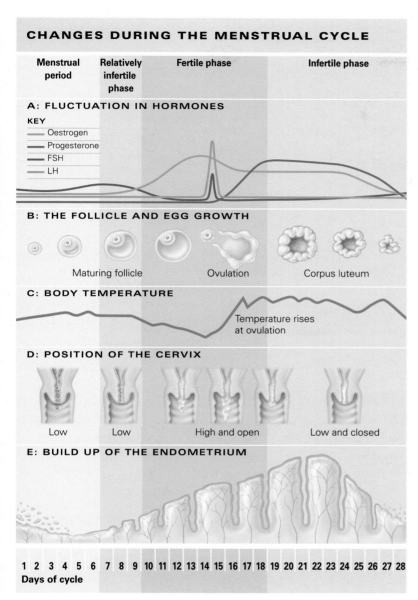

CHANGES DURING THE MENSTRUAL CYCLE

Menstrual period	Relatively infertile phase	Fertile phase	Infertile phase

A: FLUCTUATION IN HORMONES

KEY
- Oestrogen
- Progesterone
- FSH
- LH

B: THE FOLLICLE AND EGG GROWTH

Maturing follicle Ovulation Corpus luteum

C: BODY TEMPERATURE

Temperature rises at ovulation

D: POSITION OF THE CERVIX

Low   Low   High and open   Low and closed

E: BUILD UP OF THE ENDOMETRIUM

1 2 3 4 5 6 7 8 9 10 11 12 13 14 15 16 17 18 19 20 21 22 23 24 25 26 27 28
Days of cycle

Hormonal balance is the key to good fertility (**A**). In the first half of your cycle, the follicular phase, rising levels of FSH (follicle-stimulating hormone) encourage eggs to grow in the ovaries (**B**), which in turn release estrogen, a signal to reduce FSH. A surge in LH (luteinizing hormone) then triggers ovulation around day 14 or 15. Your temperature rises sharply (**C**) right after ovulation. At the same time, your cervix is high, soft, and open (**D**) and your mucus becomes "fertile," ready to receive the sperm. In the second half of the cycle, the luteal phase, the ruptured follicle produces progesterone, which halts FSH and LH production and continues the thickening of the endometrium (**E**), or womb lining, so it is ready to receive a fertilized egg.

The timings in the diagram refer to a 28-day cycle. If you have a 25-day cycle, for example, the onset of fertile mucus will be immediately after your period, about day six. If you have a 35-day cycle, ovulation may occur as late as day 21 in your cycle.

If you are in perfect balance hormonally, you won't feel the effects of estrogen and progesterone as their levels fluctuate during your cycle.

Most women have some kind of imbalance, however, which means that they feel the effects of hormonal fluctuations. Detecting these effects allows two things to happen. First, it familiarizes you with the workings of your reproductive system so that you can recognize and make the most of your fertile time. Secondly, it identifies imbalance so you can work toward correcting it by means of a program of detoxification, healthy eating, vitamin and mineral supplements, and complementary therapies (see pages 30–32 and 50–65).

If you do have an imbalance, it doesn't mean you won't become pregnant until you correct it. As I said, most women do experience some form of cycle irregularity (see pages 30–32 and 126–28). However, ovulatory problems, which in some cases are caused by hormonal imbalance, are associated with 35 percent of fertility problems, and it is thought that 10 to 15 percent of pregnancies miscarry because of hormonal imbalance. It therefore makes a lot of sense to do whatever you can to correct any imbalances that you detect.

THE THREE-MONTH PLAN

I suggest you take three months to get to know your cycle, but only if time is on your side. Keep a daily diary, noting every detail, including how you are feeling at each stage, so that you become familiar with your body's rhythms and patterns and begin to recognize any imbalances. If you have already been trying to conceive for some time, you may not feel able to take three months off. Keep a cycle diary anyway: anything you learn may help to improve your chances of conceiving.

THE BASIC PROCESS

A cycle begins with the start of your period (fresh red bleeding) on day one. The first half of the cycle lasts about 14 days, assuming you have a 28-day cycle, until ovulation. This is known as the follicular phase (see page 10), and is characterized by increasing estrogen levels. As you approach ovulation, you may experience a feeling of heightened sexuality around the middle of your cycle, when estrogen is at its peak and you are at your most fertile.

The second half of the cycle, lasting from ovulation to day 28, is known as the luteal phase (see pages 10–11). This is when—if intercourse occurs and all goes well—the released egg is fertilized and starts to implant. If fertilization does not occur, the egg is absorbed and the uterus prepares to shed its lining as a new cycle begins. The luteal phase is associated with rising progesterone levels and falling estrogen levels. In the second half of this part of the cycle you may start to experience some of the symptoms of premenstrual syndrome.

YOUR FERTILE TIME

It is important to be able to interpret your body's fertility signals for yourself. Everybody is different, however. If you're finding it difficult to recognize the signs, I recommend you see a fertility awareness nurse at a family planning clinic. She will be able to help you understand and chart your cycle.

There are several ways in which you can read your body's fertility signs. Although they can all be used individually (and you may find one method that works best for you), it's often easier to use them in conjunction with one another.

Cervical secretions Changes in your cervical secretions are the most reliable indicators of whether or not you are fertile (see pages 70–71). The start of the fertile time is signaled by secretions, so it is vitally important that you are able to recognize how these secretions change throughout your cycle.

Your cervix Estrogen and progesterone cause subtle changes in the muscle and connective tissue of the cervix. You can learn to recognize these changes by palpating (feeling) the cervix at the same time each day. Your local family planning clinic will tell you how to do this. At peak fertility, the cervix feels high, soft, and open. During the rest of the month it feels low, hard, and closed. (See diagram D on page 67.)

Body temperature Taking your temperature can be a useful indicator alongside other fertility signs, but don't become obsessive about it. Progesterone causes a rise in your BBT (basal body temperature) of at least 0.4°F (0.2°C) immediately after ovulation. This lasts until the level of progesterone falls at the start of menstruation. Your temperature may rise for other reasons, however, such as viral infections, stress, medication, drinking alcohol, or lack of sleep. Your temperature can also indicate imbalance in body systems. A temperature consistently below 96.8°F (36°C) during the follicular phase suggests a low metabolic rate, possibly caused by an underactive thyroid. Symptoms include lethargy, weight gain, and sensitivity to cold. A high temperature before ovulation may indicate an overactive thyroid. Temperature readings that remain the same may mean that you are not ovulating. This may happen after using the pill or because you have a luteal phase defect (LPD—see page 128).

The LH surge You could use a home ovulation kit to measure the surge of LH (luteinizing hormone) that takes place just before the egg is released from the follicle. But ovulation is variable and can occur at different times in different women. Some women ovulate on the same day as their LH surge, so if they wait the recommended 24 to 36 hours after the ovulation kit reads positive, they will have missed their opportunity (although LH kits only indicate the day of maximum fertility).

Cycle analysis It is important to record details of your menstrual cycle, since these will help you to work out your likely fertile time based on previous cycles. Since the fertile time may fluctuate, cervical secretions are the best indicators.

INFLUENCES ON YOUR CYCLE
Having a regular cycle that lasts, on average, 28 days will boost your chances of conceiving. Your cycle is profoundly affected by what is going on in your life, from lifestyle choices to which foods you eat. There are also some surprising influences.

Lunar cycles The cycle of ovulation and menstruation is closely linked to the phases of the moon. Scientific research has established that natural human rhythms may be influenced by the motions of the sun and the moon.

Light The influence of the heavens may not be just a matter of the moon's gravitational pull. Sunlight also plays an important role. There is evidence that fertility rates are lower in regions where people spend more time indoors and higher in regions closer to the equator, where daylight hours are longer. Animals that reproduce seasonally move into their fertile cycle when daylight patterns change with the apparent movement of the sun. This is largely because light stimuli received by the retina in the eyes are translated into hormonal signals by the pineal gland.

Some women with irregular periods have achieved greater regularity by sleeping with a light near their beds, about a yard from the head, for three days around ovulation, and by blacking out their room at night during their period.

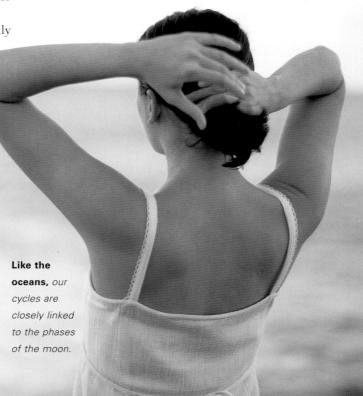

Like the oceans, *our cycles are closely linked to the phases of the moon.*

improving cervical secretions

Healthy cervical secretions are a key factor in fertility. The way in which hormones bring about changes in their feel and appearance throughout your cycle is your body's best indicator that you're about to ovulate.

STUDYING SECRETIONS

The cervix is lined with a mucus-secreting membrane. The mucus released changes in texture, color, and quantity throughout your menstrual cycle. The changes occur because of fluctuations in estrogen levels. You may notice the following:

• the entrance to the vagina may feel moist, sticky, wet, or slippery (leading up to ovulation)

• there may be a residue left on your underwear or on toilet paper

• the mucus may become very stretchy when tested between your thumb and forefinger (the fingertip test).

I ask my clients to keep a diary of their secretions, describing them at the same time each day. Most women need three cycles of observation before they are confident about recognizing the changes. It may help to abstain from penetrative sex for the first month to get an accurate record, since seminal fluid in the vagina will make it difficult to judge the condition of your mucus.

HORMONES AND MUCUS

Fluctuating hormone levels cause the changes in your mucus.

• After your period ends, you may have several "dry days" with no detectable mucus. This is the infertile phase: the vagina is a hostile environment for sperm at this time, when acidity rapidly immobilizes and destroys them.

• As estrogen levels rise as your cycle progresses, you will start to feel moist and sticky and the mucus will be white or creamy-colored. If you check the stretchiness between your thumb and forefinger, it will hold its shape but break easily.

• As estrogen levels continue to rise, the quantity of mucus will increase and it will become thinner, cloudier, and stretchier.

• As ovulation approaches, you will have a sensation of wetness and the vagina will feel slippery and wet, with copious amounts of thin, watery, transparent mucus, resembling raw egg white. On

Rising estrogen levels toward ovulation cause subtle changes in the viscosity of your cervical mucus that create an environment in which sperm can thrive. This is "fertile mucus."

CERVICAL SECRETIONS CHART

Menstrual period	Relatively infertile phase	Fertile phase	Infertile phase

FLUCTUATION IN HORMONES

KEY
— Oestrogen
— Progesterone
— FSH
— LH

CHANGES IN CERVICAL SECRETIONS

KEY
Period
Dry. No secretions seen or felt
Moist, white, cloudy, sticky
Wet, slippery, clear, stretchy

1 2 3 4 5 6 7 8 9 10 11 12 13 14 15 16 17 18 19 20 21 22 23 24 25 26 27 28
Days of cycle

finger testing, the mucus will stretch for an inch or two before breaking. This is fertile mucus in which sperm can live—usually for up to 72 hours, but sometimes for much longer. They can now move freely through the cervix. Under a microscope, you would see the long channels along which the sperm swim. Only normal sperm can fit into these channels. Women often worry about sperm leaking out after intercourse, but if fertile mucus is present, sperm will swim through it.

• The peak day for fertile mucus (directly prior to ovulation) is the last day, when mucus exhibits its most fertile characteristics. After this, you will quickly feel dry or sticky again. Thicker mucus, caused by a rise in progesterone, forms a plug at the cervix that serves as an impenetrable barrier.

PROBLEMS WITH MUCUS

If you are having problems finding fertile mucus, you may be ovulating early in your cycle, at the end of a period, so it is mixed up with menstrual blood.

The cervix responds to increased estrogen levels by opening the glands in the cervical canal to release cervical mucus. Insufficient mucus may indicate low estrogen levels (see page 30). Other causes for inadequate mucus are:
• low body weight (with a low BMI—see page 29), which can cause estrogen levels to fall and periods to stop

• rapid change in weight, which may suppress ovulation
• too much wheat bran in the diet
• deficiency in vitamin A (see page 59)
• prescribed drugs whose side effect is to dry out, thicken, or decrease amounts of mucus: these include antihistamines, cimetidine (for peptic ulcers), and clomiphene (for ovulation)
• too much exercise, which reduces circulating estrogens
• smoking, which alters the metabolism of estrogen
• high doses of vitamin C (>3 g), which may dry up mucus
• perfumed toilet paper, fabric softener, and tampons, which may distort cervical secretions
• vaginal lubricants, which may restrict the movement of sperm
• an incorrect pH balance—highly acidic mucus is hostile to sperm (see box, right)
• poor sex technique—if you are not producing arousal fluid, sex will be more difficult.

IMPROVING MUCUS

To increase the volume and health of your cervical mucus:
• eat foods containing B-complex vitamins (see pages 59–60)
• drink plenty of water
• eat foods containing PABA (see page 64).

There have been suggestions that using egg white or saliva, or drinking cough mixture, will improve cervical secretions, but there is not enough research to validate these claims.

FOODS FOR pH BALANCE

Sperm prefer alkaline conditions. Although there is no conclusive research, eating more alkaline foods and fewer acidic foods may help to improve the pH balance of mucus.

HIGH ALKALINE

Millet, almonds, seaweed, beets, artichokes, asparagus, greens, broccoli, Brussels sprouts, celery, cabbage, carrots, cauliflower, kale, cucumber, endive, escarole, leeks, kohlrabi, lettuce, onions, garlic, ginger, parsley, potatoes, sweet potatoes, pumpkins, turnips, watercress.

ALKALINE

Brown rice, apples, apricots, fresh figs, bananas, berries, melons, kiwi fruit, grapes, lemons, limes, pears, plums, peaches, mangoes, papayas, bamboo shoots, bok choy, parsnips, eggplant, okra, peppers, radishes, Swiss chard, rhubarb, spinach.

NEUTRAL

Yogurt, butter.

LOW ACID

Lamb, chicken, turkey, goose, duck, salmon, white fish, eggs, beans, barley, buckwheat, oats, rye, white rice, mushrooms, raisins.

HIGH ACID

Beef, veal, pork, ham, bacon, cheese, goat's and cow's milk, wheat, corn, tomatoes, oranges, grapefruit.

acupuncture

Although my fertility practice is grounded in Western medicine, I frequently use acupuncture to regulate the menstrual cycle or to treat other fertility problems.

TRADITIONAL CHINESE MEDICINE (TCM)

According to ancient Chinese beliefs, we all have a vital life force or energy known as *qi* (pronounced "chee"), which flows along invisible pathways called meridians (see opposite). Most of the principal meridians are named after the major internal organs through which they pass. The Conception Vessel runs up the middle of the body and has important acupoints associated with it.

Each organ plays a role in maintaining a smooth flow of *qi*, which in turn allows body systems to function well. Treatment is given to support a weak organ and restore balance. Most people have a constitutional weakness that affects their flow of *qi*. Symptoms of illness indicate imbalance in the meridian of one organ or another. Each organ exhibits a characteristic pattern of disharmony that a trained practitioner can identify from symptoms.

The meridians associated with reproduction are the kidneys, spleen, and liver. If symptoms suggest a "kidney deficiency," for example, acupuncture on specific acupoints along that meridian will support the kidneys and restore balance. According to the Chinese, the kidneys store reproductive *jing* (see below) or essence. Good *jing* means strong sperm, strong eggs, and strong and healthy children. Many women I see have a kidney deficiency, their kidney energy depleted by previous pregnancies, recurrent miscarriage, or IVF treatment.

In order to reestablish balance in a woman's body and enhance her fertility, I treat her on a weekly basis. In Chinese medicine, blood flow is considered very important, and acupoints may be used to relieve menstrual pain, encourage healthy blood flow, replenish energy by "building" the blood, boost ovulation, and encourage implantation.

YIN AND YANG

As well as *qi*, the Chinese believe in the opposing forces of *yin* and *yang*. These make up the two complementary halves of a whole, and each represents the opposite of the other in everything.

ACUPOINTS

Acupoints, or acupuncture points—365 of them in all—are located along the meridians. Acupoints resemble tiny valves through which the flow of *qi* can be regulated. Certain points are particularly relevant for fertility, as their names suggest, such

---

ACUPUNCTURE & FERTILITY

Research has shown that acupuncture may help to relieve the symptoms of many conditions, some of which may compromise fertility. These ailments include dysmenorrhea (painful periods), amenorrhea (no periods), and other menstrual cycle irregularities and reproduction system problems, including PMS (premenstrual syndrome), hormonal imbalance, anovulation (no ovulation), fibroids, endometriosis, breast pain, prostate pain, urinary and bladder pain, and menopause. **A lot of the research has been done on the use of auricular (ear) acupuncture and electro-acupuncture. It is my belief that it is also of benefit during in vitro fertilization (IVF)**. I use it twice weekly on women undergoing IVF (see page 163), when stimulation begins, and then again after egg transfer.

as Door of Infants and the Gate of Life. To find an acupoint, a practitioner will palpate along the relevant meridian until he or she locates a little dip. As the fine needle is inserted, you will probably experience a dull sensation.

DIAGNOSIS AND TREATMENT

The ancient Chinese did not have scans and blood tests for diagnosis, but instead looked to natural laws and cycles and the ways in which they are reflected in people to identify imbalances. Many details about an individual are important in diagnosis: the sound of the voice, skin tone, body odor, preferred season, food likes and dislikes, dominant emotions, and sleep patterns.

The tongue is an important diagnostic tool. Each area of the tongue represents a different part of the body: I look for color, coating, and the presence of any cracks to aid diagnosis.

Abdominal diagnosis is all about temperature. If *qi* is flowing smoothly, your temperature should be even all over. The Chinese believe that you cannot "grow" a baby in an abdomen that is cold, but many of my female clients come to me with a lower abdomen that feels cold to the touch.

The Chinese see the ear as a representation of an inverted fetus. All the major meridians cross the ear, and it has more than 120 acupoints. It is particularly useful for treating hormonal imbalance.

Finally, pulse diagnosis recognizes six pulses on the hand, each relating to specific organs. The quality of a pulse varies throughout a woman's cycle, and imbalances can be detected from these changes. Reading the pulses forms a crucial part of diagnosis.

Electro-acupuncture makes use of a machine to boost the treatment. It is particularly useful for relieving pain, boosting ovulation, and regulating the menstrual cycle.

ACUPUNCTURE FOR YOU

Acupuncture may improve your general health, alleviate underlying conditions preventing conception, or enhance the efficacy of fertility

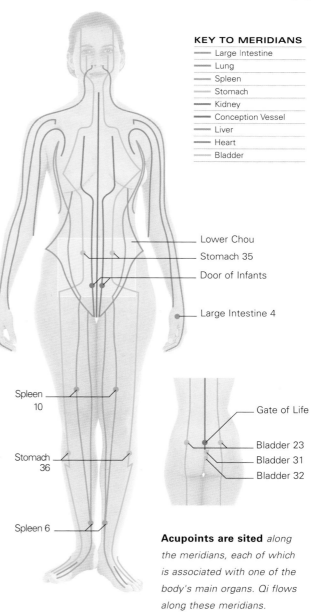

KEY TO MERIDIANS
- Large Intestine
- Lung
- Spleen
- Stomach
- Kidney
- Conception Vessel
- Liver
- Heart
- Bladder

Lower Chou
Stomach 35
Door of Infants
Large Intestine 4
Spleen 10
Stomach 36
Spleen 6

Gate of Life
Bladder 23
Bladder 31
Bladder 32

Acupoints are sited *along the meridians, each of which is associated with one of the body's main organs. Qi flows along these meridians.*

treatments. Find a practitioner who specializes in fertility, especially if you are older or you have a reproductive dysfunction. Be prepared to change many aspects of your life in order to support treatment—exercise, diet, and stress management for example. Chinese medicine treats the whole person at a physical and mental/emotional level.

improving sperm quality

It may be difficult to get your partner to work at improving his sperm quality unless he knows there is a problem, but his general health will also be improved by a few simple measures.

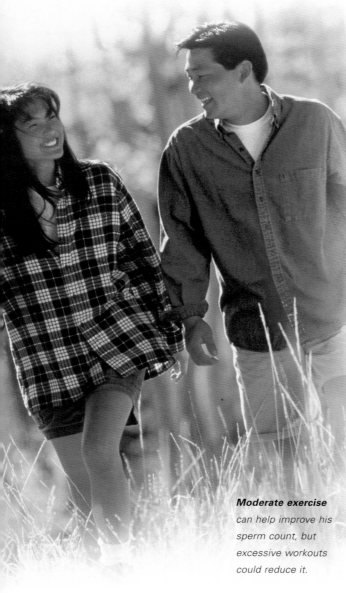

Moderate exercise *can help improve his sperm count, but excessive workouts could reduce it.*

100 DAYS TO HEALTHY SPERM

By making a few simple changes to his diet and lifestyle, your partner can make a significant difference in the quality and quantity of his sperm. But improvements don't happen overnight. It takes 100 days for sperm to develop—74 days to form and 20–30 days to mature completely. So a program to improve sperm quality and count should begin at least 100 days before conception.

WHAT CONSTITUTES GOOD SPERM?

Three essential factors are involved:
• sperm count—the average count should be more than 20 million sperm per milliliter of ejaculate
• morphology—this is the shape of the sperm
• motility—how fast sperm swim and how they progress forward

In general, the higher the count, the higher the percentage of normal sperm and motile sperm, therefore the greater the chance of conception.

LIFESTYLE CHANGES

Your partner should try to incorporate the following changes into his daily life for the next three months or so. By then, he will more than likely have improved his sperm quality (depending on why it was low in the first place), and his general health and fitness levels will be much improved. He will find he has higher energy levels, more efficient digestion, fewer headaches, and more restful sleep.

Encourage your partner to:
• eat healthily and take a good multivitamin and mineral and DHA supplements (see pages 76–79)

- go on the liver detox program for seven or ten days (see pages 50–53) to improve his liver function and hormonal balance
- find some time every day to unwind and let go of stress—he may consider learning deep-breathing techniques or meditation (see pages 42–43)
- have a weekly acupuncture treatment (on the kidney meridian) for general health and energy levels if problems are detected
- exercise and be active—taking the stairs instead of the elevator or parking farther away from his destination and walking—all these measures will improve his general fitness and reduce stress levels. But he must not overdo things, since prolonged vigorous exercise more than three times a week should be avoided
- stop smoking, cut down on alcohol, avoid recreational drugs, and reduce his caffeine intake
- drink at least two quarts (liters) of water a day—semen is made up largely of water.

NEGATIVE INFLUENCES ON SPERM FORMATION

In order to give himself the best chance of producing fertile sperm, your partner should try to avoid the following negative influences.

HIGH TEMPERATURES

Sperm cells will not develop or function well if their temperature is higher than 93°F (32°C), despite the body's normal core temperature being 98.6°F (37°C). In fact, spending a long time in a hot bath, sauna, or Jacuzzi can "cook" sperm cells. Long-distance driving also heats the scrotum.

Wearing athletic supports or tight-fitting underwear made from synthetic fibers can also reduce sperm count. If your partner wears loose-fitting, cotton boxer shorts and avoids spending too long in high temperatures, sperm recovery will take only 100 days.

STRESS

Long hours, poor diet, and high levels of stress take their toll on sperm production. Constant stress results in the body fighting on all fronts to get blood to the heart, lungs, and brain. Forget below-the-waist activity: energy is needed to make sperm, and if it is diverted to other parts of the body, sperm production suffers. Both of you should take time to relax each day.

ALCOHOL

Alcohol has many negative effects on male fertility, including interfering with the secretion of testosterone, speeding up its conversion to estrogen, lowering sperm count, and reducing sex drive (see also page 34). The breakdown product of alcohol metabolism, acetaldehyde, is toxic to sperm. As few as two drinks can have a negative effect, but damage is not permanent if your partner stops drinking now.

SMOKING

Smoking doubles the number of free radicals produced in the body every second, reduces sperm count and sperm motility, and increases the risk of sperm abnormalities and genetic defects in the embryo. Your partner should stop now.

DRUGS

The active ingredient in marijuana is chemically related to testosterone. It tends to build up in the testicles, lowering libido and causing impotence. Marijuana lowers sperm count, as does cocaine.

A number of prescribed drugs can also have detrimental effects on sperm (see pages 35–36).

ANTIOXIDANTS

Around 40 percent of sperm damage is thought to be caused by free radicals. Antioxidants vitamins C and E, beta-carotene, selenium, and zinc help to protect sperm from damage, preventing them from clumping together, increasing motility, and reducing the risk of genetic abnormalities in any offspring produced from them.

Foods that are high in antioxidants include blackberries, blueberries, garlic, kale, strawberries, Brussels sprouts, plums, alfalfa sprouts, broccoli, and red peppers.

CAFFEINE

Caffeine may impair sperm production, cause chromosomal abnormalities, and affect sperm motility (see also page 33).

MEDICAL PROBLEMS

A hernia repair, tubule infection, chlamydia, or mumps can affect sperm count. Underlying illnesses such as diabetes may affect sperm production. An acidophilus supplement will replace depleted beneficial bacteria in the gut following the use of antibiotics.

EXERCISE

Exercise is important for good health, but excessive amounts of punishing exercise, such as long-distance running, may lower sperm count and temporarily reduce testosterone production.

TOXINS AND POLLUTANTS

Toxins and pollutants, including pesticides and heavy metals, are very harmful to sperm production (see pages 37–39). Encourage your partner to include organic products in his diet as much as possible.

Many men face occupational hazards in the form of X-rays, solvents, paint products, and toxic metals (see also pages 37–39).

ENVIRONMENTAL ESTROGENS

We all take in far more estrogens than 50 years ago, leading to hormonal imbalances in both men and women (see page 31). There are traces of estrogen drugs in drinking water, for example, and livestock are given increasing amounts of growth hormones.

DIET AND NUTRITION FOR HEALTHY SPERM

A well-balanced diet is essential for sperm health, and certain key nutrients boost sperm production and neutralize damage. Your partner should take a good multivitamin and mineral supplement to maintain supplies of these vital nutrients, and he should also think about how to include them in his diet.

AMINO ACIDS

These are the building blocks of proteins and are essential if sperm are to mature properly. They are found in protein foods (see page 55), but I recommend that your partner also takes a supplement.

An important amino acid is L-arginine. In one study, sperm counts doubled after supplements were taken. The head of the sperm contains a large amount of L-arginine, and this amino acid is essential for sperm production.

Overall, clinical trials confirm its effectiveness at levels of 500 mg a day, although the benefits may be less in men with extremely low counts. Do not take arginine supplements if you have the herpes virus—it can stimulate an attack.

Other important amino acids include L-carnitine, essential for the normal functioning of sperm (50 mg a day recommended); and taurine, which is found in high levels in sperm and is needed for good motility (50 mg).

VITAMIN A

This vitamin is essential for the production of male sex hormones. Animal research shows that deficiency may produce degeneration of the seminiferous tubules (see page 14), reduced semen volume and sperm count, and abnormal sperm morphology. For good food sources, see page 59.

Take vitamin A supplements with foods containing fat or oil. Adequate protein foods, as well as vitamins C and E and zinc, and proper thyroid function, are needed to mobilize vitamin A from the liver for transportation around the body.

▶ **DOSAGE** RNI men 700 mcg/day.

VITAMIN B6

Together with zinc, vitamin B6 is essential for the formation of male sex hormones. Deficiency has been found to cause infertility in studies of animals. See page 60 for food sources of vitamin B6 and pages 59–60 for information about how to supplement B vitamins.

▶ **DOSAGE** RNI men 1.4 mg/day, but I would recommend 50 mg a day.

VITAMIN B12

Vitamin B12 is needed, together with folate (folic acid), for the synthesis of DNA and RNA. These are important compounds that are part of our genetic blueprint and are involved in the makeup of every cell in the body. B12 also helps with the uptake of folate.

Low levels of B12 are associated with abnormal sperm production, reduced sperm counts, and reduced sperm motility. Even if there is no deficiency, supplementation is worthwhile in men with sperm counts of less than 20 million/ml. In one study, 27 percent of men who had sperm counts of less than 20 million and were given B12 injections every day achieved counts in excess of 100 million/ml.

The only reliable sources of B12 are animal products, in particular lamb, sardines, and salmon. Vegans should eat fermented foods that contain bacteria, but it is better to take supplements to ensure adequate intakes. Calcium aids the absorption of vitamin B12. See pages 59–60 for information about how to supplement B vitamins.

▶ **DOSAGE** RNI men 1.5 mcg/day.

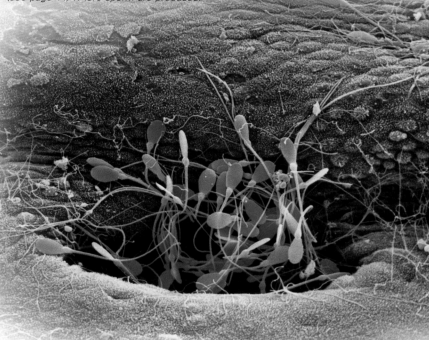

Healthy sperm emerging from a network of tiny tubes linked to the seminiferous tubules (see page 14) where sperm are produced.

FOLATE (FOLIC ACID)
Folate is very important for all rapidly dividing cells, and for the production of healthy sperm. It improves sperm count and sperm motility as well as reducing the number of morphological abnormalities. Research has shown that folic acid is just as important a nutrient for men as it is for women, and folate deficiency may be a contributing factor to male infertility in as many as 10 percent of cases. See page 61 for good food sources and information about taking folic acid supplements.

▶ **DOSAGE** RNI men 200 mcg/day, but I would recommend taking 400 mcg/day.

VITAMIN C
Vitamin C is needed for the development of healthy sperm. Research in 1991 found that men with low levels of vitamin C were more likely to have genetically damaged sperm. This may not affect fertility directly, but any genetic damage to sperm would increase the risk of a child being born with a birth defect. Vitamin C is an antioxidant. It blocks the action of free radicals, which can cause gene damage. Many studies have found that vitamin C supplementation can improve sperm motility. 15 mg/day taken for three months increases sperm count as well as motility. Vitamin C also prevents the sperm from clumping together.

See page 61 for food sources of Vitamin C.

▶ **DOSAGE** RNI men 40 mg/day, but I would recommend 1,000 mg/day.

VITAMIN E
This vitamin is important for fertility. In 1922 researchers found that male rats fed on a vitamin E–free diet were unable to reproduce, but fertility returned when wheat-germ oil was added to their diet.

As a major antioxidant, vitamin E helps to protect the high level of polyunsaturated fatty acids found in sperm cell membranes from damage by free radicals. In one study, 400 IU of vitamin E given to men twice daily for three months led to a significant improvement in their sperm's ability to bind to and penetrate an egg. Severe vitamin E deficiency can lead to degeneration of the testicular tissue. If this damage becomes permanent, vitamin E

Leafy vegetables provide many nutrients, such as folate, calcium, magnesium, potassium, iron, PABA, and vitamins A, B2, B6 and E.

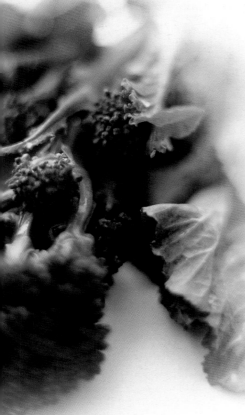

supplements are not able to repair it and a man will become sterile.

A natural (d-alpha-tocopherol), as opposed to synthetic (dl-alpha-tocopherol), supplement of this vitamin is more easily utilized by the body and retained for longer in the body tissues. Check the label when buying a supplement to see which it is. See page 61 for main food sources and information about supplementing vitamin E.
▶ **DOSAGE** RNI men >4 mg.

SELENIUM

Selenium is needed to form normally shaped sperm and to maintain a normal sperm count. Low levels of this mineral in semen have been linked to infertility. Studies on rats indicate that selenium is vitally important for the proper functioning of the epididymis (see pages 14–15), which is related to sperm maturation and motility.

Selenium also has antioxidant properties, protecting cells with a high lipid (fat) content in semen against possible damage from free radicals. See page 63 for food sources and information about how to supplement selenium.
▶ **DOSAGE** RNI men 75 mcg/day.

MANGANESE

Manganese deficiency in animals can lead to testicular degeneration and congenital malformations. Tests on animals have found that males with severe manganese deficiency exhibit sterility and an absence of libido, low sperm count, and

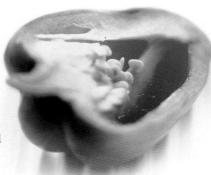

Red peppers are full of the essential vitamins A, C, and E.

increasing numbers of degenerating cells in the epididymis. A lack of manganese may inhibit the synthesis of sex hormones, and possibly other steroids (important organic compounds in the body), with consequent infertility. See page 63 for food sources and information about supplementing manganese.
▶ **DOSAGE** RNI men 1.4 mg/day.

ZINC

One of the nutrients most commonly lacking in the modern-day diet, zinc is vital for the production of healthy sperm. It is the most critical trace mineral involved in male sexual function, and is used in virtually every aspect of reproduction, including testosterone metabolism, testicle growth, and sperm production. It is also important for the motility of sperm and a good sperm count. Zinc also helps reduce excessive amounts of estrogen in male reproductive tissue, a factor that is linked to low sperm count.

Zinc is about 30 times more concentrated in sperm than in the bloodstream, and is largely found in the sperm head. Every time a man ejaculates, he loses about 5 mg of this vitally important mineral.

A lot of research has shown that supplementing zinc improves fertility, and many studies suggest that 30 mg a day will guard against deficiency, help to normalize sperm count, improve sperm motility, and increase testosterone production. See page 63 for good food sources and information about how to supplement zinc.

▶ **DOSAGE** RNI men 9.5 mg/day.

COENZYME Q10

Coenzyme Q10, a fat-soluble vitamin-like substance found in every cell of the body, is present in large amounts in seminal fluid. It helps to protect sperm from damage by free radicals and supercharges them with energy, increasing their motility.

It is difficult to obtain sufficient amounts of coenzyme Q10 from food sources (although it has been found that vegetarians have higher levels in their bodies than meat-eaters), so supplementation is the only reliable way of boosting your intake. There are no recommended intake levels for coenzyme Q10, but I usually suggest between 50 mg and 90 mg a day.

ESSENTIAL FATTY ACIDS

Essential fatty acids act as hormone regulators and the body cannot function without them. I believe it is vitally important to take them as a supplement.

Prostaglandins are made up of EFAs, and these are important for hormone regulation. Sperm contain high concentrations of omega-3 EFAs, particularly DHA (docosahexaenoic acid), the fatty acid found in oily fish. Most DHA is in the sperm tail and is thought to be important for sperm motility. Many men are deficient in omega-3 EFAs. Eating mackerel, herring, salmon, or sardines at least two or three times a week (avoid tuna because of its high mercury levels), along with a daily supplement of 2,000 mg of EFA will help to improve this situation. Flaxseed oil is a good substitute for vegetarians.

Very high levels of omega-6–derived prostaglandins are found in sperm cell membranes, and low levels of omega-6 EFAs are significantly linked to reduced male fertility. See page 64 for more details of food sources and information about how to supplement omega-3 and -6 EFAs.

EFAs are very prone to free-radical damage, and good levels of antioxidants in the body are required to reduce this risk. See pages 59–64 for antioxidant nutrients—vitamins A, C, and E and selenium.

PABA

Based on studies done as long ago as the 1940s, para-aminobenzoic acid (PABA) has been associated with male fertility—in support of the functioning of the pituitary gland and hence reproductive

hormones. A B-complex component, PABA may also be of benefit for folate production by intestinal bacteria, the production of red blood cells, and the processing of proteins. Food sources of PABA include organ meats, whole grains, brewer's yeast, molasses, spinach, and mushrooms. Folic acid and B-complex vitamins aid absorption: stress and antibiotics hinder it.

HERBS FOR MEN

Ginseng may improve levels of testosterone. Tribullus has been found to support healthy sperm production and is used to treat sexual dysfunction (impotence and lack of libido). Limited research has been done on certain herbs that are believed to have a negative effect on fertility. These include St.-John's-wort, saw palmetto, licorice, and echinacea (see also page 36).

Nuts are a valuable source of manganese and vitamin E, and release energy slowly for efficient use.

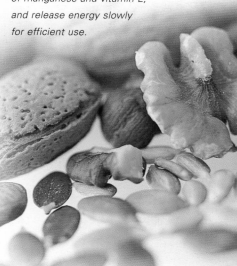

countdown to conception

Now that you have improved your fertility status and become
familiar with your menstrual cycle, you can give conception
your best shot. The following pages will guide you through each
phase of your cycle to maximize your chances of conceiving.

Massage will help you to relax
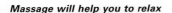
and avoid becoming overly anxious during
the next month or so as you try to conceive
and then wait to see if you are pregnant.

THE CONCEPTION PLAN

If, for the last few months, you and your partner
have adopted the changes I have recommended to
boost your fertility, you have given yourselves the
best chance of conceiving. Now that you are trying
to conceive, there are certain adjustments you can
make each week during your cycle while keeping
to the basics of healthy eating and living.

I work with clients to help them understand what
is going on inside their bodies while they try to get
pregnant. Over the next few pages, I explain these
changes and provide week-by-week guidelines on
diet, lifestyle changes, and complementary therapies
to suit your body during each phase of the cycle.

ADJUSTING THE PLAN

The average cycle is 28 days long, so the conception
plan is divided into four weeks. Every woman is
different, however, and many do not conform to
this. Use the chart opposite to help you adjust the
plan if your cycle is longer or shorter than 28 days.

CHANGING EMOTIONS

Once you and your partner decide to start a family,
everything is wonderful. Sex is fantastic because
caution (and precautions) are thrown to the wind.
But after a few months without conceiving, you
might start to think you have a problem. A cycle of
highs and lows begins—optimism around ovulation
followed by disappointment when your period
arrives. Then there is the worry that stress is
sabotaging your chances of conceiving.

ADJUSTING THE PLAN FOR LONGER OR SHORTER CYCLES

The plan is based on a 28 day cycle. If your cycle is longer or shorter, use this chart to work out how long to use the information for each week, and when you are ovulating.

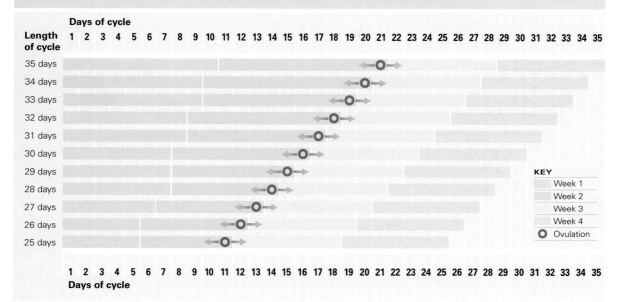

KEY
- Week 1
- Week 2
- Week 3
- Week 4
- ○ Ovulation

AVOIDING ANXIETY

If you find yourself becoming anxious, try to relax. Remember the following points.

- Don't panic. Nature has its cycles (of dormancy in winter followed by new growth in spring). Although you can try to lend a helping hand, nature generally refuses to be rushed. Try to go with the flow a little.

- Don't assume you have a problem or dwell on the negative. Limit the amount of time you spend thinking about babies and pregnancy, and don't allow yourself to think about what isn't happening. Visualize a positive outcome and distract yourself from negative thoughts.

- Before you race to a fertility specialist, take a long hard look at yourselves and think, "Have we done everything possible to conceive naturally?" If you feel you have the time, give yourselves a few more months off trying while you make any improvements you can to your lifestyle.

- Be patient. The statistics on rates of conception tell us that the average couple takes about nine months to a year to conceive.

- Keep your balance and perspective—take control of the situation (by following the countdown to conception plan on pages 82–91) rather than letting it control you.

This is an exciting time; enjoy it as much as you can. Staying positive and cheerful can only improve your chances of conceiving.

If you are older or you suspect you might have a fertility problem, it might help to pencil into your planner a date when you will call to make an appointment for you and your partner to see your doctor about fertility testing. Until that date, relax and let nature take its course. Just making that plan, knowing your alternatives, and feeling you are taking positive action (with nutrition and exercise) can make a huge difference to your anxiety levels and relieve the heavy weight on your mind.

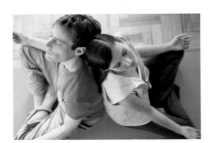

the first week

Menstruation is the beginning of the follicular phase (see page 10), when eggs begin to ripen. Chinese medicine regards the shedding of the lining of the uterus as the body cleansing itself: this is the inward and reflective *yin* phase of your cycle.

week 1
at a glance

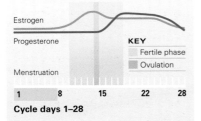

CHART YOUR CYCLE

Estrogen

Progesterone

KEY
■ Fertile phase
■ Ovulation

Menstruation

| 1 | 8 | 15 | 22 | 28 |

Cycle days 1–28

FOCUS ON

○ DIET AND NUTRITION

Eat well—this is not the week to fast or diet. Avoid alcohol but drink plenty of water. Nutrients are needed (see opposite) to regenerate the endometrium, start the regrowth of follicles, and balance hormones.

○ LIFESTYLE

In ancient cultures, menstruation was a time for women to withdraw from society and rest. You may not feel like being sociable at this time. The modern world doesn't stop for menstruating women, but in a hectic life, you should make space and time to reflect and be still.

MENSTRUATION

HORMONES

Falling estrogen and progesterone levels signal the hypothalamus to release GnRH (gonadotrophin-releasing hormone), which triggers bleeding. This, in turn, prompts the pituitary to release FSH (follicle-stimulating hormone), which will start the growth of follicles and the development of an egg inside each of them.

The majority of women begin a period at night or within the first four hours of waking. How long bleeding lasts varies from woman to woman, but it is generally between five and seven days, with the heaviest bleeding on the first day. The outer two-thirds of the lining is shed gradually. The endometrium starts to regenerate within two days of the start of menstruation and by day five is already 1/16 in (2 mm) thick.

According to traditional Chinese medicine, bleeding should last for three to five days. Flow should be not too heavy, nor too light—around 3½ to 5½ tbsp (50 to 80 ml), although the exact quantity is hard to gauge, and what some

women consider to be heavy bleeding is quite normal for others.

In the West, period pain is regarded as normal, and many women take painkillers routinely. In Chinese medicine, it is regarded as an indication of an obstruction in the flow of blood and *qi* (see page 72), both of which should be smooth. Blood should be bright red in color: dark or brown blood is old blood. Pink blood is thin and poor quality, while clots indicate stagnation in the flow.

LIFESTYLE

The body's energy naturally ebbs during a period. Don't fight this tiredness: allow yourself to rest. Soak in a warm, candlelit bath and have a few early nights, allowing your vital energy to be used for the regeneration to come.

It is good to be inward-looking rather than outgoing at this time. Use the time for reflection and visualization. Think positively about moving on to a new cycle and a new attempt to conceive. Accept the fact that for now, at least, you are not pregnant, and look at what improvements you can make for the month ahead. Make sure you keep the lower abdomen, which the Chinese call the lower *chou*, warm at all times.

Use sanitary towels rather than tampons to allow blood to flow freely (see page 39). Chinese medicine does not recommend sex during a woman's period, since it affects the blood flow. Research shows that many women, in fact, don't want sex during their period.

DIET AND NUTRITION

Continue all the good nutritional habits you have established during the last few months. Make sure that you are getting all the vitamins, minerals, and trace elements you need for this part of your cycle.

- Vitamins A and E, selenium, and bioflavonoids are all important for building up the endometrium. See pages 59–64 for dosage and good food sources.
- Eating foods rich in iron (with vitamin C to aid absorption) will help to compensate for blood loss. See pages 59–63 for dosages and good food sources.
- Take a supplement of coenzyme Q10 (see pages 59–61) to help oxygenate the blood and improve blood circulation generally.
- Vitamin B1 is also important for building up the blood. See page 60 for dosages and good food sources.

EXERCISE

Avoid strenuous or aerobic exercise during your period. Consider doing yoga, meditation, or qigong, an ancient system of movement, breathing, and meditation. Dao yin breathing (see page 44) may also be of benefit. Don't go swimming at this time because, according to traditional Chinese beliefs, the abdomen will get cold.

COMPLEMENTARY THERAPIES

Acupuncture can help to regulate the blood flow, build up your *qi*, and relieve pain. Different points will be used depending on whether blood flow needs to be increased (if it is too light) or reduced (if too heavy).

Moxibustion (the burning of small cones of dried mugwort or moxa to warm up certain acupoints) may also be used to build up the blood. In Chinese medicine, the important organs for reproduction are the kidneys, heart, and uterus. The nature and quality of blood flow is a vital diagnostic tool, and your acupuncturist will ask you about the amount, color, consistency, and degree of clotting. Pain is also significant—lower back pain, for example, is a sign of kidney deficiency. Make notes on all your menstrual details to take along.

Acupressure can also help blood flow and may be self-administered. Press gently but firmly for five minutes twice a day on the acupoints Large Intestine 4 (in the triangle formed by the thumb and index finger) and Spleen 6 (three finger-breadths above the ankle bone on the inside leg).

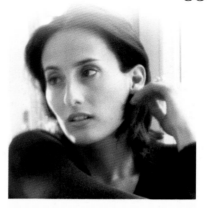

YOUR EMOTIONS

For many women, this is a difficult week because their period brings confirmation that they are not pregnant. It can be a low point, filled with despair, anger, frustration, and hopelessness. As negative as you may feel, remember that your body is cleansing itself before regenerating.

Many cultures view the period as physical renewal— the body preparing for a fresh cycle. Cleanse yourself mentally and emotionally, too. Don't feel guilty about the odd glass of wine you may have had.

You're low in energy and feel introverted, but feel a lightening from your premenstrual mood.

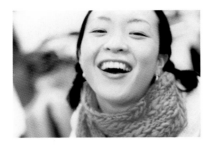

week 2
at a glance

CHART YOUR CYCLE

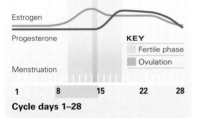

Estrogen

Progesterone

KEY
■ Fertile phase
■ Ovulation

Menstruation

| 1 | 8 | 15 | 22 | 28 |

Cycle days 1–28

FOCUS ON

○ DIET

Diet is crucially important to hormonal balance and good egg quality. Once ovulation, fertilization, and implantation occur, everything happens quickly. You need certain nutrients to ensure that the uterus is prepared and cell division is successful. If you have deficiencies, take supplements (see opposite).

○ LIFESTYLE

You will feel more energetic this week than last week and you will be much more inclined to do exercise. It's fine to keep to your normal exercise routine (see also page 86).

---

the second week

This is the most important time of the month from the point of view of fertility. Between 10 and 20 egg follicles have been developing, but only one of them will become dominant this week. The rest will gradually degenerate. By the time of ovulation, which takes place at the end of this week, only the one dominant follicle will remain.

OVULATION

HORMONES

Follicle-stimulating hormone (FSH) levels rise to further stimulate growth and ripening of the follicles. Initially these are about ⅛ in (4 mm) in diameter, but by the time of ovulation they will be five times bigger. By day nine, there will be twice as many blood vessels in a dominant follicle as in the other follicles. The rising FSH levels prompt the ovaries to release estrogen, which starts the renewal and thickening of the endometrium (ready for possible implantation). As estrogen levels rise, FSH levels fall so that no more eggs mature. Estrogen levels peak at around day 12, sending a signal to the hypothalamus to release luteinizing hormone (LH).

LH triggers changes in the ovary and follicle that will lead up to ovulation. With the LH surge on day 14, one part of the outer membrane of the follicle starts to thin. Within another 24–36 hours, the follicle membrane ruptures and the egg and its surrounding follicular fluid are released.

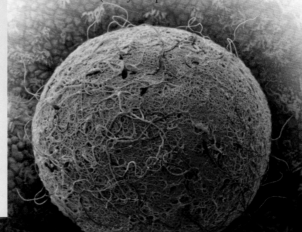

After ovulation the egg is swept into the fallopian tube to begin its journey toward the uterus. Fertilization occurs in the middle section of the tube.

DIET AND NUTRITION

Ensure that your body has all the nourishment it needs during this vitally important week of the cycle. Continue to follow the healthy eating program as you have been for the last few months, but pay particular attention to certain essential nutrients.

- All the B vitamins are important for the release of the egg, and, if it is fertilized, its implantation in the lining of the uterus and the early development of an embryo. See pages 59–61 for dosages and good food sources of all B vitamins. Vitamin B12 in particular (see page 60) is needed for the synthesis of DNA and RNA, the materials that make up the genetic blueprint of a human being and are present in the nucleus of every egg.
- Zinc, magnesium, selenium, and vitamin A are all essential nutrients for egg production, and zinc is also needed to promote cell division. Eat plenty of foods rich in these nutrients during this week. See pages 59–63 for dosages and good food sources of these essential nutrients.
- Vitamin C helps to replenish the ovaries and, together with vitamin E, selenium, and zinc, is present in the follicular fluid surrounding an egg. These essential nutrients are believed to nourish the egg during its development. See pages 61–63 for good food sources and recommended daily intakes.

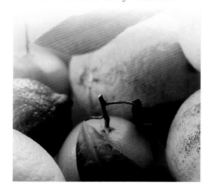

Vitamin C is an antioxidant that helps to "mop up" potentially harmful debris in the reproductive system.

YOUR EMOTIONS

Studies show that increased levels of estrogen, FSH, and LH increase your sense of well-being. Clients tell me they feel full of anticipation now, as they can "try again." You feel slimmer and more attractive. Your energy levels rise and you feel more dynamic and outgoing than last week. You are focused on goals and full of enthusiasm, positivity, and new ideas. It is a time of mental and physical activity, when ideas you may have had last week start to take on structure. Sexual desire peaks as ovulation approaches, and you feel "creative" at every level. As much as you reach a high at this point, try to focus on your secretions and what is happening to your body.

KEY INDICATORS OF OVULATION

Watch for the following signs and symptoms since they indicate that ovulation has occurred. Don't worry if you fail to pick up any of these signs: it doesn't mean you haven't ovulated.

- Abundant cervical secretions are a sign that your fertile time is approaching: the mucus will be watery, stretchy, and transparent (see pages 70–71).

- Your desire for sexual intercourse will increase markedly this week.
- A slight rise in body temperature will last from now until your next bleed (if there is one).
- Ovulation pain (or Mittelschmerz, as it is called) is something many women experience: it is a dull ache on one side of the lower abdomen, and lasts anything from a few minutes to several hours.

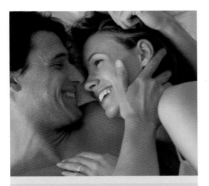

WHEN TO HAVE SEX

There are many myths surrounding sex, and a lot of confusion and misinformation about the best time to have sex in order to conceive. I am amazed to discover that many of my clients either do not have enough sex or do it at the wrong time.

Sperm can usually survive for quite a long time—up to 72 hours in alkaline secretions (and even as long as seven days), waiting for the egg to arrive. An egg is fertilizable for 12–24 hours. So the best time to have sex is during the period leading up to ovulation, when your fertile secretions are at their peak. In a 28-day cycle, with mucus peaking on day 14, that means days 11 to 13.

Some women become very anxious, thinking that the egg only lasts a number of hours, because their own work commitments or their partner's plans are not compatible with their time of ovulation. This can be very stressful for the woman desperate to conceive and a big turnoff for the man expected to "perform" no matter what.

EXERCISE

Make the most of feeling fully alive by taking brisk walks and doing regular aerobic exercise to get your *qi* circulating. Go running, swimming, power walking, cycling, or visit the gym.

COMPLEMENTARY THERAPIES

Use the aromatherapy oils sandalwood, jasmine, or ylang-ylang, which are believed to have aphrodisiac qualities. Only use these in oil burners or in scented candles, however: do not put them on your skin, either by adding oil to your bathwater or by using them as a massage oil, since this will interfere with your body's own pheromones. Male and female bodies give off natural odors that, some people believe, shouldn't be interfered with. You may not want to use perfume or other scented products for the same reason.

I recommend acupuncture as close to ovulation as possible. The acupoint is the Door of Infants on the lower abdomen (see diagram on page 73). Also in accordance with Chinese beliefs, it is very important to keep the lower abdomen warm at this time.

VISUALIZATION

Make time this week to visualize the processes of ovulation and fertilization. Picture the egg being released as the follicle ruptures (see picture on page 170). The egg

At fertilization, a sperm penetrates the egg, dissolving its outer coating in a chemical reaction.

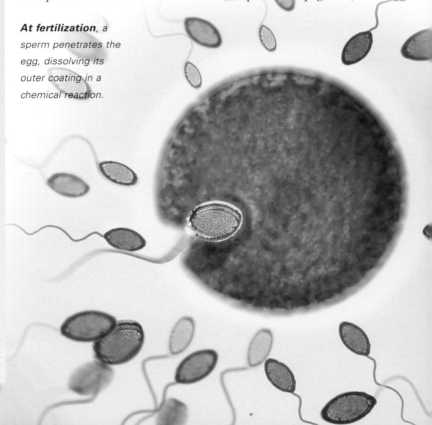

then oozes out onto the surface of the ovary. It is now sitting on the surface, surrounded by a mass of sticky cells known as the cumulus oophorous. These cells play a crucial role, making it possible for the fallopian tube to pick up the egg. The egg is gathered up by fimbria, which are fingerlike projections at the end of each fallopian tube, and swept into the tube. From here it moves toward the uterus during the next seven days, helped by cilia, tiny hairs lining the fallopian tubes. Fertilization takes place when a successful sperm, which has swum up through the cervix and uterus and into the fallopian tube, penetrates the egg. This happens in what is known as the distal third of the tube: that is, the section closest to the ovary. The fertilized egg, now known as a zygote (see page 13), continues its journey toward the uterus.

SEX UNDER PRESSURE

Sexual problems can often develop at this time. Men feel that the sexual act has become a very mechanical means to an end. Women become obsessive about having sex at just the right time so that the sperm can "get ahead" and be in place waiting for the egg. Tensions are running high, and I have often heard from my clients how all this stress can lead to arguments and hence no sex. Try not to put yourselves under such pressure, and enjoy what you are doing for its own sake.

ZITA'S TIPS

- **You cannot have too much sex.** Contrary to what many people believe, frequent sex does not somehow weaken the sperm. In fact, fertility is improved by frequent intercourse. Research has shown that couples having sex once a week have a 15 percent chance of conceiving during a cycle, while those making love every day increased that chance to 50 percent. So, aim to have lots of passionate sex at least two or three times a week.

- **Remember: you are designed** to have maximum sexual desire when you are most fertile. You will be able to detect this from your mucus (see pages 70–71). Many women try to pinpoint ovulation accurately. This is neither possible (without a scan) nor necessary. Ovulation predictor kits identify the LH (luteinizing hormone) surge about 24 hours before ovulation and temperature charts will show a temperature rise after ovulation.

- **Touch and caress each other** prior to intercourse, since sexual stimulation increases the flow of hormones and encourages fertility. Studies show that the sperm count of ejaculate from men who were turned on by a partner is higher and more potent than that of ejaculate from men who masturbated.

- **Don't use artificial lubricants in the vagina.** Oils, water-based gels, and even saliva can adversely affect the motility of sperm. The best lubrication is your own arousal fluids, which will be plentiful if you have lots of sexual stimulation prior to having intercourse.

- **Aim for sexual positions** that involve deep penetration if you want to encourage the greatest amount of contact between sperm and mucus.

- **Stay in bed for 20 to 30 minutes after intercourse** to encourage the sperm to stay in your vagina. Strong swimmers will quickly find their way through the fertile cervical secretions and move up into the uterus toward the fallopian tubes. Weaker sperm will inevitably stay in the vagina, and there will eventually be flow back from your body whatever position you adopt. There is no need to stand on your head!

- **Avoid going to the toilet** for 20 to 30 minutes after intercourse.

- **Do not use recreational drugs or alcohol.** There is mounting evidence to show that the presence of drugs or alcohol in the blood of either partner can have a negative impact on fertility and conception.

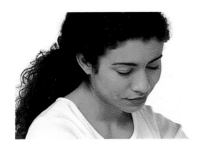

the third week

This week marks the start of the waiting period, as you wonder what is going on inside your body and hope that fertilization takes place and that implantation will occur successfully.

week 3
at a glance

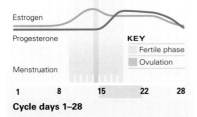

CHART YOUR CYCLE

Estrogen

Progesterone

KEY
- Fertile phase
- Ovulation

Menstruation

1   8   15   22   28

Cycle days 1–28

FOCUS ON

○ DIET

Make sure that you maintain your good dietary habits, but consider boosting certain nutrients (see right), either by supplementation or in your food. If fertilization has occurred, you may be about to be eating for two.

○ LIFESTYLE

Keep the *qi* flowing smoothly in your body (see page 72). Get at least 20 minutes of moderate exercise at least three times a week. Spend time each day calmly and positively visualizing the implantation process in your uterus (see page 43 and opposite).

FERTILIZATION

YOUR HORMONES

Last week, as soon as ovulation took place, levels of FSH (follicle-stimulating hormone) began to drop sharply and LH (luteinizing hormone) levels began to fall slowly. Now it is the time for progesterone to play an important role. This next phase of the cycle is the luteal phase (see pages 10–11). It needs to last for a minimum of nine days. If less, there will be insufficient time for implantation to take place, and even if fertilization has occurred, the pregnancy may fail.

The follicle that contained the egg, having ruptured, remained behind. It still received pulses of LH, which continue this week. This enables it to turn into a small cyst or corpus luteum (literally "yellow body"; see pages 10–11), which produces progesterone.

Progesterone has four important functions to perform at this stage of the cycle:
- it helps to build and thicken the lining of the uterus so that it can secrete nutrients that will provide the developing embryo with nourishment

- it switches off the production of FSH and LH to prevent more eggs from ripening
- it raises basal body temperature slightly in order to help prepare the uterus for receiving the embryo
- it closes the cervix and thickens the mucus, forming a plug to stop more sperm from entering the cervix after fertilization

DIET AND NUTRITION

In order for the egg to travel down the fallopian tube and divide, a good supply of nutrients is needed.
- Zinc is very important for cell division and the production of progesterone. See page 63 for dosage and good food sources of zinc.
- Vitamin A is also important for progesterone production and to protect a developing embryo. See page 59 for dosage and good food sources of vitamin A.
- Vitamin C is highly concentrated in the corpus luteum, so it is believed to be linked to the release of progesterone. See page 61 for dosage and good food sources of vitamin C.

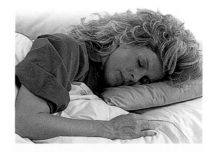

LIFESTYLE CHANGES

Many of you reading this may have been trying to conceive for months and feel as if you have put your life on hold. This might be invoking a sense of urgency in you, which may make you behave a bit obsessively. Try to practice moderation in all things and don't become obsessive about what you can and can't allow yourself to do.

EXERCISE

Traditional Chinese medicine works on the premise that it is important to get the *qi* circulating at this stage so as to get the egg moving into the uterus. Get moderate exercise, such as walking or cycling, but avoid excessive aerobic exercise.

COMPLEMENTARY THERAPIES

Acupuncture can be very effective throughout your cycle when you are trying to conceive, but especially in the six to eight days after ovulation. I treat clients to remove imbalances and promote the healthy flow of *qi*. Two points

needled at this time are Gate of Life and Door of Infants (see page 73). Your acupuncturist might use moxibustion to warm the lower chou (lower abdomen).

VISUALIZATION

Concentrate on the details of what is—you hope—happening inside of you. The developing embryo continues its journey along the fallopian tube toward the uterus. The corpus luteum continues to secrete progesterone and maintain a fairly constant level of estrogen. Progesterone levels continue to rise and influence the lining of the uterus. This thickens in readiness for receiving the embryo and supporting it once it has embedded. By about day 21 (of a 28-day cycle), the embryo—by now a multicelled blastocyst (see illustration below)—embeds into the wall of the uterus, burrowing into the nourishing cells and eventually connecting with the maternal blood supply. You may experience slight spotting a week or so after ovulation.

YOUR EMOTIONS

Hope and anticipation are familiar emotions this week, as is anxiety, as you wonder whether or not all has gone well and you could be pregnant.

Since last week, hormones have had a positive influence on your mood, making you feel energetic and positive. But if you are trying to conceive, all this good feeling may be overshadowed by the pressure of waiting until you can take a pregnancy test. Once ovulation has passed, the outgoing feelings tend to turn inward and you become reflective and emotional. Women tend to dream more vividly at this stage of the month, as if their unconscious is demanding to be listened to.

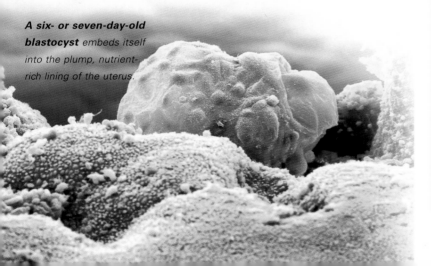

A six- or seven-day-old blastocyst embeds itself into the plump, nutrient-rich lining of the uterus.

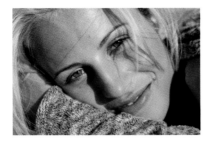

the fourth week

As the waiting game creeps toward the pregnancy test, the pressure continues to mount this week. Work on keeping yourself calm and serene. It's important to hope for the best and stay positive.

week 4 at a glance

CHART YOUR CYCLE

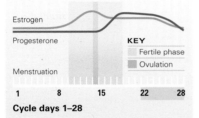

Estrogen

Progesterone

KEY
☐ Fertile phase
☐ Ovulation

Menstruation

| 1 | 8 | 15 | 22 | 28 |

Cycle days 1–28

FOCUS ON

○ DIET AND NUTRITION

As during the preceding weeks, you should maintain the healthy eating patterns you established during your program of preconception care because, if you are pregnant, you now need those nutrients (see pages 59–64) to nourish a baby.

○ LIFESTYLE

Exercise will help you focus on something other than whether or not you might be pregnant, and more holistic and reflective forms of activity might prevent you from tearing your hair out by relaxing your body and calming your mind.

DEVELOPMENT OR DEGENERATION

HORMONES

An embryo arrives in the uterus approximately 4–5 days after fertilization, and implantation occurs about 7–10 days after ovulation (in a 28-day cycle). The more developed the blastocyst before it implants, the greater the chance of a successful pregnancy. An embryo has about 30 cells by the time it reaches the uterus, and it starts to break out of its surrounding membrane, the zona pellucida. As women age, the zona becomes tougher, and it is therefore more difficult for the embryo to hatch out. (IVF fertility treatment may include assisted hatching, whereby the "shell" is broken slightly to allow the embryo to emerge.)

Once implantation has occurred, the developing placental tissues start to produce the pregnancy hormone HCG (human chorionic gonadotrophin). This maintains the structure of the endometrium and the continued existence of the corpus luteum (see pages 10–12), which produces increasing quantities of progesterone in order to sustain the pregnancy for the next 12 weeks, until the placenta has fully developed and is ready to take over pregnancy maintenance.

If conception hasn't taken place, the corpus luteum will survive for 12–16 days after ovulation, then it will degenerate. The endometrium, which is about ⅓–⅜ in (8–10 mm) thick by now, stops developing, and the uterus prepares to shed the lining. Falling levels of estrogen and progesterone trigger the hypothalamus to release GnRH (gonadotrophin-releasing hormone) and FSH (follicle-stimulating hormone), which restart the cycle of bleeding and the development of follicles.

DIET AND NUTRITION

Within your established dietary program (see box, left), you should pay particular attention to including foods with essential fatty acids (EFAs), vitamins B6 and E, zinc, and magnesium. For good food sources, see pages 60–64.

The Chinese believe that at this time you should eat plenty of warming *yang* foods. These should include as little raw food as possible and up to two quarts (liters) of water (at room temperature) a day. Any fresh juices should be made from fruits and vegetables kept at room temperature. If you eat a salad, have something warming with it, such as a baked potato, or eat the salad as an accompaniment to a hot dish. Foods should be warming and easy to digest, such as soups, casseroles, well-cooked meats, lentils, oatmeal, potatoes and sweet potatoes, papaya, ginger, and barley. Other *yang* foods include chicken, eggs, mushrooms, sesame oil, peanuts, garlic and onions, and red foods such as tomatoes and bell peppers. If, as the week wears on, you begin to suspect that you might be about to start a period, follow dietary guidelines to maximize hormonal balance (see page 126).

EXERCISE

By all means, carry on as normal with exercise this week, but, if you think you might be pregnant, don't engage in high-impact, aerobic activities that involve any bouncing. Pilates, brisk walking, yoga, cycling, or swimming are fine.

COMPLEMENTARY THERAPIES

Deep-breathing techniques (see pages 42–43) and visualization (see page 43) will encourage the embedded embryo to develop in the best possible way. The Chinese believe that wherever your mind is, *qi* will follow. Place your hand on your lower abdomen to see if it feels cold: if so, use a covered hot-water bottle to warm it up. Warmth is essential if you are to "grow" a baby.

Focus your energy on promoting inner calm as you approach the potential stress of a pregnancy test.

YOUR EMOTIONS

This can be an anxious time as you wait to see if your period will arrive and try to interpret your body's signals. Many women report feeling emotional and tearful at this time. Try to focus your energies outward rather than turning in on yourself. You need to think positively, of course—that you might be pregnant. As the week progresses, however, you may start to experience what might be your familiar premenstrual symptoms recurring or, on the other hand, what might be the first signs of pregnancy. You will need to reconcile these conflicting thoughts and then, if your period does come, you will be able to look forward (see pages 82–83). Don't forget to treat yourself kindly—have a glass of wine if you feel like it— and spoil yourself a bit.

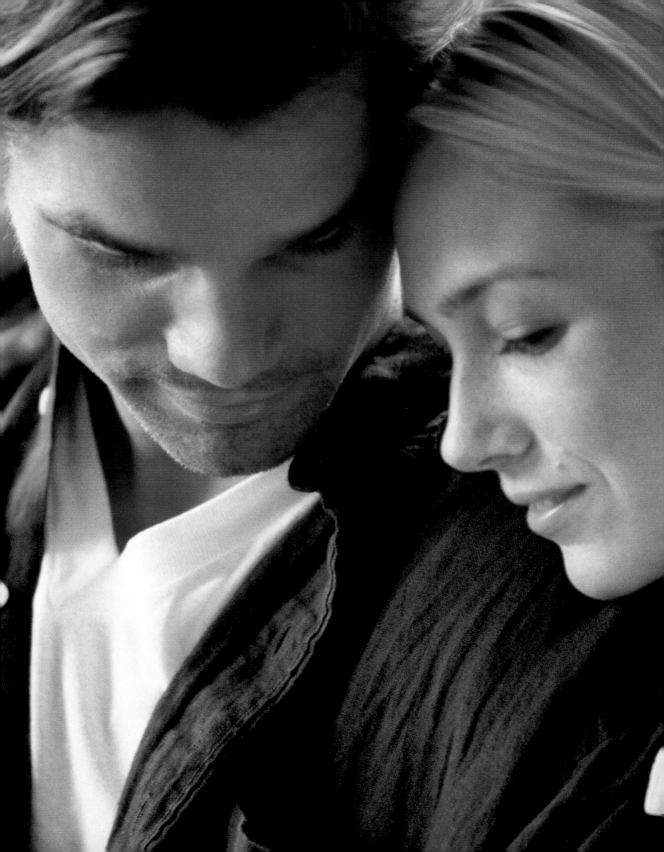

TESTING YOUR FERTILITY

OVER THE PAST FEW MONTHS, YOU MAY HAVE MADE MANY **LIFESTYLE CHANGES** TO ENHANCE YOUR FERTILITY AND BEEN MAKING A **CONCERTED EFFORT TO CONCEIVE** A BABY, BUT SO FAR **WITHOUT SUCCESS**. IF YOU FEEL THAT YOU HAVE DONE EVERYTHING TO MAXIMIZE YOUR CHANCES OF CONCEIVING AND SUSPECT THAT YOU MAY HAVE A **FERTILITY PROBLEM**, YOU HAVE REACHED THE POINT AT WHICH YOU AND YOUR PARTNER SHOULD MAKE AN APPOINTMENT WITH YOUR DOCTOR TO **DISCUSS FERTILITY TESTS. IT'S TIME FOR PLAN B.**

moving forward

If, after months of trying to conceive, you feel there is a problem, you will want to find out what it is and what can be done about it. You and your partner need to research all the options and work out a plan of action. Take things one step at a time, keep talking to each other, and prepare for what lies ahead.

THINKING ABOUT PLAN B

How long do you try unsuccessfully for a baby before approaching your doctor? If you are between ages 20 and 30, try for 12–18 months before testing; if you are 30–35, try for 12 months; and if you are over 35, try for six months.

When a couple suspects that they might have a problem that is preventing them from conceiving, they usually feel apprehensive, wondering what the problem might be and often fearing the worst. They don't know what to expect from the testing process, fearing the unknown. Feel reassured by the tests, however. Many fertility problems are minor and can be dealt with relatively easily. If you are worried, you can start testing—with blood tests and sperm analysis—while continuing to try for a baby. Generally speaking, a couple with unexplained infertility have a similar chance of conceiving a baby during a 12-month period whether or not they have fertility treatment.

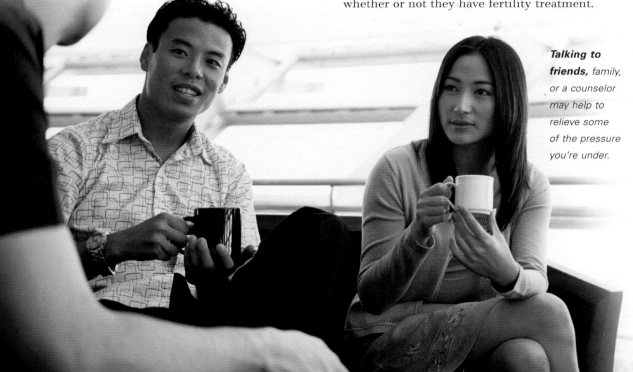

Talking to friends, family, or a counselor may help to relieve some of the pressure you're under.

WRESTLING WITH EMOTIONS

You may well be experiencing a confusing variety of thoughts and emotions (see box, right), which can increase your stress levels and take a huge toll on your physical well-being. At this stage, my clients commonly feel and express any of the following emotions:

- **shock:** "I never expected to be in this situation"
- **denial:** "This can't be happening to me"
- **fear:** "What if I never become pregnant?"
- **regret:** "Perhaps I've waited too long"
- **grief:** "I may be unable to have the one thing I feel is essential to my life"
- **responsibility:** "I've let my partner down"
- **isolation:** "I feel I don't fit in among my friends any more. I want to avoid social gatherings in order to escape thoughtless remarks and questions… and other people's babies"
- **frustration and anger:** "Other people don't seem to have any problems getting pregnant—why should it be me who has the problems?"
- **envy:** "I feel jealous of other couples when I see them with their babies"
- **failure:** "There's something wrong with me—it's as though I'm defective or disabled in some way"
- **helplessness**: "I have no control over my body and my future has been taken away"
- **anxiety**: "How will we be able to afford fertility treatment, and will I be able to take enough time off work for all the consultations and tests?"
- **apprehension**: "How will I cope with the drugs if I have to have fertility treatment?"

TALKING ABOUT YOUR FEELINGS

It is difficult for most people to appreciate what you are going through unless they themselves have been in the same situation. Explain to friends and family how you are feeling and ask them for their support and understanding. If you find it hard to tell them face to face, perhaps write them a short note or email describing how difficult it is for you both at the moment. Remind them, if you like, that stress does not cause infertility, but infertility

SUSAN'S THOUGHTS

*"I'm frustrated! I've always been healthy, but **all the time I'm not getting pregnant, I'm worrying that I don't 'work' properly**. I just want to know whether or not I can conceive. If I can't, I want to know what to do about it: if I can, then I can keep trying without the added anxiety of wondering whether or not it's possible.*

*I think the most frustrating part of this whole process is that I have no clue when it will happen, why it will happen or not, or what I can really do to make it happen. It all seems out of my control. It's difficult to manage this process because I've become obsessive about it. Pregnancy is constantly on my mind; I try not to think about it too much because I don't want to get too wound up about it, but it's hard to control my mind. It's challenging because everyone says that it will only happen when I'm relaxed about it, but it's hard not to be stressed about it when we've been trying for over a year now. **I worry that my anxiety and stress are preventing me from getting pregnant**. I don't talk about it with too many people because they all throw lots of advice at me, and I find it hard to navigate my way through all the rumors and myths."*

OTHER SOURCES OF SUPPORT

- **Check out some of the fertility websites**, and even chatrooms, on the Internet. See Useful addresses on page 187 for details.
- **Ask at your doctor's office** to see if there are any fertility support groups in your area.
- **Talk to women who are going through**, or who have been through, the same experience. This will make you feel far less isolated, and they can give you some idea of what to expect from tests and treatments.

does cause stress, and that no amount of relaxation will unblock blocked tubes or remove feelings of desperation. If you have difficulty dealing with some of your feelings, consider going to talk to a counselor. He or she might help you to be able to understand your emotions better.

LAYING GHOSTS

Also, you can explore whether or not there is anything in your psyche that might be preventing you from conceiving a baby. Such things as a previous termination, problems with or doubts about your relationship with your partner, a traumatic childhood experience, or the pressure of being the main breadwinner may all have an impact at a deep level. If there are any issues that you feel need to be dealt with, now is the time to address them. A therapist or counselor might be able to help you put your mind at rest.

A SENSE OF PERSPECTIVE

Take strength and comfort from the fact that you and your partner are not the only ones finding it difficult to conceive. Couples rarely seem to share with other people the fact that they are having problems conceiving: it remains an intensely private experience. It may appear as if everyone around you is getting pregnant, and there are mothers with babies wherever you look, but in fact, one in six couples has a problem conceiving.

UNDERSTANDING YOUR PARTNER'S EMOTIONS

Men can sometimes find it much harder than their female partners to get in touch with their feelings and then to share them. In addition, men and women often have very different attitudes to sharing private feelings with others. You and your partner may find you have reacted quite differently to your situation: while your first instinct might have been to confide in friends and family, your partner may not want to discuss the situation with anybody. It's important that you decide between you who you want to tell and how involved in the process you want family and friends to be.

The experience of not being able to have a baby exactly when you'd planned and dealing with the consequences of that, whatever the outcome, can strengthen the emotional bond between the two of you. Far from driving a wedge between you, it may bring you closer together. Many couples have admitted to me after their treatment that, with hindsight, they are grateful for this bonding experience that they would have missed had they been able to conceive right away.

NURTURING YOUR RELATIONSHIP

Despite your disappointment at the realization that conceiving a baby might be problematic, do remember that you and your partner are what matters in both the short and long term. Having a child in the future may not be a certainty for you, and, if that is the case, a mutually supportive relationship is what will help you both to come to terms with that future. Find a balance between this and other features of your life, keep talking to each other, and try also to keep a sense of perspective. As you embark on a program of fertility treatment, it's all too easy to let it dominate every aspect of your life and thinking. Limit the amount of time you spend talking about the subject each day, and refrain from referring to it at all during the course of a day or evening you have set aside and planned for togetherness.

REMEMBERING YOUR SEX LIFE

Whatever you do, don't give up on sex. Many couples, once they have been locked into fertility treatment for some time, find that they have no sex life at all, and their relationship can suffer accordingly. By now, the idea of "making love" may well have flown out the window, and sex becomes a mechanical act that happens only to an all-important schedule. The act no longer has anything to do with your feelings, but is solely dictated by the timetable of your clinic. This lack of spontaneity can be a huge turnoff for men, who are expected to perform at the optimum moment, no matter what.

Even after years of failure to conceive, it may still be possible in some instances to achieve a spontaneous pregnancy, so it makes sense to keep having regular sex—just in case.

Couples who choose to go down the IVF (in vitro fertilization) route and know that fertilization will take place in a laboratory may even start to feel that sex is obsolete. Having IVF treatment does not mean, however, that you have to give up on intimacy, fun, passion, and tenderness. Try to take time out occasionally—a weekend getaway, perhaps—to breathe life back into your sexual relationship. Remember that infertility is only temporary, and once it is behind you, you will still want your sexual relationship. So take care of it!

Don't lose sight of the fact that, whether or not you have a baby, you share a loving relationship.

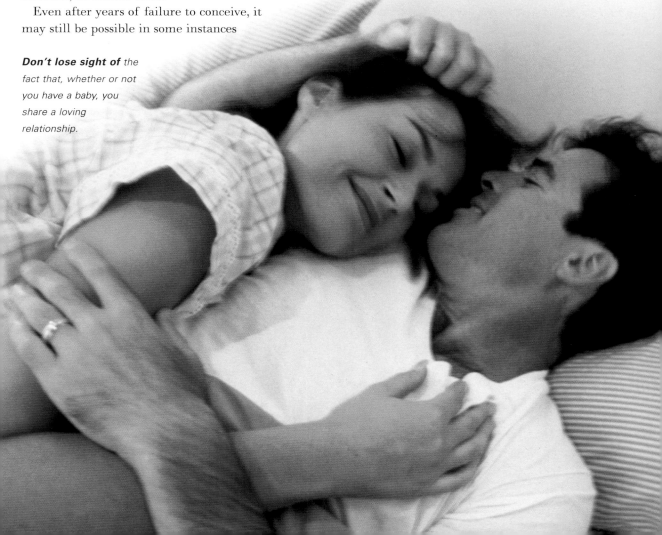

GETTING THE BALL ROLLING

If you and your partner have come to the conclusion that you might have a fertility problem, the things that will be uppermost in your mind are the possible cause of the problem and what you can do about it. Start to draw up an action plan. Make sure you discuss everything with each other as you prepare for what might lie ahead.

If you are determined to get pregnant, then it's time to make an appointment with your doctor to discuss fertility testing. If you are in your late 30s or older, visit your doctor right away or go directly to a fertility clinic. Don't be diverted: be assertive. You may be told to go away and try again for a few more months. Take your temperature chart along and describe everything that you have been doing. If you've followed all the advice in Plan A, insist that your doctor tests you now.

TAKING CONTROL

Fertility tests take the form of a progressive series of checks to eliminate possible causes of infertility in both men and women. At each level of testing, the results will determine what the next stage of testing should be, so don't expect a clear path ahead. There is no reason why testing shouldn't start at the same time for both you and your partner. It is often the woman who gets the ball rolling when it comes to fertility testing, but I often advise the couples I see to begin with sperm analysis. It is relatively straightforward and noninvasive, and it may quickly eliminate one potential problem, thus saving you time.

Although tests follow a chronological order, every case is different. Your particular experience will depend on the nature of your fertility problems and which treatment is considered to be the most appropriate for you. The testing process begins with your doctor. Depending on your age and how long you have been trying to conceive, you may be referred to a fertility clinic. The procedures can be fraught with worry because of the amount of time it takes to attend consultations and schedule tests, and then wait for the results. Take it one step at a time; focus only on what you are doing at any particular time, and be prepared to move the goalposts if something is not working for you.

Understanding the testing process will make you feel more in control of what is happening and less alarmed by it. The following pages outline the tests you might have to undergo, so that you are prepared for anything you might come across.

ZITA'S TIPS

The following tips will help you and your partner feel in control of what is happening while you test your fertility—and perhaps receive treatment—and think positively.

- **Find out all your options** and then take things one step at a time.

- **Maintain a sense of perspective:** don't put your life on hold and think of nothing but pregnancy.

- **Look at the bigger picture:** you may feel you need to take a break for a while, but consider making an appointment with a clinic in advance and then, having made a decision, you can relax for a bit.

- **Remember that your relationship is important,** whatever happens. Stay close to one another and keep talking everything through.

- **Limit yourself** to one hour per day of dealing with fertility measures, and make time for your partner.

- **Don't pester each other** about what you should or shouldn't be doing. You may be one step ahead of your partner in charting the progress of your fertility planning and treatment in the coming months. Accept that fact now.

female fertility tests

Fertility tests for women are more complicated and varied than they are for men because hormone levels fluctuate during the female cycle and their interaction is complex.

THE AIM OF TESTS

Many different factors or combinations of factors may affect fertility. Tests aim to eliminate possible causes of problems. Most tests, even the invasive, surgical ones, are quite routine and shouldn't give you too much cause for concern. You need to be prepared, however, for the possibility that some results might be inconclusive.

A series of tests may be necessary before conclusions can be reached. The sequence is as follows:

- **level one** hormone assessment—to detect any ovulation problems
- **level two** tubal and uterine assessment—to check for physical barriers to conception
- **level three** immunological screening—to assess possible reactions of your immune system.

LEVEL ONE: HORMONE ASSESSMENT

Simple blood tests can detect hormone imbalance that may be affecting your fertility. One test done on days 1–3 of your cycle will give an indication of the likely quality of your eggs and your ovarian reserve (see page 16). This is especially important for women over the age of 35. Other blood tests at this time measure estradiol, prolactin, and thyroid hormone levels if necessary.

Another blood test on day 21 (of a 28-day cycle) will measure levels of progesterone and show if ovulation has occurred. The timing will vary if your cycle is longer or shorter than 28 days.

FSH

This is the hormone produced by the pituitary gland to stimulate the growth and development of ovarian follicles. The FSH (follicle-stimulating hormone) level on days 1–3 of your cycle is used as a baseline measurement of ovarian reserve and quality of eggs. Perimenopausal and menopausal women have elevated levels of FSH (see page 17). Levels of FSH may also fluctuate if you have irregular periods.

ESTRADIOL (E_2)

This is the main estrogen hormone secreted by ovarian follicles, and is measured in a blood test on days 1–3 of your cycle. It is not routine unless it is anticipated that you will need fertility treatment. As follicles grow and mature, they produce E_2, causing the endometrium to thicken. This hormone also helps balance FSH levels, preventing

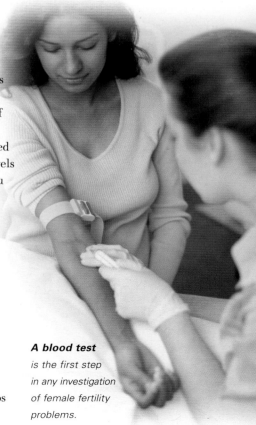

A blood test *is the first step in any investigation of female fertility problems.*

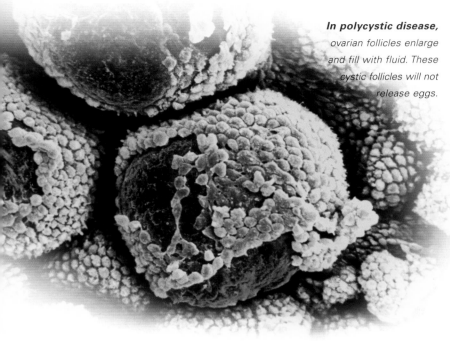

In polycystic disease, ovarian follicles enlarge and fill with fluid. These cystic follicles will not release eggs.

processes and hence the proper functioning of all body systems. TSH levels are often checked first in a fertility evaluation because an underactive thyroid is linked to infertility (see page 106). A TSH level that is beyond the expected range, combined with a level of thyroxine (T_4) that is below the expected range or even within it, is usually indicative of an underactive thyroid. If TSH levels are within the expected range but T_4 levels are below it, you are more likely to have a problem with the pituitary gland. (Low T_4 may indicate a diseased thyroid or a nonfunctioning pituitary gland that is not stimulating the thyroid to produce T_4.)

them from getting too high. As a woman approaches menopause, she does not produce enough estradiol to counteract rising FSH (follicle-stimulating hormone). Ideally, both FSH and E_2 levels should be low. High levels may indicate an ovarian cyst or a diminished ovarian reserve.

LH

Luteinizing hormone is released by the pituitary gland, stimulating ovulation (see page 10), the formation of the corpus luteum (see pages 10–11), and the synthesis of progesterone by the ovaries. A surge of LH midway through your cycle triggers ovulation. Luteinizing hormone is tested during days 1–3: high levels may indicate polycystic ovary syndrome (PCOS)—see pages 119–21.

PROLACTIN

This hormone is secreted by the pituitary gland. Its major purpose is to control milk production after childbirth, but it also stimulates the production of progesterone. Levels of this hormone also tend to be higher in the luteal phase of your cycle (see pages 10–11).

Prolactin is tested if PCOS is suspected. Levels that are higher than expected may interfere with ovulation or result in a reduced progesterone function, which will make it difficult for your body to maintain a pregnancy.

THYROID HORMONES

Thyroid-stimulating hormone (TSH) is produced by the pituitary gland and is responsible for controlling thyroid function. This is important for all metabolic

ANDROGENS

Levels of male hormones are also assessed in the blood test at the beginning of your cycle to rule out the possibility of PCOS. This might suggest a state of hormonal imbalance in which the pituitary gland produces large amounts of luteinizing hormone (LH), preventing ovulation and causing the ovaries to secrete higher-than-expected levels of male hormones.

PROGESTERONE

When a follicle releases its egg, it becomes a corpus luteum (see pages 10–11) and progesterone is produced. A blood test on day 21 of your cycle, measuring levels of progesterone, will indicate whether or not you are ovulating. This test should actually be carried out 7–10 days after ovulation has occurred, which is day 21 for women who have a regular, 28-day menstrual cycle, or seven days before your period if you do not have a 28-day cycle. If your cycle is unusual, discuss the calculation with your doctor. The test is slightly problematic since progesterone is secreted in pulses every 2–3 hours, so a single test may not give an accurate reading of the overall level and you may be required to retest. Some doctors believe the test is more accurate if it is done first thing in the morning.

This test is also used to identify a luteal phase defect (LPD—see page 30). This will reduce the role of progesterone in preparing the endometrium for implantation of a fertilized egg. If there is insufficient progesterone being secreted, the lining of the uterus will not be ready for implantation and a pregnancy will not be viable.

If your progesterone level is lower than the expected range, an endometrial biopsy may be suggested by some clinics: others will not think this necessary. It involves a small amount of tissue being taken from the uterus to double-check progesterone levels.

INTERPRETING RESULTS

If blood tests indicate that you are not ovulating, your doctor will advise you of the most suitable treatment options. Hormonal imbalance can often be adjusted by means of hormone replacement medication and/or changes to nutrition and lifestyle (see pages 30–32). If the signs are that you are not ovulating, you may be referred for ovulation-stimulating treatment (see pages 150–51).

If your FSH level is high, there are measures you can take to try to bring it down (see pages 164–65), but bear in mind that, if the level is very high, you may be menopausal. Your doctor can refer you for ovulation-stimulating treatment. It may be that in vitro fertilization (IVF) is considered to be the best route, but you will have to wait until your FSH level has come down before you can start. If the level is high, you will not respond to treatment. The last route would be egg donation.

If prolactin levels are raised, a referral to an endocrinologist may be recommended. You will be checked for a pituitary tumor, and given medication to lower the levels (see page 130).

If TSH is high, further thyroid testing will be carried out to see if you have an underactive thyroid.

If testosterone is high, further investigation will be required (fasting, blood-sugar test, and insulin test) to check for PCOS.

As far as progesterone is concerned, if the result is less than 15, the blood test will be repeated during another menstrual cycle and, if it is still low, you will be referred to a fertility specialist. If the level is higher than 15 but lower than 30, the blood test will be repeated and, if the results are the same, you may be referred for controlled ovulation. A result that is greater than 30 suggests that ovulation is adequate.

If all your hormonal levels appear to be normal and you are ovulating, further testing will be recommended to discover why you have been unable to conceive.

At some clinics, you may at this stage be advised to have a postcoital test to see if your cervical mucus can nurture and transport sperm. A mucus sample is taken from the cervix as soon as possible after intercourse and as close to ovulation as possible. This is not as widespread a procedure as it once was because it is no longer regarded to be of clinical value. Again, if your cervical mucus appears to be normal, further exploratory testing will be recommended to try to determine the nature of the fertility problem.

HORMONE LEVEL RANGES

Blood-test results relate to the expected range for each hormone. Do not worry about units: it's the numbers that count.

FSH <6 mIU/ml excellent; 6–8 good; 9–10 fair; 11–13 diminished reserve

Estradiol 25–75 pg/ml

LH <7 mIU/ml

Prolactin <24 ng/ml

Progesterone >15 ng/ml

Thyroid hormones 1.7 uIU/ml

Testosterone 6–86 ng/dl: >50 is considered to be elevated

LEVEL TWO: TUBAL AND UTERINE ASSESSMENT

Once your hormones, and hence ovulation, have been checked, the next step is to look for blockages in your fallopian tubes that could prevent the progress of egg or sperm, or uterine problems that might prevent implantation. Your doctor or fertility specialist will refer you to a lab for these tests to determine whether or not there is a blockage and, if there is, its location in your reproductive system. These procedures are usually carried out during the first half of the cycle. Some clinics prescribe a course of antibiotics first to get rid of any infection.

THE FALLOPIAN TUBES

Blocked tubes account for 20 percent of female infertility. They can sometimes be unblocked surgically. Blockages may be caused by:

- **an infection**, perhaps a sexually transmitted one (see page 108)
- **pelvic inflammatory disease** (see page 108), which is caused by a sexually transmitted infection, the insertion of an intrauterine device (IUD, or coil), or bacteria. It is a good idea for both you and your partner to be checked for STDs and to get immediate treatment if you are harboring any infection
- **adhesions** (scar tissue) from previous surgery.

HYSTEROSALPINGOGRAM

This is a routine test, known as an HSG for short, that will identify blockages in the fallopian tubes. A small tube is inserted into the cervix and liquid dye squirted through it. X-rays are taken as the dye enters the reproductive organs, picking up its course and showing up any obstructions, adhesions (scar tissue), or uterine abnormalities such as polyps (small growths that are usually harmless) or fibroids (see pages 117–19). You may experience temporary discomfort or cramping with this test, but the level of pain is variable.

Some studies indicate that the likelihood of pregnancy might increase slightly in the first few months following an HSG, possibly because flushing out the tubes removes minor blockages.

WHAT NEXT?

If there is a blockage in your fallopian tubes, your specialist will recommend a laparoscopy (see below) to determine the nature and extent of the obstruction. Minor treatment of the tubes may be required. If there are no blockages, you may still need a laparoscopy or a hysteroscopy (see below) to check the uterine cavity.

LAPAROSCOPY

This is an invasive test requiring a general anesthetic and a short hospital admission. A tiny incision is made near your navel and the abdominal cavity is filled with carbon dioxide gas, which is intended to separate the organs and enable them to be seen better. A laparoscope, resembling a small telescope, is inserted so that the doctor can inspect the abdominal cavity, uterus, and fallopian tubes for anything unusual, such as fibroids or endometriosis. The aftereffects of this procedure may include pain in the abdomen, neck, or shoulders (caused by the gas), or vaginal bleeding.

HYSTEROSCOPY

This may be done in some clinics at the same time as a laparoscopy. A hysteroscopy requires you to be mildly sedated or have a local anesthetic. A viewing instrument called a hysteroscope is inserted via the cervix into the uterine cavity to check for irregularities or adhesions. This also allows for your uterus to be "mapped" for future reference, which in many clinics is part of the preparation for in vitro fertilization (IVF).

WHAT NEXT?

If you have fibroids, your specialist can determine their size and number, and assess whether they are likely to be affecting your fertility. You may receive treatment and may be able to return to Plan A. If endometriosis (see pages 114–16) is detected, treatment may enable you to return to Plan A.

LEVEL THREE: IMMUNOLOGICAL SCREENING

This is specialist screening and will be recommended if you have a history of miscarriage or as-yet unidentified fertility problems.

Blood screening can be done by your doctor, and indeed should have been suggested if you have suffered repeated miscarriage. Usually, two blood tests are carried out six weeks apart. Alternatively, you can be referred for this testing by an autoimmune specialist or at a fertility clinic, depending on your history, or it may be part of your doctor's initial investigations into your fertility.

Certain reactions instigated by the immune system may result in your body rejecting a fertilized embryo (see pages 124–25). Your fertility consultant may suggest immunological screening if there are no apparent reasons for your fertility problems after you have undergone hormone assessment or tubal and uterine investigative procedures and your partner has had sperm analysis or other tests.

Problems with the immune system are increasingly believed to be a significant factor in some cases of pregnancy loss. Numerous studies have discovered abnormal levels of particular antibodies in women who experience either IVF failure or repeated miscarriage and have otherwise found no cause of their fertility problems.

The immunological investigative process is a complex and expensive one and involves repeat testing throughout early pregnancy once you have conceived, but it may be worth considering by couples who:

- have had two or more miscarriages
- have unexplained infertility
- have good embryos that fail to implant during IVF procedures.

DEALING WITH ANTIBODIES

If you have consistently high levels of antiphospholipid or anticardiolipin antibodies, you will have about a 10–20 percent chance of carrying a pregnancy. You may be given a low daily dose of aspirin to thin the blood. Heparin may also be offered. Thickened blood (as a result of the antibodies) increases the likelihood of miscarriage because it reduces blood flow through the placenta and increases the chance of blood clots, which have the same effect.

The presence of antinuclear antibodies may give rise to inflammation of the uterus. Inflammation of any kind in the pelvic region can put a fetus at risk. If these antibodies are detected, you may be given steroids to reduce inflammation.

If you have maternal blocking antibodies or natural killer cells, any embryos will be rejected and therefore fail to implant. Possible treatment in this instance is highly controversial, not readily available, very expensive, and carries with it other serious risks (see page 125) so you would need to research and consider this option very carefully indeed.

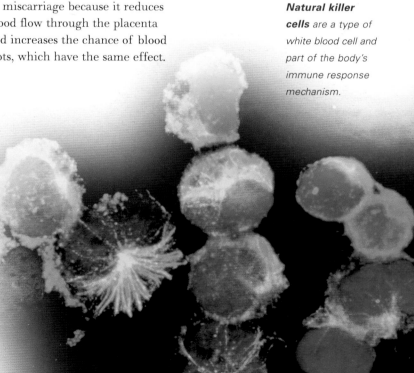

Natural killer cells are a type of white blood cell and part of the body's immune response mechanism.

female fertility problems

A diagnosis can bring with it a great sense of relief.
Now that you have identified the problem, you may feel
encouraged by the fact that there are things you can do
to alleviate it and maximize your chances of either
natural or assisted conception.

UNDERSTANDING A DIAGNOSIS

You may already be aware of a problem in your
reproductive system—menstrual irregularities, for
example—or perhaps you have just been diagnosed
with a particular condition as a result of fertility
tests. It is important to learn about your condition
and appreciate its implications for your chances of
conceiving a baby. You need to be able to recognize
symptoms; understand the causes, if they are
known; be aware of factors making you susceptible;
learn how the condition is treated; and determine
ways of improving your health and lifestyle to
make a difference to your fertility.

Some conditions that diminish fertility are
underlying general health issues; others are caused
by infections; some have to do with functioning of
the reproductive cycle and system parts; and others
are the result of physiological irregularities. They
are all described in the following pages.

I would always recommend that you combine
the advice of your conventional doctors with any
of the many complementary treatments and
remedies you might choose to try in order to
improve your condition. And never underestimate
the importance of good nutrition, too, in an
integrated plan to improve your fertility.

CAUSES OF FERTILITY PROBLEMS

Primary infertility is when a couple have being trying for their first baby for a year or more but have been unsuccessful.
Secondary infertility is when a couple have a child but have difficulty conceiving subsequently. A significant number of cases in each category are not attributable to any one cause. Figures vary from one clinic to another.

	PRIMARY INFERTILITY	SECONDARY INFERTILITY
● **ovulatory**	20 percent	15 percent
● **tubal**	15 percent	40 percent
● **endometriosis**	10 percent	5 percent
● **male problems**	40 percent	30 percent
● **unexplained**	15 percent	10 percent

underlying conditions

There are many conditions that are not directly related to the female reproductive system but have implications for a woman's fertility. Sometimes common conditions, such as anemia and thyroid problems, may be overlooked.

ANEMIA

Iron deficiency is one of the most common causes of anemia. It is estimated that more than 50 percent of women worldwide get less than the recommended intake of 10–15 mg/day. It is much harder to conceive if you are anemic and the body is, in effect, fighting on all fronts. Other types of anemia include folic-acid deficiency and pernicious anemia.

What is it? Every body cell needs oxygen, which is carried by the pigment hemoglobin in red blood cells. Anemia results when there are too few red blood cells. It can take a long time to restore normal levels once they have fallen.

What are the symptoms? Symptoms depend on the severity of the condition and include:
• shortness of breath
• dizziness and palpitations
• lethargy and weakness
• susceptibility to infection
• loss of appetite
• skin pallor
• heavy periods
• emotional fragility

What causes it? Apart from too few iron-rich foods in the diet, factors limiting iron absorption include a high zinc intake; a lack of B vitamins; too much tea and coffee; a high wheat-bran intake; antacids that are taken for heartburn; and too many dairy products. Dairy-based and iron-rich foods should be eaten separately.

Who is at risk? Women with malabsorption problems, such as celiac disease, or heavy periods are at risk, as are frequent dieters and vegetarians.

How is it diagnosed? A simple blood test. Hemoglobin levels in a healthy woman should be 11–15.

How is it treated conventionally? Iron supplements are prescribed, but are not easily absorbed. Constipation is a common side effect. It usually takes six weeks for the body to build iron supplies.

Can complementary therapies help? Specific acupoints can be treated by an acupuncturist to "build the blood."

DIET & NUTRITION

Iron, protein, copper, folic acid, and vitamins B6, B12, and C are all necessary for the formation of red blood cells. A deficiency in any of these nutrients may cause anemia. Make sure you eat lots of the following kinds of food:

• **iron-rich foods** such as organ meats, lean meat, eggs, fish, poultry, molasses, cherries, apricots, dried fruits, green leafy vegetables, parsley, pumpkin and sunflower seeds, kelp, seaweed, and nuts. Nettle tea is a tonic and a rich source of minerals. Steep a large handful of the dried herb in hot water and drink 1–4 cups daily
• **foods rich in vitamin B12**, which are principally animal products and especially lamb, sardines, and salmon
• **foods rich in folic acid** such as dark-green leafy vegetables, etc., as well as 400 mcg of folic acid in daily vitamin supplement
• **foods rich in vitamin C**—such as black currants, kiwi fruit, citrus fruits, melon, mangoes, pineapple, parsley, watercress, and broccoli—which improve iron absorption.

DIABETES

There is no direct link between insulin-dependent diabetes and fertility, but high insulin levels in the blood and impaired glucose tolerance may result in an absence of ovulation. Those with uncontrolled diabetes are six times more likely to miscarry.

What is it? This is a metabolic disorder: the pancreas fails to secrete enough insulin to help cells to absorb glucose for energy.

What are the symptoms? They may go unnoticed until you have a medical checkup. They are:

• lack of energy
• blurred vision
• excessive urination
• recurrent yeast infections
• thirst and a dry mouth

What causes it? Diabetes occurs most commonly when body cells become resistant to insulin.

Who is at risk? You are more at risk if diabetes runs in your family or you are obese.

How is it diagnosed? A simple test checks for the presence of sugar in the urine or blood.

DIET & NUTRITION

In women, diabetes is often associated with being **overweight**. Be guided by your doctor, who may refer you to a dietician for help with the condition and control of your weight. Abnormal metabolic reactions tend to generate many free radicals, so make sure you take **antioxidant supplements** (see pages 59–61).

How is it treated? Mild diabetes can be controlled by means of dietary measures alone, but more severe cases require regular insulin injections to control blood-sugar levels.

DIET & NUTRITION

A nutritional therapist can help you work out a **dietary program for managing an underactive thyroid** (but only in conjunction with advice from your doctor). Essential nutrients are needed to ensure that there are no "gaps" in the metabolic pathways and energy production is not impaired. Make sure you get enough of the following **essential nutrients** (see pages 59–64):

● vitamins B1, B2, B3, B5, and B6
● coenzyme Q10
● magnesium
● chromium
● selenium
● zinc
● iodine
● calcium

UNDERACTIVE THYROID

Thyroid hormones control the speed of metabolic processes so the body has enough energy to drive all its systems, including those that are part of reproduction. They also increase protein synthesis for the maintenance and repair of the body and are therefore extremely important for every body cell.

Thyroxine (T_4) is the main thyroid hormone, but it is inactive physiologically and has to be converted into an active form—T_3 (triiodothyronine)—to do its job.

What is it? Underlying thyroid dysfunction affects the frequency of ovulation and may even prevent it altogether (anovulation). A shortage of thyroid hormones is known as hypothyroidism. Thyroid dysfunction is commonly found to be a contributory factor in female fertility problems today.

What are the symptoms? Symptoms of an underactive thyroid vary from person to person and may be mild or debilitating. Everyone has their own physical strengths and weaknesses, depending on genetic makeup, diet, and lifestyle. As energy is depleted as a result of thyroid dysfunction, an individual's most vulnerable systems will suffer first. Symptoms may include:

• weakness and exhaustion
• memory impairment
• dry hair or hair loss
• sensitivity to cold
• skin problems and brittle nails

- depression and mood swings
- constipation
- weight gain or weight loss
- heavy or irregular periods
- PMS (premenstrual syndrome)
- muscle cramps and joint stiffness

What causes it? There are three main causes of this condition:
- failure of the thyroid gland itself
- failure of the feedback mechanisms that prompt the thyroid gland to secrete more hormones
- failure of body tissues to use thyroid hormones properly.

Who is at risk? Women are generally affected more than men, especially those who have experienced substantial weight loss or who have a history of thyroid disorders in the family.

How is it diagnosed? Often a simple blood test. You might like to investigate your thyroid status yourself. The following is by no means foolproof, but it may be able to give you an indication of whether to seek further standard thyroid testing.

Since the thyroid gland controls your metabolism, which includes temperature regulation, the Barnes temperature test may be useful. Immediately upon waking, moving as little as possible, place a thermometer beneath your arm for 10 minutes and then record the temperature. Do this on days 2, 3, and 4 of your period. The normal basal body temperature (BBT) is between 97.8 and 98.2°F (36.6 and 36.8°C). A temperature consistently lower than this may indicate an underactive thyroid.

How is it treated conventionally? A daily dose of synthetic thyroxine hormone is the drug prescribed. Conventional treatment is essential.

Can complementary therapies help? Complementary therapies cannot tackle hormone imbalance directly. Hypothyroidism is a complex disorder that must be treated with conventional medicine. Dietary measures (see box, opposite), regular gentle exercise, and other lifestyle changes may be helpful as part of a holistic thyroid treatment plan. Acupuncture may help to encourage thyroid function as part of the harmonious functioning of the body as a whole, but complementary therapies should never be substituted for prescribed drugs.

ZITA'S TIPS

Avoid contact with some widely used chemicals and pollutants that can have a detrimental effect on thyroid function.

- **Fluoride** displaces iodine in the thyroid gland, preventing the formation of thyroxine. It also interferes with the feedback between the hypothalamus and pituitary gland that controls the secretion of thyroid hormone.

- **Chlorides** block the uptake of iodine into the thyroid gland.

- **Mercury** interferes with the metabolism of selenium and zinc and can induce hypothyroidism.

- **PCBs** (polychlorinated biphenyls) are chlorinated compounds that are harmful to health. They alter the structure of the thyroid gland and may bind to thyroid hormone receptors, preventing the entry of the hormone into a cell.

- **Foods in the brassica family of vegetables** contain goitrogens, substances that compete with iodine—essential for producing thyroid hormones—for access to thyroid cells. Brassicas, such as cauliflower, broccoli, cabbage, Brussels sprouts, turnips, kale, kohlrabi, rutabagas, and watercress, contain vital nutrients, however, and cooking usually deactivates goitrogens. Millet, peanuts, pine nuts, cassava, corn, and sweet potatoes also contain goitrogens.

- **Some prescription drugs** interfere with hormone function. Your doctor will advise you.

pelvic disorders

Any disorders of the female reproductive system may ultimately affect a woman's fertility, including pelvic infections, which are very common. If you think you may have an infection, get it checked out as soon as possible.

PELVIC INFLAMMATORY DISEASE (PID)

Many women may have had PID in the past without knowing it because of a lack of symptoms. Longstanding or serious infection may cause scar tissue to build up around a fallopian tube, preventing the passage of an egg. Ectopic pregnancy or miscarriage may also occur as a result.

What is it? PID is an umbrella term for any inflammation of the pelvic organs. Since there are often no symptoms, it is not known how many women are affected.

What are the symptoms? Many women are unaware they have PID until they start trying to conceive a baby. When there are symptoms, they can be acute or chronic and include:

• foul-smelling vaginal discharge
• fever, chills, and nausea
• pain in the lower abdomen
• bleeding between periods
• painful intercourse
• a need to pass urine more frequently than usual
• painful urination

What causes it? PID is usually the result of a chlamydial infection (see page 110) or another sexually transmitted infection (STD), such as gonorrhea (see pages 110–11), spreading upward from the vagina to the uterus and tubes.

Who is at risk? Women (or their partners) who have had a number of different sexual partners are at most risk from pelvic infections.

How is it diagnosed? Swabs can be taken in your doctor's office or at the public health department for analysis.

How is it treated conventionally? Antibiotics treat the infection; surgery can remove scar tissue.

Self-help measures include: dietary measures to fight infection (see page 111) and complementary remedies to aid the reproductive system (see pages 145–49).

GENITO-URINARY PROBLEMS

Fertility is easily compromised by inflammation and other consequences of genito-urinary problems. Studies at one infertility clinic in the UK found that some 69 percent of their patients suffered from GU infections.

Certain pelvic infections in women can lead to PID (see above), blocked tubes, ectopic pregnancy, and early miscarriage, and in men to damaged sperm and blocked ducts in the testes. If you or your partner have had a number of sexual partners, it is a good idea to get a sexual health screening to make sure you have no sexually transmitted infections (STDs). If either of you has, then you must both get treatment. Some STDs have a direct effect on fertility (see below). They can be bacterial, viral, or mycoplasmal in origin. Other conditions, such as hepatitis, are passed on during intercourse and affect general health, which in turn impacts on fertility.

Many women today receive abnormal Pap smear results as a result of cervical dysplasia. This may have a number of causes. Any treatment required may lengthen the time it takes to conceive.

CANDIDA (DYSBIOSIS)

Any condition that compromises your general state of health and leads to nutritional imbalances can have a negative effect on fertility. An overgrowth of certain micro-organisms in the vagina may make intercourse painful and create a hostile environment for sperm.

What is it? *Candida albicans* is a yeast that occurs naturally in the gut, on the skin, and in the vagina as part of a network of micro-organisms keeping the body healthy. If the yeast proliferates, dysbiosis, more commonly known as candida or candidiasis, may result. It is a very common complaint.

ZITA'S TIPS

- **Buy a good probiotic supplement** (acidophilus) to recolonize the gut with beneficial flora.

- **Eat a daily portion** of "live" yogurt containing *Lactobacillus acidophilus.*

- **Wear loose-fitting cotton** underwear to promote a cooler, less moist environment.

- **Avoid using bubble bath**: put a handful of salt in the bath water, or a few drops of antifungal tea tree oil.

- **If candida varies in degree,** try a candida diet, but this will need to be supervised.

What causes it? Candida is usually kept under control by "friendly" bacteria in the gut. In certain circumstances, however, the good bacteria are compromised and candida organisms proliferate.

Who is at risk? Several factors may contribute to a proliferation of candida:
- poor nutrition
- a diet high in refined sugars
- taking broad-spectrum antibiotics
- hormone treatments, such as the contraceptive pill
- long-term use of steroids
- surgery, especially gastrointestinal
- disease or illness
- stress
- hormone imbalance with an excess of oestrogen
- poor adrenal function

What are the symptoms? There are many symptoms associated with this condition and often there aren't any obvious or separate characteristics. They may include:
- food cravings, especially sugars
- bloating and flatulence
- vaginitis or cystitis
- vaginal thrush
- changes in bowel habits
- irritable bowel syndrome (IBS)
- depression or lethargy
- impaired absorption of nutrients
- alcohol intolerance

How is it diagnosed? Testing for candida overgrowth is not easy, and there is great debate among

DIET & NUTRITION

Diet is probably the best way to deal with candida, both as a preventative measure and as a cure. A completely sugar-free diet is almost impossible to achieve, but try the following:

- **cut out refined sugars and** natural sweeteners such as honey and maple syrup
- **reduce consumption of yeasts** and fermented food and drinks such as bread and beer
- **avoid moldy foods** such as blue cheese
- **avoid alcohol**

You may notice that symptoms initially get worse before they improve, as a reaction to candida die-off (dead yeast organisms).

medical practitioners about its efficacy. Some believe there has been a tendency for complementary health practitioners to diagnose this condition too readily.

How is it treated conventionally? Antifungal creams and pessaries can be applied to affected areas.

Can complementary therapies help? Many people benefit from an antifungal and anticandida diet. Certain herbal tinctures, including marigold (*Calendula officinalis*) and coneflower (*Echinacea angustifolia*) may soothe: consult a qualified herbalist. Constitutional homeopathic treatment may also be helpful.

CHLAMYDIA

Tubal damage caused by acute inflammation of the fallopian tubes (salpingitis) or other forms of pelvic inflammatory disease (PID, see page 108) is the most common cause of female infertility. Research suggests that as many as 66 percent of cases of salpingitis and 30 percent of other pelvic inflammatory diseases are caused by *Chlamydia trachomatis*. Some women suffer little, if at all, as a result of having this bacterial infection, while others experience extensive damage to their reproductive systems—with long-term implications for fertility—from a minimal level of infection.

What is it? A microorganism found in the genito-urinary tract, chlamydia causes mild to severe infection. Believed to be the most common sexually transmitted, disease-carrying organism in the Western world, it infects the cervix first, causing chlamydial cervicitis, then spreads to the endometrium. If left untreated, it can move into the fallopian tubes, causing acute salpingitis or PID. Chlamydia is now a widespread complaint: as many as 15–20 percent of sexually active people show evidence of previous chlamydial infection, and the number of reported cases is on the increase.

What are the symptoms? You may develop a slight vaginal discharge for a couple of weeks, but if the infection attacks the cervix, there may be no outward indications at all. Chlamydia is known as a "silent infection" because of this: it has been estimated that more than 70 percent of infected women exhibit no symptoms at all.

Who is at risk? Women are at greater risk of having contracted this disease if they have had a number of sexual partners. At least one country—the UK—is pursuing the idea of a national chlamydia screening program (based on urine tests), but there are many issues to be resolved before this becomes a reality.

How is it diagnosed? A swab is taken from the cells of the cervix to identify any infection. A hysterosalpingogram (see page 102) will reveal the extent of any tubal damage. Both partners should be tested for infection.

How is it treated conventionally? Antibiotics—usually a 10–14 day course of treatment—almost guarantee a cure. It is advisable to use a condom during sexual intercourse to protect you from any further infection.

Self-help measures include: nutrition and dietary measures to help fight infection (see opposite).

GONORRHEA

It is estimated that well over half a million people in the US alone become infected with gonorrhea each year. The disease is much less widespread than it used to be, however, as a result of early detection, improved methods of treatment, and safe-sex practices, but it is still one of the most common STDs. Twice as many men as women are infected.

Early treatment of this sexually transmitted infection is crucially important: if it is detected almost immediately, there is little chance of lasting damage. Undetected infection in women, however, can spread up through the uterus, eventually infecting and damaging

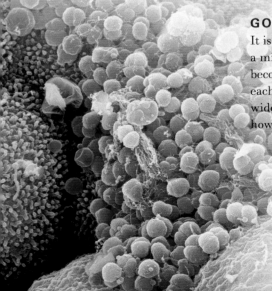

Gonorrhea bacteria
(red) are surrounding other cells (green) in this image.

the fallopian tubes, causing them to become misshapen and blocked. In addition, untreated gonorrhea increases a woman's chances of an ectopic pregnancy.

What is it? A bacterial infection (*Neisseria gonorrhoea*), gonorrhea is one of the most infectious diseases there is. It is one of the major causes of pelvic inflammatory disease (PID) and leaves women more susceptible to contracting chlamydial infections.

What are the symptoms? Within five days of intercourse with an infected partner, a man will have a creamy discharge from the urethra, and it may hurt to pass urine. Abdominal pain and high fever will follow. A woman may have similar symptoms, but more than 70 percent of infected women exhibit no symptoms at all.

Who is at risk? Unprotected sex with many different partners will put you at increased risk.

How is it diagnosed? A swab is taken from the infected area and tested for the bacteria. Both partners should be tested.

How is it treated conventionally? Cefatriaxone effectively kills the bacteria, and the infection should clear up within four or five days, but you should be retested about 10 days after treatment to make sure you are clear of infection before having sex again.

helping fight infection

Boosting the immune system by eating a nutrient-rich diet and taking a good multivitamin and mineral supplement is the best way of preventing infections from spreading. Eliminate foods containing yeast and sugar to help fight yeast infection.

If you are on antibiotics, take a probiotic (disease-destroying bacteria) supplement, such as *Lactobacillus acidophilus* (three capsules a day usually) or eat a small carton of live yogurt that contains "active" bacterial cultures. Other supplements known to be helpful for vaginal infections include:

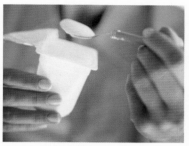

Eat a portion of live yogurt every day to help restore "friendly" bacteria in the gut and vagina.

- **vitamin C**—helps the formation of collagen. If the collagen matrix (the main component of the body's connective tissue) is intact, infection will be less able to spread, you will develop less scar tissue, and damaged tissue will repair more quickly
- **beta-carotene**—a powerful antioxidant that is vital for the functioning of the immune system and the normal growth of vaginal tissue. It also helps to fight infection
- **vitamin E**—increases resistance to chlamydial infections. As well as taking it orally, you can open a capsule and apply the oil directly to the inflamed area to soothe and heal. Yeast-free capsules may also be inserted into the vagina

- **B vitamins**—needed to fight infection. Women with vaginal infections are very often found to be deficient in B vitamins
- **zinc**—boosts immunity, encourages healing and prevents recurrence of infection
- **garlic**—has strong antibacterial properties to help fight infection
- *Lactobacillus acidophilus* supplement (containing at least 4 billion beneficial bacteria)—this is antagonistic to unfriendly bacteria and toxic to *Gardnerella vaginalis*, the bacteria responsible for many infections of the vagina and vulva. Acidophilus is usually taken orally, but capsules may be inserted into the vagina.

HERPES

This condition is widespread. Many people who have it are reluctant to talk about it, however.

What is it? Genital herpes is closely related to herpes type 1, which causes cold sores on the lips. The virus can lie dormant for years before the first outbreak.

What are the symptoms? A burning sensation on the labia is followed by itching and a crop of small blisters. These crust over and heal in about a week, but you might be infectious for another five days.

What causes it? After the initial attack, the virus lies dormant rather than disappearing, although the body produces antibodies that help prevent further attacks. The virus may be reactivated by stress, menstruation, depression, anxiety, a suppressed immune system, lack of sleep, or poor diet. Outbreaks occur less frequently over time.

Who is at risk? Those having unprotected sex with multiple partners are most at risk.

How is it diagnosed? A swab taken from an active herpetic sore can be analyzed, or a blood test may identify herpes antibodies.

How is it treated conventionally? An anesthetic ointment and some pain relief is usually prescribed. The drug acyclovir (Zovirax) may reduce the severity of symptoms if applied early enough.

Can complementary therapies help? Acupuncture may help to boost the immune system, for example, but conventional drugs are needed to treat the infection.

Self-help measures include:
- avoiding sex during an attack
- taking multivitamins and minerals, especially vitamin C, bioflavonoids, and zinc
- avoiding arginine-rich foods
- applying tea tree oil or calendula ointment to the blisters
- exposing the area to the air
- taking garlic capsules at onset

BACTERIAL VAGINOSIS

Studies have shown that couples with fertility problems are more likely than fertile couples to have high concentrations of some of the minute microorganisms that normally inhabit the genital tract. These include *Gardnerella vaginalis*, *Mycoplasma hominis*, *Ureaplasma urealyticum*, and Group B *Streptococcus*.

What is it? Although some of these are the smallest disease-carrying organisms, if they are allowed to proliferate, the balance between all the microorganisms in the genital tract is altered, causing a variety of genito-urinary problems, especially if your general health is poor and the immune system is weakened. Rarely, women may go on to develop pelvic inflammatory disease (PID, see page 108).

What are the symptoms? There may not be any, but some women experience a vaginal discharge or vulvovaginitis—inflammation of the vagina and vulva.

What causes it? The reasons for overgrowth of organisms are not fully understood, but the condition may be associated with another sexually transmitted infection.

Who is at risk? Those having unprotected sex with multiple partners are most at risk.

How is it diagnosed? Bacterial vaginosis may be obvious from the symptoms, but a swab will often be taken to confirm the diagnosis. Both partners should be checked.

How is it treated conventionally? A course of antibiotics will clear up the infection within a couple of days, but the condition does tend to recur.

Self-help measures include: nutrition and dietary measures to help fight infection (see page 111).

Can complementary therapies help? Complementary therapies may help to boost the immune system and help fight infection.

reproductive organ dysfunctions

Problems with the basic functioning of the female reproductive system range from physical problems in parts of the reproductive organs to malfunctions of the processes of egg production, fertilization, implantation, and development.

ECTOPIC PREGNANCY

This is an implantation problem: a fertilized egg implants not in the lining of the uterus, but in tissue outside it. The egg then begins to develop into an embryo, but it is not able to grow normally and will not survive.

What is it? An ectopic pregnancy develops outside the uterus, usually in one of the fallopian tubes. About one in 100 pregnancies is ectopic.

What are the symptoms? Common signs include:
• abdominal pain, often on one side
• vaginal bleeding, often with dark blood, "like prune juice"
• a missed period and symptoms of pregnancy
• faintness and lightheadedness
• shoulder pain (referred pain)

What causes it? Damage to a fallopian tube may restrict the passage of an egg to the uterus, but the cause is not always known.

Who is at risk? There is an increased risk of having an ectopic pregnancy if you have:

• previously had a pelvic infection
• had surgery on the fallopian tubes or ovaries
• had a previous ectopic pregnancy, which increases the risk of having another one 20-fold
• used an intrauterine device (IUD, or coil) as a contraceptive
• had in vitro fertilization (IVF) treatment

How is it diagnosed? As well as a pregnancy and blood test, you may be referred for:
• an ultrasound scan
• a laparoscopy (see page 102)

How is it treated conventionally? An ectopic pregnancy is usually dealt with surgically as soon as possible. The tube is opened up, the embryo removed, and the tube repaired using laparoscopic surgery, or, if it is badly damaged, removed altogether. A larger cut above the pubic hairline may be necessary in an emergency situation or if laparoscopic surgery is not possible.

Following an ectopic pregnancy, there is a higher risk of another one in subsequent pregnancies. It

CASE HISTORY

Tara, age 32, conceived within a few months, but soon developed spotting and pain. A scan revealed an ectopic pregnancy and evidence of a previous pelvic infection. Tara did not want to go straight to IVF (in vitro fertilization). Despite there still being a risk of an ectopic pregnancy because of tubal scarring, *she opted to improve her diet for six months before trying again.* If she had no success, she would then try IVF.

is advisable to have an early scan to ensure that implantation is in the uterus. Your fertility may be slightly reduced by having a fallopian tube removed, but most women conceive and deliver subsequently with no complications.

DIET & NUTRITION

Good nutrition is vitally important in treating the underlying causes of endometriosis. Consider a detox program—see pages 50–53—to help balance estrogen levels:

- **increase your intake of dietary fiber,** especially whole grains, legumes, brown rice, flaxseed, fruits, and vegetables
- **eat bitter foods** such as chicory and radicchio, and vegetables such as cabbage, cauliflower, Brussels sprouts, broccoli, and turnips, to aid estrogen clearance via the bowel
- **reduce your saturated fat intake** and cut down on meat and dairy produce
- **avoid foods containing** sugar, chocolate, caffeine, and alcohol
- **eat foods containing** natural phytoestrogens (see page 31)

To help reduce inflammation:

- **eat fruits rich in vitamin C and bioflavonoids,** especially the pulp and inner peel of citrus fruits, grape skins, and berries
- **take a daily multivitamin and mineral supplement** containing vitamins B-complex, C, and E, zinc, magnesium, and selenium (see pages 59–63)
- **take a daily supplement of** omega-3 essential fatty acids and evening primrose oil (see also pages 63–64)
- **avoid partially hydrogenated oils,** including margarine

ENDOMETRIOSIS

A large number of women who undergo a laparoscopic procedure (see page 102) to investigate the possible causes of their fertility problems are found to be suffering from endometriosis. This condition is not the direct cause of infertility, but it may be a major contributing factor. The root cause of it may also be responsible for the woman's failure to conceive.

If the extent is mild-moderate to severe and there are adhesions (scar tissue) and tubal and/or ovarian damage, ovulation and fertilization will obviously be affected. If the condition is mild, with only a few scattered implants, the link with infertility is more difficult to establish. It may be because more prostaglandins (hormonelike substances) are produced in the pelvic cavity. These may interfere with ovulation and affect the muscles in the fallopian tubes, preventing transportation of the egg along the tube. It may be because there is an increased number of white blood cells attacking and destroying foreign bodies, including sperm or embryos. Tackling the underlying causes of endometriosis is therefore perhaps the best option.

What is it? The migration and implantation of endometrial tissue, which forms the lining of the uterus, in other parts of the body, usually in the pelvic region (ovaries, fallopian tubes, uterine muscles, colon, and bladder) but occasionally outside it. These "implants" are stimulated by hormonal changes, so they build up and then bleed in the same way as the lining of the uterus does, causing scarring and adhesions.

Estimates of how common a complaint this is range from 4 to 17 percent of all menstruating females, but the figure could be higher. Endometriosis is believed to be the cause of as much as 80 percent of pelvic pain.

What are the symptoms? The severity of symptoms is not related to the severity of the condition. You may have no symptoms or a combination of several, including:

- severe pain or cramp in the pelvis, abdomen, leg, or lower back
- pain during bowel movements or urination
- pain during intercourse
- abnormal menstruation
- spotting between periods
- heavy bleeding with thick clots
- severe premenstrual syndrome (PMS—see pages 126–27) with bloating, sore breasts, cravings, and headaches
- mood swings, anxiety, irritability, depression, and a feeling of being overwhelmed
- fatigue, exhaustion, and low energy levels

What causes it? The cause is not known, but there are a number of theories. It is probably due to a

combination of factors, including:
- excess estrogen (see pages 31–32)
- menstruation starting at an early age or delayed pregnancy
- retrograde menstruation, in which blood and tissue flow back into the fallopian tubes
- a weakness that some women have in their pelvic area, making them vulnerable to infections and conditions such as candida overgrowth (see page 109)
- a weakened immune system (as a result of chronic stress, poor diet, nutritional deficiencies, etc.)

In traditional Chinese medicine (see page 72), endometriosis is believed to be the result of a blockage in or "stagnation" of the flow of energy around the body.

Who is at risk? Several factors may combine to increase the risk of endometriosis, including:

- regular heavy periods that last more than seven days
- an immediate family member— a mother or a sister—who has endometriosis
- strenuous physical activity while menstruating (although regular exercise reduces the risk)
- using an intrauterine device (IUD), which may increase the amount of retrograde blood flow

How is it diagnosed? If your medical history reveals a number of the symptoms that are usually associated with endometriosis, you will be given a pelvic examination. Depending on the findings, you may then be referred to a lab for an MRI or an ultrasound (which uses high-frequency sound waves to create images of the pelvic cavity). Alternatively, you may have

a laparoscopy (see page 102), which is another means of confirming a diagnosis of endometriosis.

How is it treated conventionally? Conventional Western medicine uses the following methods:
- painkillers
- synthetic hormones, usually the contraceptive pill, synthetic progesterone or gonadotrophin-

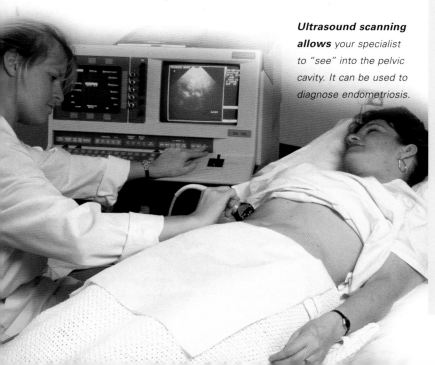

Ultrasound scanning allows *your specialist to "see" into the pelvic cavity. It can be used to diagnose endometriosis.*

ZITA'S TIPS

- **Get regular exercise**, especially first thing in the morning, and avoid strenuous activity during a period.

- **Make sure you get** plenty of rest when you need to.

- **Use painkillers that do not contain codeine**, but try to cut down on using analgesic drugs altogether.

- **Relax in an Epsom-salt bath** to relax the muscles deeply and release emotions and stress. Dissolve a tub of salts in hot water and immerse yourself for 20 minutes or so. When you are dry, lie down quietly for another 20 minutes.

- **Do not use tampons** or, if you must, make sure they are 100 percent cotton. In Chinese medicine, tampons are believed to interfere with the free flow of blood from the body.

releasing hormone (GnRH) to arrest the further development of endometrial lesions

- surgery: the laparoscopic removal of lesions or small cysts from the endometrium may be possible (see page 102), but sometimes microsurgery will be necessary to remove adhesions from less accessible locations within the pelvic cavity or fallopian tubes. Laser surgery may also be used (during a laparoscopic procedure) to destroy small areas of endometrial tissue, increasing

your chances of conception for about 4–6 months until the condition recurs.

Can complementary therapies help? A combination of dietary and lifestyle changes together with specific complementary treatments can be used to tackle the underlying causes of the condition, reduce the severity of the symptoms, and minimize the chances of recurrence. Every individual is different, so you need to work out the right program

for you with the help of a complementary practitioner. Treatments to try include:

- herbal remedies, such as chaste-tree berry (*Vitex agnus-castus*) to encourage ovulation
- acupuncture, to restore balance between the body's systems, improve the flow of vital energy, and relieve pain
- homeopathy: constitutional remedies recommended might include cimicifuga, coffea, or folliculinum, depending on your particular symptoms.

CASE HISTORY

Rosy, aged 38, used the Billings method of natural contraception for four years before actively trying to conceive. After eight months without success, she visited a gynecologist who diagnosed severe (grade 2) endometriosis. Rosy had always suffered very heavy, painful periods with a lot of clotting, but she had taken this for granted as "normal" for her. After reading an article by a fellow endometriosis sufferer, she cut out wheat, dairy products, and caffeine from her diet. Although this was not easy to do, she was very determined and noticed an improvement almost immediately: her next period was lighter and less painful. On the recommendation of a friend, she started

coming to me for acupuncture. After weekly treatments throughout one cycle, Rosy conceived her daughter Agnes, who is 16 months old as of this writing.

Rosy breast-fed Agnes for ten months, during which time she had no periods. Two months after her periods resumed, she discovered she was pregnant again. Sadly, she miscarried this baby at 13 weeks. During both pregnancies she says she "never felt healthier."

She has been advised to try to conceive another baby as soon as possible because of her age. She has been taking a preconception multivitamin and mineral supplement for many months, follows a healthy diet, and avoids alcohol.

FIBROIDS

Fibroids growing on the walls of the uterus won't necessarily stop you from getting pregnant, but even small fibroids can interfere with endometrial development and implantation (see page 12). Fibroids any larger than about 1½–2 in (4–5 cm) in diameter may cause problems during pregnancy as they push against blood vessels, possibly preventing the fetus from developing normally.

Some fibroids grow outside the uterus, but if they are larger than 2½ in (6 cm) in diameter, they may get in the way as the fallopian tube tries to pick up an egg after ovulation, and this could affect your ability to conceive. However, once you are pregnant, small fibroids will not hurt your developing baby. Many women go to term without their fibroids causing any problems.

What are they? Fibroids are benign tumors that grow in the uterine cavity, in the muscular walls of the uterus, or on the outside of the uterus. Only very rarely, in less than 0.5 percent of cases, do they become malignant. Fibroids vary enormously in size, from microscopic to the size of a soccer ball, and are made of a hard, white, gristly tissue. Their size often fluctuates during the menstrual cycle, growing after ovulation and shrinking after a period, with hormonal changes. They usually shrink rapidly after

menopause. Fibroids are the most common structural abnormalities of the uterus, and it is estimated that between 20 and 50 percent of women between the ages of 35 and 50 have them. They are more common in black women than Caucasians, although it is not understood why.

What are the symptoms? It depends on the size and location of the fibroids, but many women have no symptoms at all and may be quite unaware that they have them. Possible symptoms caused by large fibroids include:

- heavy or irregular bleeding if the fibroids are growing in the uterine lining
- menstrual cramps and/or pelvic pain, if there is also endometriosis present
- extremely heavy bleeding, almost hemorrhaging, leaving you exhausted and anemic
- pain, if the fibroid has outgrown its blood supply and started to degenerate, in which case the nerve at the center of the fibroid registers the lack of oxygen as pain. As the fibroid shrinks and the nerve adjusts, the pain usually decreases
- a feeling of fullness or pressure in the lower abdomen, if the fibroid is quite large and is pressing on internal organs
- constipation
- the need to pass water frequently and urgently, especially during

DIET & NUTRITION

Fibroids are estrogen-sensitive, so a high-fat, high-protein, low-fiber diet will put you at greater risk of developing this condition, or exacerbating it, because more estrogen will be circulating in the body as a result of eating these types of food. Changing to a low-fat, high-fiber, mostly vegetarian diet for at least three months may help to reduce the pain and bleeding associated with this condition.

- **Eliminate refined sugars**, wheat products, saturated fats, dairy products, chocolate, caffeine, and salt from your diet as much as you can.
- **Include large quantities of** green leafy vegetables (such as spinach) and cruciferous vegetables (such as cauliflower and broccoli), whole grains (excluding wheat), and legumes.
- **Cut down on** red meat, poultry, and alcohol.
- **Take an iron supplement** daily to prevent or relieve anemia if you have heavy bleeding, together with a high dose of vitamin C and bioflavonoids to enhance iron absorption (see pages 57 and 61).
- **Take a good multivitamin and mineral supplement daily**: of particular importance are vitamin B-complex (especially its choline and inositol components), vitamin E, calcium, magnesium, potassium, and the amino acid methionine (see pages 59–64).

ZITA'S TIPS

- **Do regular aerobic exercise** such as swimming, cycling, or running for at least 20 minutes three times a week.

- **Practice yoga** to reduce pelvic congestion, improve blood circulation, relax the muscles of the uterus, and relax you generally, as well as improving your sense of well-being.

- **Use stress-reduction techniques** such as meditation, deep breathing, aromatherapy, and massage (see pages 42–43).

- **Try herbal formulas** containing chaste-tree berry (*Vitex agnus castus*), dong quai, wild yam, licorice root, or sarsaparilla (see page 31), for example, but always make sure that you consult a qualified herbal practitioner before taking any herbal remedies.

the night, because the fibroid is exerting pressure on the bladder
- recurrent bladder infections or irritation.

What causes them? The cause is unknown.

Who is at risk? The following factors may increase your risk of developing fibroids.
- If a close female relative (your mother or a sister) has fibroids, it may mean you have a genetic predisposition to the condition, but dietary and environmental factors are believed to be more significant.
- A high-fat, low-fiber diet that encourages the circulation of estrogen and contributes to constipation, which prevents the elimination of estrogen.
- Obesity, possibly because of the production of non-ovarian estrogen in fatty tissue.

How are they diagnosed? Fibroids are often detected during a routine pelvic examination. If they are growing inside the uterus, the diagnosis can be confirmed by means of an ultrasound scan. If they are located on the outer surface of the uterus, they will also be revealed on a scan or during a laparoscopic procedure (see page 102).

How are they treated conventionally? There are various methods of treatment, depending on the seriousness of the condition.
- If the fibroids aren't causing any problems, a wait-and-see policy may be adopted.
- Hormone therapy (synthetic or natural progesterone or gonadotrophin-releasing hormone—GnRH) may be prescribed to reduce levels of estrogen and control bleeding, inducing temporary menopause.

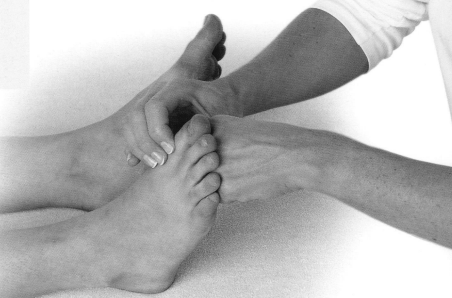

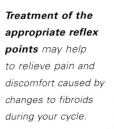

Treatment of the appropriate reflex points may help to relieve pain and discomfort caused by changes to fibroids during your cycle.

• Fibroids can be surgically removed (myomectomy), usually by means of a hysteroscopic procedure (see page 102) via the cervix or by making an incision in the abdomen. Embolization (or uterine artery embolization procedure, to give it its full name) is a relatively new method of treating fibroids that is based on the principle of blocking off the supply of blood to a fibroid. This procedure is, however, still regarded as being in the experimental stage, and is probably not suitable for those women with fibroids who are planning to have children.

Can complementary therapies help? Several therapies may help women with fibroids, either alone or in combination, by relieving the symptoms of excessive bleeding and pain and helping to reduce the size of fibroids so that myomectomy becomes a practical option. Complementary therapies may also help to tackle underlying causes of fibroids, especially the energetic and emotional patterns contributing to their development.
• Acupuncture, including moxibustion, can release blocked energy in the liver and pelvic area as well as relieving pain.
• Homeopathy may be helpful at

a constitutional level to resolve both physiological and any emotional problems associated with this condition.
• Herbal remedies may help to reduce the size of fibroids and redress hormonal imbalance.
• Shiatsu or massage can increase the flow of life energy to the pelvic region.
• Reflexology, particularly on the reflex points for the uterus and liver, can release blocked energy.
• Counseling or psychotherapy can help you deal with underlying emotional issues and concerns that might be aggravating your state of health.

POLYCYSTIC OVARY SYNDROME (PCOS)

PCOS is responsible for many of the fertility problems in the women I see. The underlying cause is the inability of the ovaries to produce hormones in the correct relative proportions. In addition, abnormally high levels of insulin may reduce egg quality. Women with PCOS tend to produce many small follicles, so there is an added risk of ovarian hyperstimulation syndrome (OHSS) if these women choose to go down the IVF (in vitro fertilization) route.

What is it? PCOS is a chronic condition in which the ovaries develop lots of tiny cysts just beneath the surface, caused by egg follicles that haven't matured properly. It is accompanied by hormonal imbalance and a variety

of other characteristics such as a low level of progesterone and a high level of luteinizing hormone (LH). These abnormalities in hormone levels make it much more difficult for eggs to mature and to be released. Nonsteroidal anti-inflammatory drugs, such as ibuprofen and adult-strength aspirin, may contribute to the occurrence of PCOS.

It is estimated that 20 percent of women have a tendency to polycystic ovaries and 5–10 percent have full-blown PCOS.

What are the symptoms? Symptoms often begin during adolescence or a woman's early 20s. They vary in severity and may include:
• irregular or absent periods

DIET & NUTRITION

Eating a **nutrient-rich diet** will help your body to restore **hormonal balance**. Cut down on animal fats, but increase amounts of **essential fatty acids**. Replace processed foods with **whole foods**. Eat plenty of **vegetables and fruits**, preferably organic. Take a good multivitamin and mineral supplement.

• the absence of ovulation
• fertility problems or recurrent miscarriage
• rapid weight gain or difficulty losing weight
• increased amounts of facial hair, caused by the overproduction of androgens as well as raised levels of testosterone
• skin problems such as acne or oily skin

ACUPUNCTURE

More research has been carried out into the effectiveness of acupuncture in the **treatment of PCOS** than for any other female reproductive problem. It includes **auricular acupuncture** (which uses acupoints located on the ear) and **electro-acupuncture**, in which a low-intensity pulsing electric current is applied through the needles to stimulate acupoints. Acupuncture has long been recommended for improving cycle irregularities and relieving pain.

Acupuncture treatment impacts on B-endorphins, which in turn affect levels of **gonadotrophin-releasing hormone** (GnRH), and has been used in an attempt to regulate hormonal imbalance and specifically to adjust **FSH and LH levels**.

• thinning hair or male-pattern hair loss
• insulin insensitivity leading to raised blood-sugar levels.

What causes it? PCOS is caused by a hormonal imbalance—overproduction of luteinizing hormone (LH), androgens, or estrogen, and underproduction of follicle-stimulating hormone (FSH) or progesterone. It is not known, however, whether the problem originates in the hypothalamus or the ovaries. Sometimes only one ovary is affected, which would suggest that the problem is ovarian.

Who is at risk? You are more at risk if you:
• are overweight or obese
• are a smoker
• have a family history of diabetes

• have close female relatives with the condition, which would suggest a genetic link

How is it diagnosed? On an ultrasound scan, the ovaries will appear enlarged because of multiple small cysts formed from undeveloped eggs. A blood test will detect hormonal imbalances (raised LH and low FSH levels). Blood pressure and blood-sugar levels should also be checked.

Self-testing is possible, but results are unreliable because high levels of LH sometimes give a false positive in an ovulation-kit test. Your BTM (basal temperature measurement) may be erratic and difficult to determine accurately.

How is it treated conventionally? Since the causes are not always obvious, conventional drugs aim to

ZITA'S TIPS

• **Lose weight.** If you are obese, a weight reduction of 10 percent of your body weight will boost your fertility (and regulate your cycle) as effectively as any assisted reproductive technique. Slow and gentle weight loss, with a gradual change in the types of food you eat, is a better method than crash dieting and calorie counting.

• **Women with PCOS** often have higher glucose levels and so are prone to diabetes. Losing excess

body fat will increase your insulin secretion, leveling out your blood sugar and reducing excess androgens. You may be prescribed drugs to help with this.

• **Weight loss** is particularly difficult if you have PCOS. Try not to be too discouraged or depressed, even if it is a long haul.

• **Balancing blood-sugar levels** is also very important for this condition. Choose foods that have a low glycemic index—that is,

"slow-release" or complex carbohydrates (see page 57 for examples)—and introduce protein into each meal (see page 55).

• **Stress management** is vitally important if you suffer from PCOS, since the adrenal glands react to stressful situations by releasing more testosterone, which further upsets hormonal balance.

• **Exercise regularly**: go for a brisk, 30-minute walk at least three times a week.

reduce the symptoms of PCOS by:

- reducing the chances of cancerous changes in the endometrium (by prescribing the contraceptive pill or progesterone)
- improving fertility problems by inducing ovulation (antiestrogen drugs such as Clomid)
- reducing the masculinizing effects of the androgens (anti-androgen hormones or estrogen).

Women are advised to lose weight if necessary, although this can be difficult for women with PCOS, since weight gain is symptomatic of the condition. Insulin-sensitizing medication such as metformin may be prescribed as part of a calorie-controlled diet, but this antidiabetic drug may have side effects (in 20 percent of women) such as nausea, diarrhea, abdominal discomfort, or cramps.

Can complementary therapies help? If the condition is severe, natural remedies must only be used in a supportive capacity, accompanying conventional drugs prescribed to redress hormone imbalance. Treatments and remedies might include:

- acupuncture (see box, opposite)
- herbal medicines, which should always be prescribed by a qualified practitioner
- constitutional homeopathic remedies, which should also be prescribed by a qualified practitioner and preferably one with experience of treating fertility problems

CASE HISTORY

Elaine was diagnosed with PCOS in her early 20s. She conceived her two sons after a short course of Clomid, but when she tried for a third child, at the age of 34, she suffered unpleasant side effects from the drug, "feeling lousy with awful skin and horrible bloating." Ovulation tests did not look promising, so after six months Elaine came off Clomid and tried a natural progesterone supplement instead. Again, there were unpleasant side effects, including manic mood swings, an erratic cycle with constant spotting, and a feeling of being drained of energy. By this point she had given up all hope for a third child and simply wanted her erratic cycle to be evened out. Her doctor recommended the contraceptive pill, but Elaine wanted to try a more natural route. She decided to try acupuncture. Her first treatment eased the spotting, and the second cleared it completely. Elaine continued to have weekly appointments, and a month later she had a "normal" period. Concurrently, at Zita's suggestion, Elaine visited a nutritionist who put her on vitamin and mineral supplements to redress various nutritional deficiencies. She cut out red meat and drank a minimum of two quarts (liters) of water a day. Acupuncture at this stage was geared solely to regulating her cycle, not starting ovulation, but her next period failed to appear. A pregnancy test was negative and there were no symptoms of pregnancy. A second test proved positive, however, and to her enormous surprise and delight, Elaine now has a daughter.

DIET & NUTRITION

Certain nutritional deficiencies are thought to be linked to miscarriage. If you are at risk, be sure to include certain key vitamins and minerals in your diet or take supplements.

- **Low levels of magnesium** are believed to be a factor. Oxidation, a process that damages cell membranes, can result in a loss of magnesium. Include magnesium-rich foods in your diet or take a supplement (see pages 61 and 63).
- **The antioxidant mineral selenium** protects cell membranes, helping to maintain magnesium levels. Women who miscarry have been found to have lower levels of selenium than women who go to term. Make sure you increase your dietary sources of this mineral (see page 63) or take a supplement.
- **Research suggests that levels of coenzyme Q10** (see page 63) are lower in women who have miscarried. Production of co-Q10 in the body also depends on folic acid, vitamin B12, and betaine.
- **Vitamins A and E and beta-carotene levels tend to be** lower in women who have miscarried. Take a prenatal multivitamin supplement to raise your levels (see pages 59 and 61).
- **Vitamins B6 and B12 and folate** (see pages 60–61) are also essential. Deficiencies have been linked to miscarriage.

RECURRENT MISCARRIAGE

Although losing a pregnancy is not the same as an inability to conceive, the impact of either can be devastating, both physically and emotionally. Too often, couples are advised to "just keep trying," especially if they have already had a successful pregnancy. They won't be sent for tests until they have lost at least three pregnancies. New studies of immunology show, however, that if a miscarriage is the result of an autoimmune problem, subsequent pregnancies only serve to make the condition worse. Unfortunately, few HMOs will pay for tests after just one miscarriage.

Roughly half of all the eggs fertilized never progress to a viable pregnancy. Most women never know that they were pregnant, let alone that they have miscarried. More than 25 percent lose a baby during the first trimester, and about one in 200 couples have two or more consecutive miscarriages.

What is it? Miscarriage is the loss of a pregnancy during the first 24 weeks of gestation. The loss of a pregnancy after 24 weeks is termed a stillbirth.

What causes it?
- The most common cause of a miscarriage—in at least half of cases—is a chromosomal abnormality of that pregnancy.
- Abnormal female anatomy, such as distortion of the uterine cavity or adhesions (scar tissue) caused by surgery or infection, is responsible for up to 10 percent of miscarriages.
- Luteal phase defects (LPDs), such as inadequate progesterone production, are responsible for about a fifth of miscarriages.
- In as many as 15 percent of cases of miscarriage, the cause is unknown.
- Other possible causes may include certain immune-system factors, endocrine (hormonal) disorders—such as poorly controlled diabetes or an under-active thyroid—defective sperm, infections of the reproductive tract, or a problem with the time of implantation of an embryo.

Who is at risk? Women most at risk include those who:
- have had a miscarriage before
- are over the age of 35
- have anorexia
- are smokers
- have more than two alcoholic drinks a day
- drink coffee. Caffeine stays in the body of a pregnant woman much longer than in that of a nonpregnant woman. One study of 3,135 pregnant women showed that moderate to heavy coffee drinkers were more likely to have a late-first- or second-trimester miscarriage than non–coffee-drinkers.
- are exposed to X-rays or who spend long periods in planes

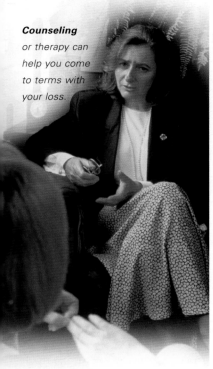

Counseling
or therapy can help you come to terms with your loss.

- are excessively exposed to environmental toxins such as lead, mercury, or organic solvents
- handle cytotoxic agents or whose partners do
- have a serious illness
- use cocaine

Other risk factors include:
- eating fish contaminated with pollutants
- using laxatives, such as senna, that stimulate smooth muscles, including the uterus
- drinking chlorinated water containing CBPs (chlorination by-products). These are formed when chlorine reacts with organic material in the water

How is it diagnosed? Medical advances mean that 80 percent of the causes of miscarriage can be identified, and most problems can be corrected or overcome. The order of testing is usually:
- structural abnormalities
- problems with the luteal phase
- immune abnormalities (see also pages 124–25)
- genetic diseases

How is it treated conventionally? There have been huge advances in the field, but there is also huge controversy surrounding certain forms of treatment.

Antibodies that might cause the autoimmune disorder systemic lupus erythematosus (SLE)—which is inflammation of the body's connective tissue, causing damage to internal organs—can be treated with the drug Prednisone.

Raised levels of natural killer (NK) cells may be treated with an immunoglobulin G (IgG) infusion—a preparation of human-derived antibodies—to prevent rejection of an embryo.

Most structural defects can be corrected surgically. In the case of luteal phase defects, progesterone may be prescribed during the first 12 weeks of a pregnancy. This hormone is responsible for maintaining the endometrium, which sustains the embryo/fetus until the placenta has developed.

If there is a problem with blocking antibodies, the mother may be immunized with concentrates of the father's white blood cells, but this is a highly controversial form of treatment and is not widely available.

Women with abnormal blood-clotting often carry the genes for a tendency to encourage blood clotting. Clotting problems may be treated with low-dose aspirin, but some clinics use heparin injections to thin the blood, starting before pregnancy occurs and continuing until 4–6 weeks after the birth. This is, however, another controversial form of treatment.

Can complementary therapies help? As well as physical treatment, you also have to deal with the emotional devastation of miscarriage. Feelings of guilt, depression, failure, separation, loss, envy, and rage are all common. Losing a baby can be especially traumatic if you have had fertility problems or you've miscarried before. You need to work through your feelings at your own pace and with the right support (therapy, counseling, or a support group), and learn how to deal with the accompanying stress and anxiety.

ZITA'S TIPS

- **Seek advice** from a specialist miscarriage clinic.

- **Talk things through** and explore all the treatment avenues very carefully.

- **Acupuncture** may strengthen the kidneys. In Chinese medicine, weak kidneys are linked to miscarriage.

immune problems

About 40 percent of "unexplained" infertility and 80 percent of "unexplained" pregnancy loss (miscarriages that aren't the result of chromosomal defects, hormonal imbalance, or abnormalities of the uterus) are probably caused by immunological dysfunction.

RESEARCHING THE PROBLEMS

The medical world's understanding of reproductive immunology has increased significantly over the last few years, and a great deal of work is currently being done in North America and Europe. There is still disagreement among experts, however, about the causes of immune problems, and treatment remains controversial.

The area is a complex one, and specialists often work in narrow fields of research, so that it's hard to assess the whole picture. There is a lot of information published on the Internet, but inevitably some of it is contradictory and even alarmist. If you have been diagnosed with an immune problem, my advice is to examine the evidence very carefully as it relates to you, and seek out a second opinion or even a third.

Immune problems are increasingly believed to be a factor as far as some fertility problems are concerned, and may be the cause in cases of unexplained infertility. Antiphospholipid antibodies (APAs) are the most common example of abnormal immune reactions (see below).

What causes immune problems?

The body naturally produces antibodies to fight off invasive and potentially harmful organisms. An embryo consists of tissue and genetic material from both you and your partner, and they combine to create a genetic structure and tissue type that is different from your own. The body's normal reaction is to reject "foreign" tissue, but during pregnancy your body should respond differently, forming a sort of protective blanket around the developing baby.

Some women's bodies are unable to do this, however. Their immune system behaves abnormally, either producing an autoimmune response, rejecting and attacking the developing embryonic cells as if they were an invading illness, or producing an alloimmune response, rejecting the father's genetic contribution (although this may not necessarily happen with a different partner). What this means is that the body does one of the following:

- produces antiphospholipid antibodies (APAs). These attack the cells that build the placenta and its blood supply. This may cause problems initially with implantation, affect blood circulation between mother and embryo, and increase the risk of miscarriage, intrauterine growth retardation, and preeclampsia
- produces antinuclear antibodies (ANAs). These attack the nuclei of cells in the uterus and placenta, causing inflammation and putting an embryo at risk. This may particularly affect women who suffer from conditions such as rheumatoid arthritis or systemic lupus erythematosus (SLE)
- fails to produce blocking antibodies. Maternal blocking antibodies stop the immune system from attacking the fetus. Without them, the fertilized egg will be rejected and fail to implant. Sometimes the signal to switch on the maternal blocking antibodies is never triggered, perhaps because both parents have very similar genetic and tissue makeup
- produces an overabundance of natural killer (NK) cells. These aggressively attack any rapidly growing or dividing cell in order to protect you from life-threatening diseases such as

cancer. Unfortunately, however, they may be lethal as far as a developing fetus is concerned.

How are immune problems diagnosed? Blood tests are taken at six-week intervals to assess your immune status.

How are they treated conventionally? Anticoagulants help to counteract clotting caused by APAs, so you may be prescribed low-dose aspirin to be taken daily or a combination of aspirin and injections of low-dose heparin (an anticoagulant derived from animal tissue). Treatment may be most effective if it is started before you conceive and then continued during the pregnancy.

Antinuclear antibodies can be treated with prednisone, a corticosteroid drug administered orally twice a day. This medication suppresses the inflammatory process and stabilizes the cell.

An absence of maternal blocking antibodies can be treated by immunizing the mother with her partner's white blood cells. This is known as leukocyte immunization therapy (LIT). It is a highly controversial treatment option and there is conflicting evidence about its success. Its availability is currently limited.

Overproduction of natural killer cells can also usually be controlled by LIT (see above), and a low dose of prednisone may also be given. If this doesn't work, injections of immunoglobins (antibodies) may be given to suppress the production of killer cells and enhance the production of "helper" cells. This is very expensive treatment, however, and it carries with it a risk of infection similar to that during a blood transfusion.

CASE HISTORY

Andria, a 35-year-old British woman, started trying to conceive four years ago. She got pregnant after nine months but miscarried at six weeks. Her doctor advised her to keep trying. Ten months later she conceived, but she miscarried at seven weeks: a third pregnancy ended at eight weeks. Still her doctor did not recommend investigations. Andria's husband is American, so she had tests in the US. No obvious cause of the miscarriages was identified. Immune therapy was discussed but dismissed as too controversial.

Back in the UK, Andria was impatient to conceive and embarked on IVF. The first cycle was successful but she lost the baby at seven weeks. She wanted to keep trying and begin another IVF cycle but her FSH (follicle-stimulating hormone) levels were consistently too high.

Meanwhile, Internet research led her to fertility experts in Chicago and London. She was found to be positive for antibodies and was therefore a good candidate for immune therapy. While waiting for her FSH levels to come down, Andria had acupuncture. Following a vacation, she learned she had conceived naturally. At five weeks, the optimum time for treatment, she was injected with her husband's white blood cells and began daily low-dose injections of a blood thinner. At the time of this writing, Andria is eight months pregnant.

hormonal imbalances

All aspects of a woman's reproductive life are influenced by the relative levels of the different female sex hormones in her body. Imbalances between them are responsible for a number of disorders.

DIET & NUTRITION

In most cases of hormonal and menstrual irregularities, dietary changes can improve the condition.

- **Eliminate all dairy products** from your diet (but make a point of taking a calcium supplement).
- **Cut down** as much as possible on animal fats, processed foods, and refined sugar.
- **Give up coffee**—even if you only drink one cup a day—and other drinks or foods with caffeine.
- **Increase the amount of fiber** in your diet to help eliminate excess estrogen (unless you already consume a lot of fiber) and eat more foods containing phyto-estrogens (see page 31).
- **Avoid alcohol** altogether if you can, or limit yourself to an occasional drink.
- **Take a good multivitamin** and mineral supplement daily. Make sure you have sufficient intakes of calcium, magnesium, and vitamin B6 in particular (see pages 60–68).
- **Ensure that your diet contains** enough essential fatty acids (see pages 63–64): sources include oily fish, nuts and seeds, evening primrose oil, flaxseed oil, sesame oil, walnut oil, and sunflower oil.

CYCLE PROBLEMS

There is no direct link between certain menstrual irregularities and fertility problems (with the exception of luteal phase defects), but it follows that underlying hormonal, nutritional, or emotional imbalances that contribute to cycle problems may also be a factor in reduced fertility. Until a balance has been restored, it may be difficult to conceive. The nature of hormonal imbalance varies, but it is closely linked to nutritional deficiencies and high intakes of processed foods, fats, and caffeine. A good diet is an essential part of any treatment plan (see box, left).

PMS

Between 25 and 100 percent of women are believed to suffer from premenstrual syndrome; 10 percent are seriously debilitated. It is more common in women of 35–45, but certain symptoms may be signs of perimenopause.

PMS includes a range of symptoms that recur cyclically, usually between 12 and 5 days before menstruation. They disappear once a period starts. Symptoms are the result of a complex interaction of emotional, physical, and genetic factors, but are generally related to estrogen and progesterone imbalances. Depending on the type of PMS you have, symptoms may include headaches, cravings, fatigue, dizziness and fainting, abdominal bloating and cramping, breast tenderness, back pain, mood swings, insomnia, irritability, tearfulness, social withdrawal, depression, and forgetfulness.

PMS is often triggered by hormonal changes—for example if a woman stops taking the Pill, if she is approaching menopause, or if she has had a serious emotional trauma. Women may also be at risk if they have a diet high in processed foods, refined sugar, dairy products, and animal fat but low in whole grains, fruit, and vegetables; they have low levels of magnesium, selenium, and vitamins B-complex, C and E; they are overweight; they don't exercise enough; or they suffer chronic stress leading to adrenal exhaustion and estrogen dominance.

Conventional drugs such as painkillers, antidepressants, diuretics, or synthetic progesterone may relieve symptoms, but they do not tackle the underlying cause and may have unpleasant side effects.

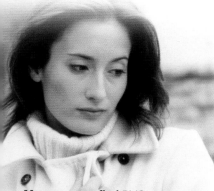

Many women find PMS symptoms are worse during fall and winter.

Rather than addressing specific symptoms, complementary medicine views PMS as a wake-up call to alert you to underlying imbalances. Acupuncture or constitutional homeopathy may help tackle the underlying causes of hormonal imbalance. Herbal remedies such as chaste-tree berry may relieve symptoms, but should only be taken under supervision.

MENORRHAGIA

This describes excessive menstrual bleeding that may be the result of an estrogen or progesterone imbalance. Periods are regular but blood flow is extremely heavy and may be long-lasting and contain large clots. Menorrhagia can lead to anemia and chronic fatigue. It is most common in women in their 40s, and may be related to endometriosis (see pages 114–16), ovarian cysts (see pages 119–21), pelvic inflammatory disease (PID, see page 108), thyroid problems (see pages 106–107), or fibroids (see pages 117–19).

Conventional treatment varies, depending on the cause, but may take the form of prostaglandin inhibitors (such as ibuprofen) or synthetic progesterone. A number of self-help measures may help to improve this condition, including regular exercise and stress relief, as well as good nutrition (see box, opposite). Herbal medicine may be useful to help regulate bleeding or clear estrogen. Homeopathy or acupuncture may also help.

DYSMENORRHEA

This describes severe pain and cramping during menstruation, felt in the lower back, abdomen, and inner thighs. It is thought to be related to an estrogen and progesterone imbalance. If it is related to endometriosis or other pelvic disease, it is felt more as a dull ache in the lower back and pelvic area (and is known as secondary dysmenorrhea). Up to 60 percent of women suffer from menstrual cramps, some of them being severely debilitated.

ZITA'S TIPS

- **Allow yourself time for self-nurturing**—to be alone to rest quietly, reflect, and switch off from daily stresses and strains. The reduction of stress is important for the relief of many cycle problems, preventing adrenal exhaustion and the resulting estrogen dominance.

- **Do at least 20 minutes of aerobic exercise** at least three times a week to help relieve stress, improve general circulation, and release endorphins.

- **Eat small meals at regular intervals** so that blood-sugar levels do not fall too low.

- **Try to get at least two hours of bright light** or sunshine every day.

- **Try homeopathic remedies** to relieve your particular symptoms, especially those of PMS. Take every 12 hours for 3 days before the onset of symptoms:
  Sepia 30c if you are irritable, tearful, emotionally flat ,or craving sweet or salty foods.

Pulsatilla 30c if you are tearful or nauseous and you have painful breasts and irregular periods.
Natrum mur 30c if you are low and irritable and have water-retention and swollen breasts.
Calcarea 30c if you are tired, lethargic, and clumsy and your breasts are swollen and painful.
Lycopodium 30c if you are bad-tempered and crave sweet things.
Causticum 30c if you are pessimistic and oversensitive, with urinary problems and colicky pains.

Conventional treatment takes the form of anti-inflammatory drugs or the contraceptive pill, which is obviously not a good idea if you are trying to get pregnant. Gentle exercise prior to a period, stress-reduction techniques, and good nutrition (see box on page 126) are useful self-help measures.

AMENORRHEA

As with other menstrual problems, amenorrhea is an indication of hormonal and nutritional imbalance. Periods stop for several months, not because of pregnancy or menopause but as a result of temporary failure of the ovaries and the pituitary gland.

The condition is sometimes accompanied by an underactive thyroid (see pages 106–07), and may be a symptom of polycystic ovary disease (see PCOS, pages 119–21). You may also be at risk

if you suffer great weight loss, do intense physical exercise, come off the Pill, have extreme emotional stress, are obese, take certain drugs that increase prolactin levels, or have nutritional deficiencies.

Diet is the best place to start with this problem, especially maintaining a good balance of carbohydrates, fat, and protein, eating plenty of whole grains and legumes, and taking a multivitamin and mineral supplement (see also box on page 126). Estrogen replacement therapy is the conventional treatment.

LUTEAL PHASE DEFECT (LPD)

This is technically an ovulation disorder resulting from hormonal imbalance and causing conception difficulties. If the luteal phase (see pages 10–11) is shorter than normal, insufficient progesterone is available to maintain a fertilized

egg until it implants. Progesterone deficiency may be associated with the faulty secretion of luteinizing hormone (LH) and hence failed ovulation. Drug treatment may include ovulation stimulation or progesterone supplementation.

PREDICTING OVULATION

Women who have **irregular menstrual cycles** may find it hard to predict when they ovulate. Many use **ovulation kits** to identify the LH surge (see page 10). Women with long or short cycles may need **follicular tracking**. This is the use of **ultrasound scanning** at weekly intervals during a woman's cycle to determine when ovulation has taken place. The advantage of this is that a woman doesn't have to take medication to regulate her cycle.

ZITA'S TIPS

There are several self-help measures that may encourage your FSH levels to come down.

- **Get regular, gentle exercise** but nothing too strenuous.

- **Try to lose excess weight** if you are overweight.

- **Practice** meditation and deep-breathing techniques on a regular basis in order to reduce stress and improve relaxation.

RAISED FSH LEVELS

Levels of follicle-stimulating hormone (FSH) tend to fluctuate during a woman's monthly cycle throughout her 30s and early 40s as perimenopause approaches (see pages 16–17). Few women have any idea about their FSH levels, however, until they start trying for a baby. I see many women who wait from month to month for their FSH levels to come down, having discovered that they have problems conceiving and while they wait to start IVF (in vitro fertilization) treatment.

What is it? FSH is a hormone released by the pituitary gland to encourage an egg to ripen and mature (see pages 10–11). FSH levels give a good indication of ovarian reserve (see page 16). If levels are raised, as your body tries to stimulate ovulation, it is likely that egg quality will be poor.

What causes it? FSH levels do fluctuate naturally, especially in reaction to stress, but raised levels may indicate that perimenopause or menopause is imminent or has already started. This condition may also indicate that ovulation has not occurred. Some women do, however, go on to have a successful pregnancy, although this is uncommon. It is possible for a 45-year-old woman to have good-quality eggs (for her age) and still be fertile. On the other hand, a 25-year-old can have poor-quality eggs and be infertile—unless she uses donor eggs. These are extreme examples, admittedly, but the point is that egg quality tends to decline significantly in a woman's 30s and at an even faster rate during her early 40s, but egg quality in an individual may be average for her age, better than average, or worse than average.

What are the symptoms? There are no symptoms of raised FSH levels, and very often the first thing a women knows about the significance of her FSH levels is following the results of a routine blood test that she might have as part of fertility testing procedures (see page 99) if she finds she is having difficulty conceiving.

How is it diagnosed? A routine blood test is done on days 1–3 of the menstrual cycle (or, if a period has been missed, at any time). This test is used to diagnose or evaluate disorders of the pituitary gland or reproductive system.

How is it treated conventionally? There is currently no conventional treatment for raised FSH levels.

Can complementary therapies help? I use acupuncture to help lower raised FSH levels with some degree of success, but it does depend on how high the levels are to start with. I treat a number of important acupoints for hormone regulation and reproduction.

There are a number of general lifestyle factors to be considered (see box, opposite), and diet is important (see box, right).

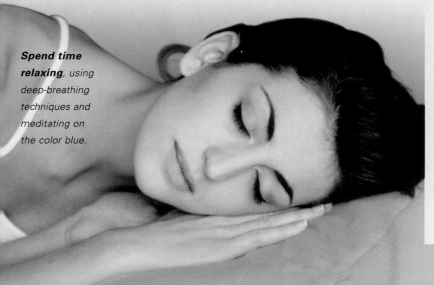

Spend time relaxing, using deep-breathing techniques and meditating on the color blue.

DIET & NUTRITION

There are a number of dietary measures you can put into effect to try to bring down your FSH levels.

- **Put yourself on a detoxifying program,** including drinking at least two quarts (liters) of bottled or filtered water a day, cutting down your salt intake, and avoiding coffee, tea, and sugary and carbonated drinks. Drink hot water and lemon juice instead. (See also pages 50–53.)

- **Consult a qualified herbalist** about taking a daily supplement of chaste-tree berry (*Vitex agnus-castus*), which may help to lower elevated FSH levels.

- **Take a B-complex supplement,** containing 50 mg of B6, and a zinc supplement to help regulate hormones generally.

- **Take 1,000 mg of essential fatty acids a day,** either evening primrose oil or fish oils.

- **Eat legumes, onions, and garlic** to help the liver to break down estrogen, and cabbage to increase the rate at which the liver converts estrogen into its water-soluble form so that it can be excreted from the body.

- **Eat foods containing phyto-estrogens**—such as legumes, flaxseed, alfalfa sprouts, oats, cabbage, and Brussels sprouts—which bind to estrogen receptors, causing a weak estrogen-like response (see also page 31). This will help to balance hormones.

RAISED PROLACTIN LEVELS

Prolactin levels are usually high during pregnancy and lactation (see also page 100). Abnormally high prolactin levels may upset hormonal balance and interfere with normal ovulation and the luteal phase following the release of an egg (see pages 10–11). This is the reason why nursing mothers rarely become pregnant. Once prolactin levels are normalized, ovulation resumes in most cases.

What is it? Prolactin is a hormone that is produced by the pituitary gland, principally to prepare the breasts for producing milk after childbirth. Levels are normally low in non-pregnant women. The release of prolactin is suppressed by dopamine, a neurotransmitter produced in the brain. Any reduction in the production of dopamine not only allows prolactin levels to rise but

also interferes with the production of gonadotrophin-releasing hormone (GnRH). This in turn affects the manufacture of follicle-stimulating hormone (FHS) and luteinizing hormone (LH). The result of this hormonal imbalance is menstrual dysfunction (irregular periods) and disrupted ovulation.

What causes it? High levels of prolactin, or hyperprolactinemia, can be caused by or associated with:
- certain drugs, including blood-pressure medication, antidepressants, and anesthetics
- prolonged periods of stress
- excessive amounts of exercise
- an underactive thyroid (see pages 106–07)
- polycystic ovary syndrome (PCOS)—see pages 119–21
- small, noncancerous tumors (prolactinomas) in the pituitary gland that either cause more prolactin to be secreted or prevent dopamine from reaching prolactin-producing cells

What are the symptoms? These include menstrual irregularities, such as absent periods, and ovulatory dysfunction, the inappropriate production of breast milk, and a loss of libido.

Who is at risk? Anyone suffering from high levels of stress, hypothyroidism, or anorexia, or taking certain drugs (see above) is at risk of raised prolactin levels.

DIET & NUTRITION

Dietary measures recommended for lowering raised prolactin levels include **increased amounts of zinc and vitamin B6**, both of which are necessary for the normal synthesis of dopamine. **Good food sources** of zinc include lean meats, fish and seafood, chicken, eggs, pumpkin and sunflower seeds, rye, oats, and whole grains, while for **B6, which aids the absorption of zinc**, they are green leafy vegetables, whole grains, molasses, nuts, brown rice, egg yolks, organ meats, fish, poultry, legumes, and seeds.

How is it diagnosed? A blood test will measure prolactin levels.

How is it treated conventionally? Levels can be brought down with the drugs bromocriptine (brand name Parlodel), a synthetic form of dopamine, or cabergoline (brand name Dostinex). If a tumor is responsible for raised levels, it can often be treated successfully with drugs and will only occasionally require surgery.

Can complementary therapies help? The herb chaste-tree berry (*Vitex agnus-castus*) has been shown to mimic the action of dopamine and may help to lower prolactin levels after use for about three months. Make sure you consult a qualified practitioner. Acupuncture may help to balance hormone levels.

ZITA'S TIPS

There are several self-help and lifestyle measures that may help lower raised prolactin levels.

- **Use relaxation** and stress-management techniques to reduce the impact of stress.
- **Avoid strenuous exercise** for prolonged periods.
- **Avoid alcohol**, especially beer

herbs for hormonal imbalance

Some herbs act as hormonal regulators, while others are good uterine tonics. You should never self-subscribe herbal remedies: always seek the supervision of a qualified herbalist, and stop taking any remedies once you become pregnant.

A number of herbal remedies might be recommended by a practitioner. These include:

- **chaste-tree berry** (*Vitex agnus-castus*), a hormonal regulator that stimulates the release of luteinizing hormone (LH) and prolactin, decreases the secretion of follicle-stimulating hormone (FSH), and promotes ovulation. This herb is the most extensively researched in connection with the treatment of hormonal problems in women. It is particularly useful for luteal phase defects (see page 128), anovulation (no ovulation), and polymenorrhea (very frequent periods). It should be taken every morning of your cycle, starting on day one. Do not use it if you might be pregnant or if you have polycystic ovaries.
- **Siberian ginseng** (*Eleutherococcus senticosus*), which can help to regulate hormones and promote general health and vitality. It supports the adrenal glands and helps to reduce stress levels.
- **dong quai** (*Angelica sinensis*), which can tone a weak uterus and regulate hormones and the menstrual cycle. This should be taken under supervision, since too much can cause heavy periods.

- **red clover** (*Trifolium pratense*), which contains estrogen-like compounds.
- **licorice** (*Glycyrrhiza spp.*), which can help women who have irregular periods and those who have elevated testosterone and low levels of estrogen. This herb has a high sodium content and intake must be supervised.
- **black cohosh** (*Cimicifuga racemosa*), which stimulates the release of LH and contains isoflavone constituents that have estrogen-like activity—that is, they bind to estrogen receptors. Do not confuse with blue cohosh.
- **Mexican wild yam** (*Dioscorea villosa*), which contains components of progesterone and encourages the release of this hormone after ovulation.
- **red raspberry leaf** (*Rubus idaeus*) is a uterine tonic and hormone regulator. Take this before conception but not during the first six months of pregnancy.

***Red clover blossom** contains estrogen-like compounds.*

- **motherwort** (*Leonurus spp.*), a uterine tonic that tones the female reproductive system.
- **squaw vine** (*Mitchella repens*), a uterine tonic that provides a calcium- and iron-rich remedy for hormonal imbalance and irregular periods.

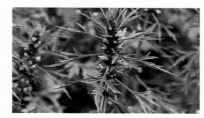

***Motherwort** tones the uterus and the female reproductive system.*

male fertility tests

In as many as half the couples who are unable to conceive, it is the man who has a fertility problem. It is important, therefore, that your partner is involved in the diagnostic process. Many conditions affecting male fertility (see pages 138–41) are symptomless, so skilled investigation is necessary in order to identify them.

CHECK SPERM FIRST

I always suggest to couples that a sperm check is one of the first tests to have: it's relatively quick and straightforward. Men are often reluctant to take action before a specific problem has been found and to take a test that may identify them as the one with the problem. Your partner will have to be prepared to give a detailed personal and medical history to your doctor or a consultant, including his previous sexual activity. Coping with a negative result and finding somebody to talk to about it, other than you, isn't easy, even though the problem is far more common than most people, especially men, imagine. You will need to be prepared to handle all these issues sensitively.

Just as for women, there are many different factors and combinations of factors that give rise to fertility problems in men. The sequence of tests for a man is as follows:

- **level one** physical examination and analysis of a semen sample
- **level two** hormone assessment
- **level three** further tests including physical examination, scanning, biopsy, and genetic tests

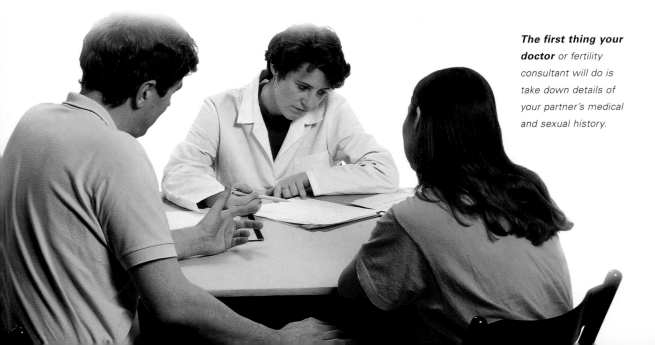

The first thing your doctor or fertility consultant will do is take down details of your partner's medical and sexual history.

LEVEL ONE: PHYSICAL EXAMINATION & SEMEN ANALYSIS

LOOKING FOR THE OBVIOUS

On your partner's first visit to the doctor, your doctor will check the testicles visually and manually for varicocele (see page 139), undescended testicles, or any other visible evidence of physiological problems (see pages 140–41).

ANALYZING SEMEN

Semen assessment is a simple and convenient way of measuring a man's potential fertility. There are many different reasons why he might have abnormal sperm; semen analysis may pinpoint the cause (see pages 138–41).

One common misconception about semen quality is that male fertility is linked to virility. If a man receives a poor semen assessment, he may feel crushed on two counts—the implications for his prospects of becoming a father, and the perceived reflection on his status as a man. Many men are reluctant to admit the problem to their peers, and make other excuses for having to give up alcohol, for example, in order to improve their sperm count.

PROVIDING A SAMPLE

At a fertility clinic, your partner will be asked to ejaculate into a sterile container. The sample is examined under a microscope. It sounds simple, but masturbating to order is not always easy, especially in that environment. It can be easily perceived as an embarrassing, uncomfortable, and humiliating experience, the ultimate invasion of privacy.

If your partner has difficulty producing a sample for whatever reason, or your religion forbids masturbation, it is possible to use nonspermicidal, nonlatex condoms at home. He will need to get the sample to the clinic within an hour for immediate assessment, however. Also, semen needs to be transported at body temperature, since cold kills sperm. Your clinic will advise you how to do this. Consider asking them to freeze and bank a supply of semen in case your partner is unable to produce a sample at a critical point in a procedure. If his difficulty is the result of impotency caused by a physiological or a psychological problem (if he was abused as a child, for example), specialist counseling may help.

Your partner should refrain from ejaculation for two to four days before providing a sample. In specific cases, he may be asked to give a urine sample immediately after ejaculation: this will be used to check for retrograde ejaculation (see page 141). Bear in mind that sperm can take up to 100 days to mature (see pages 14–15), so it is worth mentioning any illnesses he's had in the last three months that may have affected the condition of the sperm, any medication he has taken or is taking, excessive heat he has experienced (for example, in a sauna), and excess weight he is carrying. Clearly, it might be dangerous to stop taking certain prescribed drugs. The fact is that doctors do not know the cause of some sperm problems, but discuss all medication with the consultant.

The results of semen analysis are usually available quickly, so make an early followup appointment to discuss them with

LAB ANALYSIS

It is essential that the semen assessment is done properly. This can mean that lab tests are done at a fertility clinic or even an **andrology lab**. Specimens sent to regular labs may not get immediate attention, and the morphology assessment in particular may be inadequate, giving false or misleading results. It is also vitally important that the results are **properly interpreted**— not all doctors or even gynecologists have the necessary training or experience. Valuable time can be wasted if a couple is told their sperm is fine when a faulty test or misinterpretation has failed to reveal a problem. Going to a reputable fertility clinic is essential. (In some cases, health insurance covers this, but check your policy carefully to be sure). It is not hugely expensive and is definitely **money well spent**.

your doctor. Sperm quality is easily affected by variables such as health and stress, so your partner may have to give further samples over the next few months, even if the first test is normal or borderline. Do not be in too much of a hurry to retest. Allow time for lifestyle or dietary improvements to take effect.

UNDERSTANDING THE RESULTS

There are several different aspects of semen analysis, each with its parameters with regard to what is considered "normal" fertility.

Appearance Normal semen is opalescent and grayish. Yellow semen might indicate high intakes of vitamin supplements, which is not a problem; high levels of flavoproteins resulting from long abstinence, which is easily remedied; or, rarely, jaundice. A reddish color may mean there are red blood cells in the semen. This may indicate an infection, so further investigation will be necessary (see page 137).

Volume The average ejaculate is less than half a teaspoon (about 2 ml). Many men are surprised and apologetic about this. A high volume means a diluted concentration of sperm. Less than 1 ml may indicate a pathological problem, such as a current or past infection (for example, a sexually transmitted infection, or STI) which has blocked the ejaculatory ducts producing seminal fluid. Low volume may mean retrograde ejaculation or problems with accessory glands, seminal vesicles, or the prostate. Low volume as well as no sperm might indicate a condition such as congenital bilateral absence of the vas deferens (CBAVD—see page 141). Your partner might then be referred to a urologist for treatment or for another referral for an assisted reproductive technique (ART—see page 144).

Viscosity and liquefaction

Normal ejaculate is initially very viscous but becomes runny after about 10 minutes due to the action of enzymes. If this does not occur within about an hour, sperm find it difficult to swim up the cervix. This is not a serious problem: sperm can be washed and re-suspended in a special solution before being injected into the uterus.

Acidity Semen is normally quite alkaline (with a pH rarely below 7; the norm is between 7.2 and 8.0). Ejaculate that is acidic and without sperm is probably the result of CBAVD (see above).

Agglutination This means that motile sperm stick to one other. It usually indicates the presence of anti-sperm antibodies (see page 140 and below)—proteins that coat sperm and bind to cervical mucus, preventing sperm from moving toward an egg or fertilizing it. This is a common cause of failed IVF. Some antibodies are cytotoxic, which means they destroy sperm. A MAR (mixed agglutination reaction) test (see below) will be necessary if sperm are sticking.

Antibodies Antibodies are not usually present in semen. They are caused by injury or surgery, such as vasectomy reversal or hernia repair, when a breakdown in the blood–testes barrier allows blood and testicular tissue to come into contact. Anti-sperm antibodies may be present in semen even if there is no agglutination (see above). It is only when they are present on sperm at relatively high levels that fertility may be affected. As well as preventing sperm from moving, antibodies may coat the sperm heads, making it difficult for them to recognize an egg and fertilize it.

Antibody tests are expensive and tend not to be done routinely until other factors have been eliminated. In vitro fertilization (see pages 154–81) with intra-cytoplasmic sperm injection (ICSI, see page 174) or intra-uterine insemination (IUI, see pages 152–53) may be suggested, depending on test results. Steroid treatment is another option.

MAR (mixed agglutination reaction) This test (also known as an immunobead test) is very important for antibodies but is often overlooked in standard semen analysis, and you may need to pay for it to be done at a fertility clinic. If it shows less than 50 percent binding, antibody levels should not affect your partner's fertility.

Round cell concentration

Round cells are either immature sperm cells or white blood cells. A concentration of more than 1 million per 1 ml white blood cells or 5 million round cells may indicate an infection. Prognosis depends on severity: a course of antibiotics may clear up the problem, but a serious infection can result in permanent damage.

Sperm concentration This is the number of sperm in semen. A count of at least 20 million per ml is considered to be normally fertile (the average is 60–80 million/ml). A lower count is termed oligozoospermia. No sperm in the semen is known as azoospermia. Frequent ejaculation reduces the concentration. Well-documented evidence shows that sperm count is hugely affected by lifestyle factors—intakes of caffeine, tobacco, alcohol, and recreational drugs, diet, exercise, and stress levels. Lifestyle changes can make a big difference and may be all a man needs to do to increase the count. Numbers of sperm may also be affected by a previous STI. A concentration of less than 5 million per ml

SEMEN ASSESSMENT

Patient: John Smith	DOB: February 3
Address: 2 Long Lane	Reference No: JS209W
Newtown	Referring Practitioner: Zita West
Tel: 555-6789	Date: April 6

Duration of abstinence (days): 3
Interval between ejaculation and start of analysis (min): 20

	Sample	Normal Range
Appearance	Normal	
Volume (ml)	3.2 ml	2 ml or more
Viscosity	Normal	
Liquefaction	Complete	Complete within 60 min
pH	8.0	7.2 or more
Agglutination	Some	None
Round cell concentration (10^6/ml)	0.3	5×10^6/ml or less ($<1 \times 10^6$/ml leukocytes)
Sperm concentration (10^6/ml)	47	20×10^6/ml or more
Total no. of sperm (10^6)	150	40×10^6 per ejaculate or more
Motility (% a + b + c)	62	50% or more (a + b) or 25% or more (a)
(a) rapid progression	42	
(b) slow progression	16	
(c) nonprogressive motility	4	
(d) immotile	38	
Morphology (% abnormal forms)	92	multicenter studies now in progress
– normal	8	current values 15% or more
– head defects	89	
– neck or midpiece defects	43	
– tail defects	12	
– cytoplasmic droplets	2	
Teratozoospermia index (TZI) (total no. defects/no. sperm with defects)	1.59	1.6 or less

Comments *High proportion of abnormal forms (teratozoospermia) – multiple defects; most sperm have round or amorphous heads. All other parameters within normal reference range.*

Semen analysis *The results your partner gets back may look something like this, although forms vary from clinic to clinic. Your consultant will explain the findings very carefully, but ask questions if you do not fully understand the implications.*

CASE HISTORY

Stephen, 35, had been trying to conceive a baby with his wife, Wendy, for more than a year. He wasn't expecting anything untoward from his sperm analysis and was devastated when the count was zero. Stephen became depressed as further testing revealed hormonal imbalance and testicular failure. His doctor was rather abrupt when outlining the couple's options—donor sperm or adoption. After counseling, Stephen and Wendy opted for donor insemination and now feel much more positive, having made the decision.

indicates that your partner may have a genetic chromosomal defect, which might result, for example, in a miscarriage. If your partner has a Y-chromosome deletion, it affects the way sperm are made and cannot be corrected. An assisted reproductive technology (ART) with pre-implantation genetic diagnosis may be recommended. Donor

insemination is also a possibility. If the count is very low or zero, your partner will be referred to a urologist for blood tests (see Level 2, right) or a testicular biopsy.

Motility Sperm need to be good swimmers and move rapidly in straight lines. Motility describes the proportion of moving sperm and is affected both by lifestyle and frequency of ejaculation. After a long period of abstinence, semen will contain many dead and immotile sperm, so a man needs to have intercourse within three days of a sperm test—but not on the same morning or else the concentration will be lowered. Poor sperm motility is known as asthenozoospermia.

Progression describes the way in which the sperm are moving and is graded as follows:
- rapid progression in straight lines
- slow progression with erratic movement
- nonprogressive motility—the sperm are twitching but not moving forward
- immotile

Normal, fertile sperm usually includes at least 50 percent first and second progression categories, or 25 percent first category. If a man's sperm are mainly third and fourth categories, he may have a serious fertility problem.

Many men mistakenly believe that the occasional alcoholic binge does not affect the quality of their sperm. In fact, just one evening of heavy drinking will

seriously damage sperm, and it could take three months for the sperm count to be restored.

Morphology This refers to the shape of sperm. Abnormalities include large or small heads, irregularly shaped heads, two heads, or coiled tails. Poor morphology is known as teratozoospermia. According to the World Health Organization, 15 percent or more normal sperm constitutes normal fertility. Levels below 15 percent may indicate subfertility, and less than 5 percent, a severe problem. Morphology is affected by lifestyle and occasionally genetic defects. Age is also significant: sperm quality deteriorates beyond 40, and the number of abnormal sperm increases over time. Men can, however, produce healthy sperm all their lives.

ASSESSING MALE FERTILITY

Fertility (or subfertility) is a matter of degree. Suboptimal parameters do not mean a man is infertile, but he might find it difficult to conceive naturally. It is almost impossible to predict whether or not a man can become a biological father: absolute sterility (the absence of sperm in either ejaculate or testes) is rare.

The next step will depend upon the results of semen analysis. If sperm count is low and does not improve after a few months of lifestyle changes, further testing will be recommended.

LEVEL TWO: HORMONE ASSESSMENT

This is not often necessary. A simple blood test will indicate levels of the key sex hormones—FSH (follicle-stimulating hormone), LH (luteinizing hormone), prolactin, and testosterone. LH stimulates the production of testosterone—necessary for the development of healthy sperm—in the testicles. Prolactin can interfere with LH-induced testosterone production. FSH is essential for sperm development. Results falling on either side of the expected range indicate hormonal imbalance, which has a number of causes (see page 140). Treatment is by hormone-replacement drugs.

UNDERSTANDING THE RESULTS

The interpretation of hormone results is complex: the following examples are simplified. If your partner has high levels of FSH and LH and low testosterone levels, he may have testicular failure (see pages 140–41). A biopsy can determine whether or not it is possible to retrieve sperm for ICSI (intra-cytoplasmic sperm injection; see page 174), a procedure in which sperm are injected into an egg. Another option would be the use of donor sperm (see page 182). Low levels of testosterone and FSH may indicate hypothalamic dysfunction (see page 140).

The hormonal control of sperm production may also be affected by underlying medical conditions, such as liver disease. If your partner's hormone levels appear normal, his consultant may recommend other, specifically targeted tests.

LEVEL THREE: FURTHER TESTS

Further investigation may be recommended to determine whether or not there is damage to the testes, any other physiological damage, or genetic defects.

Cell culture This can identify infection. Testicular inflammation may lead to reduced testosterone and therefore no sperm production. On the other hand, severe infection may cause a permanent obstruction, leading to azoospermia.

Ultrasound scanning This is used to examine the scrotum, testes, epididymis, prostate, and seminal vesicles. It can detect infection and inflammation, the absence of the vas deferens (CBAVD), obstruction, and tumors. Varicocele diagnosis uses Doppler ultrasonography. Surgery to unblock an obstruction may be helpful in some cases, but the benefits of surgery for solving fertility problems are still open to debate. Alternatively, sperm may be removed surgically from behind the obstruction and used in an assisted reproductive technique such as ICSI (see above).

Testicular biopsy This is used to determine whether or not there is any sperm development in the testicular tissue. This test is useful if all other tests are normal and yet there is an unexplained absence of sperm in the semen.

Chromosome testing Genetic evaluation may be offered to men who have sperm counts of fewer than 5 million per ml. About four percent of men with such a low count, and up to 15 percent of those with no sperm, have a chromosomal abnormality. Chromosome testing will also be offered to men with CBAVD because of its association with cystic fibrosis, which could be inherited by any offspring.

If your partner has severe oligozoospermia (see page 135), nonobstructive azoospermia (see page 141), or an absence of sperm due to a blockage, the cause may be a chromosomal abnormality. Other genetic causes for male infertility include Young's syndrome, Kartagener's syndrome, or Klinefelter's syndrome (see page 141). Potential genetic problems are investigated by means of blood tests. Depending on the results, you may be offered an assisted reproductive technique (see page 144) and genetic counseling.

male fertility problems

Fertility has traditionally been considered the woman's "responsibility." In fact, female factors alone account for 35–40 percent of fertility problems, male factors are the cause in 30–35 percent of cases, and in the rest there is a combined problem. Sperm-quality problems can often be improved.

SPERM AND FERTILITY

In order to impregnate a woman naturally and successfully, a man must first produce sperm that are capable of finding their way to the egg and the are able to fertilize it. For this to be possible, sperm need to be produced in sufficient quantities, be of good enough quality, and be fit enough to complete what amounts to a herculean task. If a man's production of healthy sperm is compromised in any way, it may affect a couple's fertility. In most cases, the reason for poor sperm quality is not known (idiopathic).

DECLINING SPERM COUNTS

Average sperm counts are in decline. They have decreased rapidly in the last 50 years (from 113 million per ml to around 70 million per ml). The percentage of sperm with abnormalities has increased 12-fold and sperm motility has decreased. As a practitioner, I've noticed increasingly over the last few years that greater numbers of men are coming to me with fertility problems. There are many theories about the cause of the decline: It is probably the result of a combination of factors.

THE CAUSES OF MALE INFERTILITY

Generally, male infertility can be grouped into four major categories: abnormal sperm; defective hormone production; damage to the testes and other physiological problems—such as ejaculation problems; and genetic problems.

In at least 30 percent of male infertility cases, the cause is never determined; in 3–5 percent of cases, the cause is hormonal in origin; in at least 30 percent, problems are thought to be due to the effects of varicocele; 10–20 percent result from infections; 6–7 percent of cases are due to sperm obstruction; and 6–7 percent of problems are ultimately found to be of genetic origin.

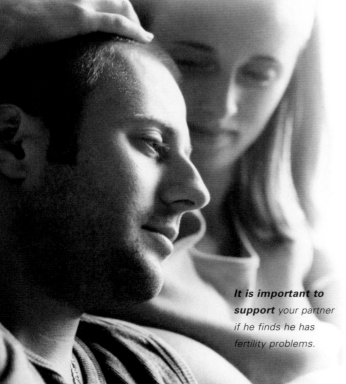

It is important to support your partner if he finds he has fertility problems.

ABNORMAL SPERM

In some men with apparent fertility problems, their hormonal balance and testes appear fine, but the sperm they produce are abnormal. Sperm can be damaged in a number of ways. Some men have great-looking sperm—a high count, excellent motility, and a good shape—yet the sperm are not able to fertilize an egg. There are so many events occurring at the molecular level that are required for normal fertilization to take place, that if there is a problem with any one of them, fertilization will be compromised. At this level, it is almost impossible to diagnose the cause, and in most cases the reason for infertility remains unexplained.

Immotile sperm Kartagener's syndrome, also known as immotile cilia syndrome, is a condition in which normal quantities of sperm are produced but their tails do not enable them to move. Even though they cannot move, as long as the sperm are alive and healthy in all other respects, they can be removed from a man and injected into a woman's eggs in order to fertilize them.

Environmental toxins We hear a lot about the impact of toxins on sperm (see pages 75–76). Some of them, including cigarette smoke, contain what are known as reactive oxygen species. These molecules are also produced by white blood cells in response to infection and by damaged sperm themselves. The oxidizing effects of reactive oxygen species are thought to be responsible for greater numbers of abnormal sperm. Taking an antioxidant supplement (see pages 59–63) may help to reduce the amounts of these molecules in semen.

Varicocele Varicocele is a condition that is similar to varicose veins in the testicular area. Some men with varicocele experience no fertility problems, while other men do. Varicocele is found to be quite common among infertile men. The condition results in poor blood flow and is generally believed to be responsible for sperm damage.

YOUR PARTNER'S FEELINGS

*Receiving a poor diagnosis, and particularly the discovery that he has a low or nonexistent sperm count, can have a devastating effect on a man. He may feel inadequate and have low self-esteem. **If he receives a poor semen assessment, as well as thinking his virility has been undermined, he may blame himself for letting you down.** These feelings will be accentuated if the quality of his sperm cannot be improved and as a couple you need fertility treatment to conceive. He will have to stand by while you undergo drug therapy and invasive procedures, while the worst he will have to endure, except in a few unusual cases, is to ejaculate repeatedly into a cup. **He may be withdrawn or lose interest in sex: he may even suffer from erectile dysfunction.***

*It is important that you keep talking to each other, although he may find it difficult under the circumstances. **Don't misinterpret his reactions as lack of concern.** Remember that more than 40 percent of all fertility problems occur in males: two percent of men produce no sperm at all. There has been a marked decline in sperm quality, and male infertility is a growing problem.*

Antibodies In some cases, the inability of sperm to fertilize an egg may be due to antibodies in the semen. Antisperm antibodies only affect fertility, however, if they actually coat the sperm and occur in relatively high concentrations. This is known as immunological infertility. Surgery, such as for hernia repair, or vasectomy reversal, usually results in the presence of antisperm antibodies.

DEFECTIVE HORMONE PRODUCTION

Men often associate hormones with women's reproductive cycles, little realizing that hormones have a huge impact on their own fertility (see pages 14–15). Specific hormonal imbalance can affect a man's fertility. Follicle-stimulating hormone (FSH) and luteinizing hormone (LH), the gonadotrophin hormones, are released from the pituitary gland to stimulate testosterone production. A lack of these hormones means a lack of testosterone and impaired sperm production. This is known as hypogonadrotropic hypogonadism. It may be the result of a genetic defect, such as Kallmann's syndrome, or damage to the pituitary gland or hypothalamus as a result of another medical condition, such as a brain tumor. It may even be caused by malnutrition or fasting.

General hormonal imbalance may be caused by certain medical conditions, such as chronic liver disease or chronic kidney failure. These illnesses are unrelated to fertility, but they can affect the whole body, including the reproductive system, upsetting the balance of reproductive hormones and even causing testicular damage and a loss of libido. Although thyroid disease is a rare cause of male infertility, men with an overactive or underactive thyroid are susceptible to fertility problems. The hormonal control of sperm production may be affected by diabetes. There has long been a belief that men with diabetes were less fertile. Research shows that, in fact, their sperm swim in straighter lines than those of nondiabetics, therefore reaching the egg more quickly. Men with diabetes do tend to have other fertility problems, however.

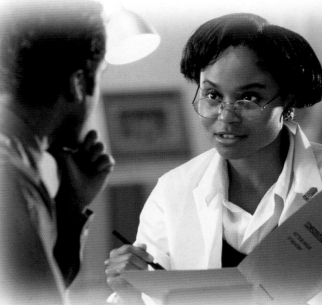

Be sure to ask your doctor or fertility consultant all the questions you have about your condition.

Age also has an impact on hormonal balance in men. This is a major factor affecting fertility and is not just confined to women (see pages 16–17). Men experience what has been termed andropause, which is similar to menopause in women, when hormone levels change and sperm quality may be adversely affected as a result.

Being overweight or doing an excessive amount of physical exercise may also affect hormone levels, as can the amount of stress in your lives and other aspects of your lifestyle (see pages 33–43).

DAMAGE TO THE TESTES

If the testes themselves are damaged, the release of the hormones they produce is also affected. As a result, gonadotrophin hormone levels increase to try to compensate. Men with testicular failure produce either no sperm or very few. In some cases, the damage may be so great that there is a complete absence of germ cells from which sperm are derived (Sertoli cell–only syndrome). Testicular failure may be due to any of a number of reasons.

Genetic defects Klinefelter's syndrome is a genetic condition that results in a man having an extra X-chromosome. This is a leading cause of testicular failure, which can also occur in men who have an extra Y-chromosome. Some genetically normal men (that is, they have XY-chromosomes) produce testosterone, but none of the cells in the body recognize it, so the men develop as females. This is known as testicular feminization. In about six percent of men who have permanently low sperm counts (fewer than 5 million per ml), small amounts of the Y-chromosome responsible for the normal functioning of the testes are missing.

Alterations in chromosomes other than the sex chromosomes may also adversely affect male fertility (autosome disorders). These conditions are known as balanced translocations and inversions. In addition, testicular failure may be associated with other problems as a result of a genetic disorder, such as celiac disease and sickle-cell disease.

Birth defects Cryptorchidism, or undescended testes, is a birth defect that frequently leads to testicular failure. Men who have one normal test is are more likely to be fertile.

Inflammation of the testes Known as orchitis, testicular inflammation does not always affect fertility, but at worst it may lead to a reduction in the release of testosterone and an end to sperm production. Sexually transmitted infections (STDs) such as herpes, syphilis, chlamydia, and gonorrhea are leading causes of inflammation, as is mumps if it occurs after puberty. Orchitis also occurs with tuberculosis, typhoid, and some tropical diseases. In addition, any condition such as influenza, which causes a fever with a temperature of more than 101.3°F (38.5°C), may damage sperm production for up to six months.

Physical traumas Accidents such as a kick in the groin are only likely to damage the testes if the trauma is severe. Twisting of the testis (torsion)

can block the blood supply to the testis. If this condition is not treated quickly—within six hours—it can result in permanent damage.

EJACULATION PROBLEMS

Retrograde ejaculation This occurs when the muscles that pump the semen through the penis do not work properly. Instead, semen is pushed back into the bladder. This condition may be caused by ailments that damage nerves, such as diabetes or paraplegia, and sometimes surgery to remove the prostate. It is possible to recover sperm from your partner's urine, and prepare it for intra-uterine insemination (IUI, see pages 152–53).

Erectile dysfunction This may be caused by conditions such as diabetes, paraplegia, or other diseases of the nervous system, as well as previous surgery that has affected parts of the male reproductive system. In most cases, however, the roots of the problem are of a psychological nature. The condition can usually be treated by counseling.

Obstruction Blockages in the male reproductive system may also give rise to infertility, as they do in females. In some cases, surgery such as a hernia repair may result in an obstruction, but by far the most common cause of inflammation and subsequent blockage are sexually transmitted infections (see pages 108–11).

If there are no sperm present in the semen, either your partner is not producing any sperm (nonobstructive azoospermia) or he has a blockage in the reproductive system preventing the sperm from being ejaculated (obstructive azoospermia).

Absence of the vas deferens Some men have no vas deferens, the tubes linking the testes to the penis. This condition is known as congenital bilateral absence of the vas deferens, or CBAVD. It has been associated with cystic fibrosis, so men with CBAVD should be tested for cystic fibrosis to prevent the possibility of their passing it on.

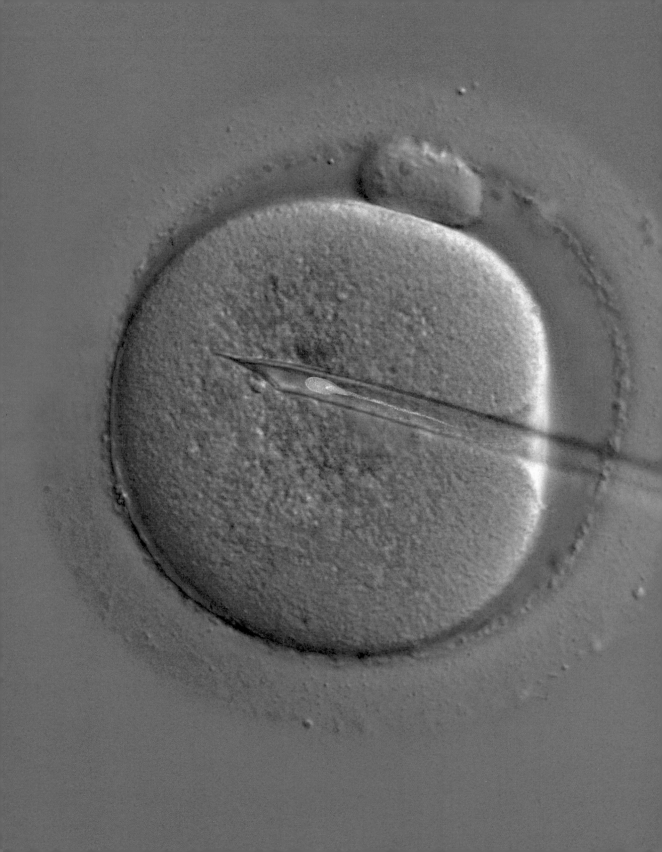

ASSISTED CONCEPTION

BY NOW, YOU WILL KNOW WHETHER OR NOT YOU

HAVE A FERTILITY PROBLEM. YOU WILL PROBABLY

HAVE IDENTIFIED THE CAUSE AND BE CONSIDERING

THE USE OF **ASSISTED REPRODUCTIVE TECHNOLOGY**

TO HELP YOU CONCEIVE. THIS CHAPTER DESCRIBES

THE **OPTIONS** THAT YOUR FERTILITY CONSULTANT

MIGHT OFFER YOU—IN PARTICULAR, IN VITRO

FERTILIZATION. FERTILITY TREATMENT DOES NOT

HAVE TO BE A DAUNTING PROSPECT IF YOU PREPARE

YOURSELVES PROPERLY, AND YOU CAN **IMPROVE**

YOUR CHANCES OF SUCCESSFUL TREATMENT

THROUGH AN APPROPRIATE DIET AND LIFESTYLE AND

THE USE OF CERTAIN COMPLEMENTARY THERAPIES.

your treatment options

Now that you and your partner have had a variety of fertility tests, you will have a clearer idea of how best to proceed to the treatment stage of Plan B. There is likely to be a range of options for you both to consider in consultation with your clinic.

WEIGHING EVERYTHING UP

Armed with test results, you will be able to discuss with your doctor or fertility consultant how to adapt the most appropriate treatment for you to suit your particular needs and circumstances, bearing in mind, for example, your age, specific blood-test results, and your feelings about and reactions to what you have learned so far about your fertility. Do not agree to proceed with anything that you are not completely happy about, and keep doing your own research. The Human Fertilization and Embryology Authority (HFEA) is a good source of information. You might also like to visit websites for information or support (see page 187).

Many couples who discover that they have fertility problems have to consider assisted reproductive techniques (ARTs). These make use of high-technology procedures to bring together sperm and egg. In vitro fertilization (IVF), for example, involves the removal of eggs from the ovary. They are fertilized in a laboratory dish before being placed in the woman's womb.

ACCEPTING INTERVENTION

The thought of intervention in conception may be a daunting prospect. If it is possible, start with less interventionist procedures and build up. No procedure will seem as frightening once you are underway. Where you start, however, will depend upon the results of fertility testing. It might be ovulation induction (OI), intrauterine insemination (IUI), in vitro fertilization (IVF), or a combination of treatments.

Various treatment protocols are discussed in the pages that follow, in a format that makes it easier for you to understand what will be happening on various days of your cycle, when to take drugs, and when you will need an ultrasound scan or a blood test, for example. Procedures may be helped along their way by using complementary remedies and changing aspects of your lifestyle.

ZITA'S TIPS

● **Do your research methodically and logically:** after you have received a diagnosis, work out a plan of action, find out exactly what is involved, decide which clinic you would like to attend, and calculate how much any treatment is likely to cost.

● **Beware of information overload:** it may seem that everyone is telling you what you should do; which treatment you should have; the best clinic to visit; the latest research you should know about. Others may have sound advice to give you, especially if they have also been through fertility treatment, but remember that your situation is unique, and you and your partner need to take time to find the solutions that are right for you.

● **Stay focused on one thing at a time:** there may be several treatment options to consider. Don't panic and careen off in different directions at once.

complementary therapies

The wealth of complementary therapies available offers varying degrees of help and hope to couples with fertility problems. Although you do need to be realistic about how much these treatments might be able to help, there are many good reasons for giving them a try. Do be wary of some overenthusiastic therapists, however, making unproven claims and offering false hope.

CHOOSING A THERAPY

Choosing to go down the complementary route does not mean forgoing conventional medicine. We are talking *complementary*, not *alternative*, therapies. Most will help to increase your general state of health by improving the functioning of all your body systems.

There is little hard evidence to support most complementary therapies, and few doctors are willing or able to give extensive advice. Unproven doesn't necessarily mean ineffective, however, and there is plenty of anecdotal evidence. Remember that every individual's case is unique, and there is no guarantee that what has worked for one person will also have a positive outcome for you.

Find out as much information as you can about all the individual therapies you are considering—from support groups, books, magazines, the library, the Internet—before making your choice. Find out how long the treatment has been in use and how widespread it is. Some therapies, such as herbal medicine and acupuncture, have been around for thousands of years. Trust your instincts if you feel particularly drawn to one type of therapy.

Always get a full medical diagnosis first, and don't abandon mainstream medicine. Keep your doctor fully informed about which complementary therapies you are having, and tell your therapist about any conventional drugs you have been prescribed by your doctor or a fertility consultant. Ideally, you should all be able to work together: collaboration is the key.

COMPLEMENTARY BENEFITS

Most complementary treatments and remedies, while not solving your fertility problems, will contribute to an integrated healthcare plan that will make assisted reproductive techniques more likely to succeed. Complementary therapies provide a range of benefits:

- **a sense of control** and direct involvement in your treatment program
- **control over who you see** and when you see them
- **sympathetic treatment** that engenders a real sense of being listened to
- **plenty of time to ask questions** and discuss your fertility problems in greater depth
- **holistic treatment** that addresses the mental and emotional as well as the physical aspects of your case
- **a greatly reduced risk of unpleasant** or dangerous side effects
- **physical and emotional support** to help you tolerate the protocols of IVF
- **encouragement to take responsibility** for your own healthcare and treatment program
- **help with mental and physical relaxation** so that you can cope with stress
- **an opportunity for your partner** to become more involved, depending on the therapy
- **nutritional advice** and recommendations about lifestyle changes to encourage successful treatment
- **improved health generally**, accompanied by an enhanced sense of well-being.

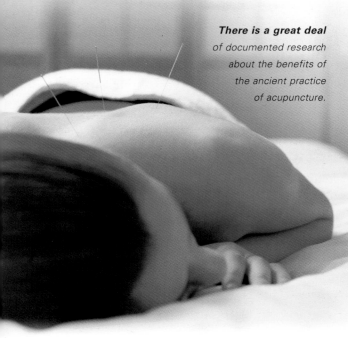

There is a great deal of documented research about the benefits of the ancient practice of acupuncture.

CHOOSING A PRACTITIONER

As with fertility clinics and specialists, nothing beats the combination of thorough research and personal recommendation. Try to get several word-of-mouth recommendations. Support groups are useful for this, or ask another practitioner whose opinion you value.

Talk to a therapist before committing yourself to a particular course of treatment—it is important to feel confident and comfortable and to establish a good rapport. A good practitioner should be empathetic and receptive to questions, so don't feel shy or embarrassed about asking them.

Find out how much experience they have in the field of fertility, what training they have had, how long they have been practicing, what their fees are, and if they are affiliated with the appropriate professional body. Be wary of anyone who makes wild promises or asks for money up front. Trust your instincts. If at any point you feel uneasy or unhappy, say so. If your issues are not addressed satisfactorily, go to another practitioner.

It is important that you do not feel as if you are being controlled by a practitioner and that you like him or her. You must be realistic about your expectations and not develop false hope. This is especially important if your FSH (follicle-stimulating hormone) levels are high or if you are older. You cannot afford to wait very long in hope before going down an interventionist route.

ACUPUNCTURE

My own speciality is acupuncture (see pages 72–73) so I'm naturally somewhat biased in its favor. I work closely with doctors and specialists at various clinics and have had a great deal of success in helping women to conceive naturally or supporting them through fertility treatment. There is a great deal of documented evidence on acupuncture and electro-acupuncture. A Swedish study in 1996, for example, established that electro-acupuncture improved uterine blood flow in infertile women. Many studies have shown that it can help to:

- improve male fertility by improving sperm quality—count, concentration, and motility
- lower raised FSH levels sufficiently for an IVF cycle to commence
- relieve symptoms of endometriosis (see page 114)
- induce ovulation in women with polycystic ovary syndrome (PCOS, see page 119)
- balance hormone levels
- regulate the menstrual cycle, especially shortening a long cycle
- improve general health

If you have rejected acupuncture because you are needle-phobic, I can tell you that the needles used are very fine—little thicker than a hair—and that the discomfort is minimal.

CHIROPRACTIC

Chiropractic has been found to improve fertility, possibly by releasing pressure on the spinal nerves connecting with the uterus. It can also address neck and pelvic problems and hormonal dysfunction caused by a restriction of the sphenoid bone or its membrane attachments, which may affect the functioning of the pituitary gland.

The approach is holistic and takes into account posture, lifestyle, diet, work conditions, and even the height and hardness of your bed. It is important to find out not only what has gone wrong but why, so that bad habits can be corrected and the problem is less likely to recur. A treatment usually lasts about 45 minutes and is totally safe and noninvasive.

CRANIAL OSTEOPATHY

Cranial treatment may help the pituitary gland to function properly if there is a hormonal imbalance. A treatment usually lasts for about 40 minutes and you may find you feel slightly light-headed for a short while afterward.

FLOWER REMEDIES

Flower remedies deal with a particular emotional state or aspect of personality, and are described by their indications (for example, for shock, anxiety, or resentment). They are also recommended for depression, irrational thoughts, and fear, and to help you adjust to change. There is, however, no research supporting the claims of these remedies.

Up to six or seven remedies may be taken together, depending on need. You cannot overdose and they can be taken quite safely with other medication. They are preserved in brandy, so it is recommended that they are diluted in water. Put two drops from each selected remedy in a 1-oz (30-ml) bottle and top off with mineral water. Take four diluted drops at least four times daily.

There are flower remedies from all over the world. She oak, an Australian bush flower essence, is one that is specifically indicated for fertility problems, particularly any emotional blocks, conscious or subconscious, that may be preventing you from conceiving a baby.

HERBAL MEDICINE

Herbs have been used medicinally for thousands of years. The whole plant, including the roots, is used, not just the active constituent, so herbs tend to have a much gentler impact on the body than conventional drugs, and they have few unpleasant side effects. Always choose sources of organically grown herbs if you can.

There are a number of herbs that can help with fertility problems, hormone imbalance (see page 131), and specifically female dysfunctions, but I do not recommend that you self-prescribe. Consult a qualified herbalist, preferably with experience in treating women who have fertility problems.

HOMEOPATHY

There are homeopathic remedies to treat both male and female fertility problems. In some cases, homeopathic preparations may help to eliminate hormonal imbalance and disorders, correct menstrual irregularities, and improve a variety of reproductive functional disorders. Homeopathic remedies are available over the counter at many drugstores and health-food stores, but I would strongly recommend that you have a consultation with a qualified and experienced practitioner to determine the appropriate constitutional remedy for your particular needs.

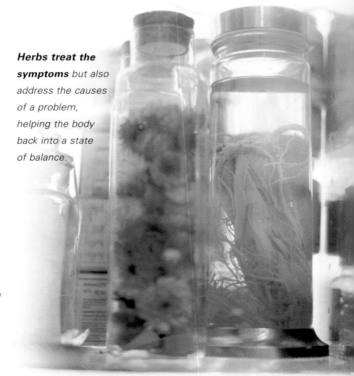

Herbs treat the symptoms but also address the causes of a problem, helping the body back into a state of balance.

A first appointment can last between one and two hours. Details of your temperament, medical history, habits, likes and dislikes, hopes, and fears are noted, allowing the practitioner to build up a complete picture of you and identify the right remedy. Lifestyle changes may be recommended. Symptoms may get slightly worse initially, or old ones briefly resurface, before your condition improves. Once there is a marked improvement, you should stop taking the remedy. The number of consultations needed varies from person to person. It is quite safe to take homeopathic remedies while being treated with conventional drugs.

HYPNOTHERAPY

Hypnotherapy has gradually gained the respect of the medical establishment. It has had a degree of success in treating some cases of unexplained fertility. It can remove subconscious mental blocks that may be preventing you from conceiving, and

The choice of homeopathic remedy will be based on your constitutional make-up and your specific fertility problem.

also help you to relax about the issue of fertility. Stress levels can be reduced by hypnotherapy, and some patients have reported that, as a result, high prolactin levels have also been lowered. Women who have suffered termination, miscarriage, abuse, or violence can be helped to let go of the grief and guilt associated with a trauma in their past.

Under hypnosis, the conscious part of the brain is temporarily bypassed, allowing the subconscious part, which influences mental and physical functions, to take control. In this state of profound relaxation you are extremely receptive to suggestion, and you can be desensitized as far as phobias and deep-rooted fears are concerned.

Ninety percent of the population is thought to be capable of entering hypnosis. The state is pleasant and comfortable and, despite myths to the contrary, can only work with your consent, so you always remain in control. If you find it difficult to relax into a meditative state, a hypnotherapist can teach you how to quiet the mind and relax t he body for visualization and affirmations, as well as work with you to improve your positive outlook. There are no side effects.

OSTEOPATHY

Osteopathy can help to correct some of the structural problems that lead to infertility by restoring and maintaining balance in the neuro-musculoskeletal systems of the body. There are three main areas of structural and postural strain: the mid-cervical, dorso-lumbar junction, and sacro-iliac joint. Misuse or trauma can upset the fine balance between muscles, joints, ligaments, and nerves, resulting in ovarian and uterine irritation and dysfunction. Osteopathy tries to restore and maintain this balance. There has already been much research in this field, and more investigative projects are underway in the UK using osteopaths within the national health service.

Osteopaths assess the whole person and do not just study a condition or its specific symptoms. At your first appointment the practitioner will take a full case history. You'll be asked to undress to your underwear, and the osteopath will make detailed observations of your posture, weight distribution, mobility, and so on before making a diagnosis and suggesting a treatment plan. Treatment is usually weekly until symptoms improve. There are few side effects, though you may feel tired after a treatment and the symptoms might get worse for 24 hours or so before they get better.

REFLEXOLOGY

Reflexology is a technique of foot massage. It is used to a lesser extent on the hands. The nerve endings are stimulated by massage to effect changes in other parts of the body: the feet are believed to represent a map of the whole body. Although reflexology is not a diagnostic tool, it may detect signs of disorder or disease. It aims not to treat illness specifically, but to stimulate the body's own ability to rebalance and heal itself. There is little research data on reflexology and fertility, but it is a particularly successful treatment for stress relief and relaxation and works well as a "complement" to orthodox treatment.

Treatment can take up to an hour or more, and six weekly sessions are usually recommended. The therapist moves his or her thumbs across your feet, covering every minute point, including those corresponding to the ovaries, uterus, hypothalamus, and pituitary gland. The aim is to activate the body's self-healing capacity by stimulating the reflex points, or to calm and relax zones where there are indications of acute disturbance.

LYMPHATIC DRAINAGE

This procedure helps to rid the body of toxins by encouraging the action of the lymphatic system. Light pressure is applied to the skin in gentle rhythmic movements that manually assist the flow of lymph. The lymph system is a vitally important part of the immune system: it is, in effect, the body's waste disposal system, clearing away toxins, bacteria, and cell debris. If it is not functioning

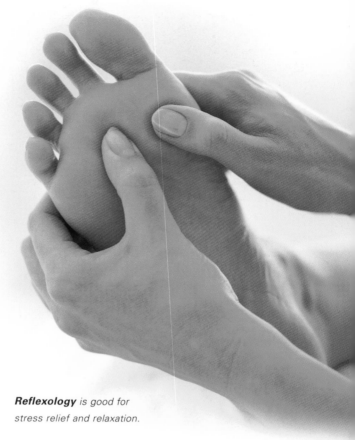

Reflexology is good for stress relief and relaxation.

properly, blockages in the waste-disposal system may occur. There are many lymph nodes located in the groin area, and clearing these will improve blood supply to the whole pelvic area. A lymphatic drainage session usually lasts for about an hour.

I sometimes suggest lymphatic drainage to some of my clients as part of a fertility treatment program. It is particularly useful prior to an IVF (in vitro fertilization) cycle or in between other specific courses of fertility treatment.

Any complementary treatment that involves deep-breathing techniques or is meditative has a calming effect on the body and helps you to relax and relieve stress. It may also help to build up reserves of energy by focusing your mind and clearing out a lot of the "clutter" in your head.

ovulation induction

Ovulation induction (OI), or ovarian stimulation, is a way of regulating your menstrual cycle by kick-starting ovulation in order to increase your chances of conceiving naturally.

Q&A

○ What is the success rate for clomiphene?

Eighty percent of viable pregnancies that come about following the use of clomiphene occur during the first three months of stimulation. Very few pregnancies occur among women who have taken clomiphene for six months or more without a break.

○ How is it taken?

Clomiphene is taken orally (in tablet form), usually for five or more days each month, starting with a dose of 50 mg, on days 3–7, 4–8, or as late as 5–9 of your cycle. It induces ovulation on day 13 or 14 if you have a regular 28-day cycle. The dosage may be increased to 100 mg the following month if you have not ovulated, but doses higher than 150 mg are not often recommended. Protocols vary from clinic to clinic.

○ Is it an expensive treatment?

Cost varies according to the combinations of drugs used.

○ Are there any side effects?

Some women suffer headaches and nausea, weight gain, and bloating. Doses higer than 150 mg may cause hot flashes, breast tenderness, or migraines.

○ Is there anything I need to do while I am on the treatment?

There is a limited amount of research to suggest that 500 mg of vitamin C a day may boost the action of clomiphene.

WHO IS IT SUITABLE FOR?

Ovulation induction is recommended for women whose periods are irregular as a result of an inadequate or unbalanced production of FSH (follicle-stimulating hormone) or LH (luteinizing hormone). These women's ovaries and hormonal systems are functioning, but they need help to ovulate regularly and develop follicles to maturity.

OI is also recommended for women who have polycystic ovary syndrome (PCOS—see pages 119–121) or a luteal phase defect (LPD—see page 128). In the case of the latter, insufficient amounts of progesterone are produced in the luteal phase of the cycle (see pages 10–11). The drug used in OI (see below) enhances progesterone production by making multiple follicles, although there is still some debate about its use for women with an LPD.

HOW THE DRUGS WORK

The drug used in OI is clomiphene citrate (brand names Clomid or Serophene). HCG (human chorionic gonadotrophin) injections may also be given (see below). Clomiphene binds to estrogen receptor sites in the brain, fooling the body into thinking that the amount of estrogen in the blood is too low. This stimulates the hypothalamus to release more GnRH (gonadotrophin-releasing hormone), prompting the pituitary gland to release more LH and FSH. This causes a follicle to start maturing an egg ready for ovulation.

There is a certain amount of debate about the safety of clomiphene. Apart from the side effects that some women suffer (see box, left), in about

15 percent of cases, too many eggs are produced. This is known as ovarian hyperstimulation. Regular monitoring of women taking this drug is essential. Ultrasound scans check the number and development of follicles in the ovaries. If more than three large follicles are found to have developed, treatment may be suspended because of the increased risk of multiple births.

In addition, clomiphene has a drying effect on cervical mucus and results in a thinning of the endometrium over time, reducing the chances of implantation. The drug should not be given unless tests have shown evidence of an ovulation disorder because of this effect on mucus, and it should not be taken for more than six cycles (months). A month's break after three months is advisable: this is important if you are going to have further treatments. There are links between the prolonged use of clomiphene (a year or more) and ovarian cancer, and the drug is associated with a higher rate of miscarriage. It is important to take the lowest possible dose, but you may be advised that it needs to be increased, of course, depending on your circumstances. Discuss all these potentially worrisome issues with your fertility consultant.

Figures show that, after a course of clomiphene, about 80 percent of women with irregular or no ovulation will ovulate, and about 40 percent of those who do ovulate will conceive within six months of treatment. Twenty percent of women have no response to clomiphene: those over the age of 40, in particular, may not respond well to it.

CLOMIPHENE AND HCG

If ovulation induction using clomiphene alone has not been successful, the next step may be to have an injection of HCG to encourage the final maturation of the follicle and the release of the egg. This drug is generally administered when one follicle reaches a diameter of at least 18 mm. Sexual intercourse or intrauterine insemination (IUI—see pages 152–53) will be timed for 36–40 hours after the injection has been administered.

CASE HISTORY

Lee, aged 34, first realized she had a problem at the age of 18, when her periods stopped and then became very erratic. She also found herself losing weight. She married in her early 20s and tried unsuccessfully for a family for 18 months before seeking medical help. *Following a laparoscopy, she was diagnosed with PCOS and was prescribed Clomid.* Treatment was successful, and within two months she was pregnant. Lee's periods continued to be erratic following the birth of her son. *When she decided to try for another child 18 months later, she was given Clomid and her second son was born two and a half years after the first.*

A mature ovarian follicle containing a ripe egg.

intrauterine insemination

The aim of intrauterine insemination (IUI), or artificial insemination as the procedure used to be called, is to place active sperm close to an egg to assist fertilization.

WHO IS IT SUITABLE FOR?

IUI may be the next step for women for whom ovulation induction using clomiphene alone has not been successful. It is a way of assisting natural fertilization when there is a problem with sperm quality, there are reduced numbers of antisperm antibodies, the cervical mucus is hostile, or FSH (follicle-stimulating hormone) levels are high, or in some cases of unexplained fertility or endometriosis. The procedure is not recommended for women who have blocked fallopian tubes or whose partners have a very low or nonexistent sperm count or poor sperm quality (a minimum of 1 million washed sperm per milliliter is required for this procedure).

HOW IUI WORKS

After ovulation, a sample of washed sperm is injected directly into the uterus by means of a catheter through the cervix. IUI treatment may involve the use of clomiphene to stimulate the follicles, or injections, depending on clinic protocols. Ovulation may be induced by means of an HCG (human chorionic gonadotrophin) injection (see opposite). The procedure is performed as near as possible—ideally within six hours—to ovulation, which is determined by an ultrasound scan or by using an ovulation predictor kit. Two IUIs may be scheduled by some clinics—one just prior to ovulation and the other around ovulation. Protocols will vary from clinic to clinic.

IUI PROTOCOL

Days of cycle	1–5 Menstrual period	6–10	11–13
Stage of egg development			
Drugs	● Clomiphene, usually on days 2–6		● HCG injection if needed
Scans, tests, and procedures		● Ultrasound scan on day 10 to see if follicles are developing	● Ultrasound scan ● Home ovulation kit to detect LH surge to check if ovulating

IUI WITH DRUGS

With IUI alone, there is a 10 percent rate of success per cycle. IUI with clomiphene increases this figure to 10–15 percent. The latter option is usually recommended when the use of clomiphene alone hasn't been successful in a previous attempt. IUI combined with an HCG injection—to encourage follicle maturation and the release of an egg—is another option.

With each stage of IUI treatment, the necessary medications get stronger in order to increase the chances of success. As a consequence of the strength and cost of the drugs involved, however, I do advise choosing the gentlest options first and building up only if you are unsuccessful. Having acupuncture at weekly intervals while you are going through IUI may be of benefit, as may other complementary treatments (see pages 145–49).

I would also recommend that you choose a clinic for IUI treatment that is open on weekends. I have seen many disappointed women who have known they are ovulating during a weekend, but have been unable to do anything about it because their clinic was closed at the time.

CASE HISTORY

Sandra, age 35, and her partner tried for *a baby for two years before seeking help.* *Clomid was prescribed, with few side effects,* *and* *Sandra had three IUIs in consecutive* *months.* *The third was successful, and Sandra now has a baby boy. "The procedure was uncomfortable and unpleasant; it was cold and clinical, and so far removed from how I imagined my baby would be conceived. Also, the clinic gave me hardly any time to lie down after the procedure, and I've since learned that this is very important.* *So I was* *amazed and absolutely delighted when it* *worked—third time lucky!"*

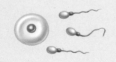

14

● Washed sperm injected into uterus via cervix

Q&A

○ What is the success rate of IUI?
It's about 10 percent per cycle, but drugs can improve this (see above).

○ How long does it take and is it a painful procedure?
It takes a few minutes and usually causes little or no discomfort; you may feel wet as a result of the cervix being washed beforehand. Cramping is occasionally felt afterward.

○ Do I need to rest after having IUI?
Yes. Clinics generally don't allow you long enough after the procedure.

Remain lying down for at least 30 minutes after the procedure and then take it easy for a while.

○ How many IUIs should we try before moving on to IVF?
In general, three IUIs using clomiphene, followed by three attempts with injections, should bring success. If not, discuss IVF with your clinic. Take your age into account, however. Three cycles of IUI might "delay" you for 4–6 months before moving on to IVF.

in vitro fertilization

Embarking on IVF is a major decision and one that you should not rush into. It requires a great deal of research and thought, and then mental and emotional preparation.

BEING PREPARED

With IVF, you are "bringing in the big guns." You need to be very sure about what you are doing, why you are doing it, the possible effects, the time it will take, the costs involved, and the emotional roller coaster you will have to endure. Be prepared to have your life turned upside down!

WHAT IS IVF?

IVF stands for in vitro fertilization: in vitro means "in glass." It involves an egg being fertilized in a petri dish in a laboratory under very carefully controlled conditions.

In a normal, natural cycle, usually only one egg ripens within a growing follicle. The egg is released and, if fertilized (penetrated by a sperm) in one of the fallopian tubes, it travels to the uterus, where it implants and grows. With IVF, the aim is to cultivate multiple follicles to harvest many eggs, which are surgically extracted and fertilized outside the body. They are then placed in the uterus, which has been prepared by hormone treatment to be ready to receive an embryo.

PLANNING YOUR TIME

There are key stages in the IVF process when you must put aside adequate amounts of time and give priority to the treatment above all your other commitments. In the first week, blood tests and scans may take up at least a day throughout the week. Don't be surprised if clinics run late. Bear all this in mind when planning your work schedule for that week. Even when consultations run according to schedule, results may not, and you need to be prepared to be called unexpectedly. Discussing the consequences of your results may take time. And do not be surprised if some tests or procedures have to be repeated.

The egg retrieval process doesn't take very long, but you may feel some effects afterward. You may feel groggy, for instance, if you have had an anesthetic. I always recommend a rest afterward to allow the body to heal. Following the transfer of embryos, you should take at least three days to rest. Carry out only light duties in order to give implantation the best chance of success.

DECIDING WHO TO TELL

If you are still working full time, you must face the difficult decision about whether or not to confide in your boss or other colleagues, given

Human embryos are stored frozen using liquid nitrogen before they are transferred to the uterus.

that treatment can demand a lot of time out of your working week and you have no guarantee that the treatment will work on the first attempt. My advice would be not to broadcast what you are doing, but find a friend in whom you can confide, preferably one who's had a similar experience and who can understand what you are going through.

THINKING IT THROUGH

The procedures and drugs used in IVF place huge demands on your body. You are putting very powerful medications into your system. Some of the risks and side effects, such as irritability, hot flashes, and other menopausal symptoms, are well documented. The immediate effects of the medication last only as long as you are taking the drugs. It may be some time, however, before we become aware of all the long-term health implications of IVF: a possible link has been made, for example, between an increased incidence of certain female cancers and IVF treatment, and scientists are now investigating this.

Discuss the IVF route thoroughly with your partner and medical advisers, and be sure to take into account your medical history and that of your family—particularly close female relatives. Use every means at your disposal to find out what the latest research and contraindications may be, since new information is emerging all the time. There are plenty of websites and support groups out there (see page 187) that can give you information and the "other" side of the story from the one you may hear at your clinic or from drug companies. You may, of course, come across alarming reports, such as the claims about IVF babies having a higher incidence of genetic conditions or abnormalities and being at a greater risk of cancer than naturally conceived children. Discuss all your worries with your fertility specialist.

Don't be pressured or influenced by others. You are the one who will have to put up with the discomforts of testing, the uncertainty of waiting for results, and the aftereffects of treatment.

KEY CONSIDERATIONS

Think long and hard before answering these important questions, and make sure you do so with total honesty.

- **Can I change my day-to-day routine to make enough time in my life to meet the demands of this treatment?**
  Do not underestimate the impact that treatment will have on your and your partner's normal routines.

- **Will I get the support I need, physically, emotionally, and mentally, from my partner?**
  You both need to understand the commitment involved, not just procedurally while you are undergoing tests and treatments, but also when you have to take essential rest at certain key points in the cycle. When I point this out to my female clients, they often say to me, "I wish you would tell my partner that."

- **Can I make time not just for the treatment but for other important aspects of life?**
  Remember that you have to have a relationship at the end of all of this, whether or not you have a baby.

- **How will we get through if I am very stressed?**
  Each of you will react in your own way to the problems that IVF treatment throws up along the way. The direct experience that each of you has will be different, and the way in which each of you reacts to your experience may be different, too. Accept this and get used to the idea now in order to avoid conflict later.

- **Do I need another family member or friend in whom I can confide—particularly someone who has gone through the process herself?**
  You will need a lot of support while you are undergoing IVF, particularly if your partner finds it hard to cope with all the ups and downs, or he is unable to be there at important moments. It may useful at times to have the perspective of someone who isn't directly involved.

getting ready to go

If you have weighed up all the pros and cons and are ready to go ahead with IVF, you must begin to prepare yourself physically and mentally well in advance. This will increase your chance of success so that the number of cycles you may need can be kept to a minimum.

DECIDING WHEN TO START

Age is one of the key factors in the success of IVF, and you should bear this in mind as you decide when to start the treatment. Unless you have already had preliminary fertility tests carried out, your chosen clinic will need to investigate the reason why you have not conceived in order to plan the right course of treatment for you. Consider having the necessary investigations done in consultation with your clinic or doctor while you are waiting for an appointment to start IVF.

Whatever decisions you make and whatever the eventual outcome of those decisions, you need to be able to look back without regret. Once IVF has begun, you will probably find that the treatment is not as bad as you had anticipated. You will quickly

become familiar with the regimen of blood tests, scans, nasal sprays, and self-injection that treatment involves. I never cease to be amazed at how quickly women acquire detailed knowledge about every aspect of the process. You may know nothing when you first start out, but I promise you that you'll soon be an expert. This knowledge is important because it increases how much control you feel you have over what is happening to you. Men on the whole do not tend to gather as much information as their partners.

CHOOSING THE RIGHT CLINIC

Research, research, research! I cannot overstress the importance of doing your homework before you select a clinic. Some people put more effort into choosing a vacation than their IVF clinic. Research will save you time, money, and heartache. Word of mouth is important, but do not rely solely on this: what is right for one couple may not be right for you. Also, IVF techniques are constantly changing, so their experience may be out of date.

Neither should you depend exclusively on your doctor's recommendations. Treatments can vary enormously from clinic to clinic, and where you go may make all the difference to your success. Many clinics have open days and evenings. Canvas the views of other fertility professionals.

Knowledge is key—it
*increases your participation
in the process and makes
you feel more in control.*

YOUR CHANCES OF SUCCESS

The pregnancy rate per treatment cycle is about 30 percent. The clinic you choose can affect the outcome of treatment, and you are likely to respond better at your first attempt.

In addition, your chances will be greater if:

- you, the female partner, are under the age of 40
- at least one ovary is responding to the stimulation drugs
- your FSH (follicle-stimulating hormone) level is 10 or less (see page 164) on days 2–3 of your cycle and estradiol, prolactin, and LH (luteinizing hormone) levels are at their optimum (see pages 99–100)
- you have had a pregnancy in the past
- your partner has healthy sperm

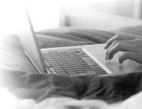

Your choices may be limited, depending on your health insurance policy or HMO, so be sure to investigate your plan before making any calls. If you are paying for your own treatment, on the other hand, you will have lots of good choices. Making the right choice is more important than worrying about offending people. So, if you feel you're at the wrong clinic or that another clinic can offer you something better, don't hesitate to move.

ASKING QUESTIONS

Contact at least two clinics and compare what they have to offer. Read their brochures, decide what your priorities are, and draw up a list of questions. Look carefully at costs, which vary enormously. Price should not be the overriding factor, but multiple IVF cycles can be very expensive. Talk to the staff. Feel free to ask anything you think is important. Never feel that question is trivial or inappropriate. You'll be in contact with your clinic several times a week, so find out the name of the person you'll be talking to and how available nurses and doctors are to take calls and answer questions. I strongly recommend you look at the

Society for Assisted Reproductive Technology (SART) website—www.sart.org—for their guidelines on clinics and for information such as their success rates, and RESOLVE—www.resolve.org—for firsthand support and feedback for couples undergoing IVF. The Internet is also a good source of information about other assisted reproductive techniques that may be relevant to your treatment but not available in your area. Traveling long distances for treatment can be very expensive, but it may be worthwhile to see a specialist who will tailor the treatment to your needs.

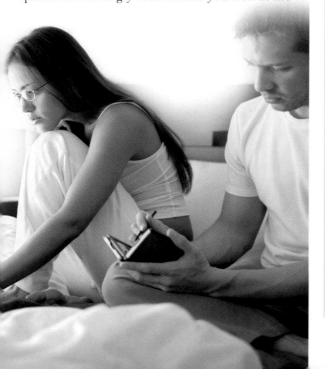

ASSESSING A CLINIC

- **Location**—be prepared to go out of your way to get to a clinic that has a particularly good reputation.
- **Opening hours**—choose a clinic that operates seven days a week so that it can work with your body clock and not just within office hours.
- **Reputation and success rates**—what are the statistics for your age, particular fertility problem, etc.?
- **Specialist expertise**—do they treat older women, those who have high FSH levels, or those who have had multiple IVF failures or recurrent pregnancy loss?
- **Reviews after failed cycles**—check if these are included in the basic price for the IVF cycle.
- **Which stimulation protocols are used**, especially the use of drugs such as Viagra, baby aspirin, heparin, or ritrodine?
- **Are the appropriate treatments** to suit your particular requirements available?
- **What is the level of general care:** does the staff put you at ease? Will they be accessible if you have questions or concerns?
- **Availability of counseling**—some clinics have a better reputation for providing counseling than others (see box, page 158).
- **Waiting times**—bear in mind that it may be worth going on the waiting list of your chosen clinic in advance of when you want to start treatment.

MEETING YOUR CONSULTANT

Having researched and chosen your clinic, you will meet your doctor to discuss in detail your medical and surgical history and any previous fertility treatments, and to talk about and decide upon the appropriate course of action for you.

Clinics usually collect certain information (names, dates of birth, medical details), which is confidential.

Before treatment begins, you and your partner will have consent forms to read and sign. These forms vary from clinic to clinic. There are no federal guidelines regulating these documents. Sign them only when you are satisfied that you understand completely the details and implications of what you are agreeing to. Consent forms usually include your agreement to:

• the storage of any gametes or embryos created for your future use; also, how you may choose to allow them to be used—for example, to be donated or to be used for research

• the procedures of treatment, such as egg collection and embryo transfer

SCREENING FOR INFECTIONS

There are a number of routine tests (blood tests and swabs) to check for infections before an IVF cycle begins. Following positive tests, antibiotics will be prescribed. You will be re-tested to see if you are free of infection. The tests vary depending on the clinic (some clinics have added West Nile virus and syphilis) but usually include:

Gonorrhea (see pages 110–11) This may, among other things, lead to blocked fallopian tubes.

Chlamydia (see page 110) This causes inflammation of, and perhaps even permanent damage to, the fallopian tubes.

Ureaplasma (see Bacterial vaginosis, page 112) This is a microorganism that does not normally cause symptoms, which can be present in either partner and may interfere with implantation.

HIV Many clinics feel they do not have the expertise to treat HIV-positive patients. Some clinics, however, will treat you, and use various methods to attempt prevention of passing on the infection.

Hepatitis B and C Many clinics will not treat you if you test positive for hepatitis. Again, it depends on the clinic.

Rubella Exposure to rubella during pregnancy may cause birth defects in the baby. If you do not have rubella antibodies, you need to be immunized before embarking on IVF. You will be rechecked for immunity a few months later.

THINKING POSITIVELY

Try to enter every treatment cycle with a positive attitude. Think of IVF, as with all assisted reproductive techniques, as a course of treatment.

COUNSELING

Find out if your fertility clinic has professional counselors on staff. Couples undergoing assisted reproduction should be offered counseling to discuss any concerns before, and during, treatment. The quality of counseling varies enormously and may cover various issues including:

○ IMPLICATIONS COUNSELING

to help those considering the use of donated sperm, eggs or embryos, or surrogacy. It should include genetic counseling, and is recommended for women 35 and older.

○ SUPPORT COUNSELING

to give emotional support, especially if treatment fails

○ THERAPEUTIC COUNSELING

to help couples to cope with their fertility problems and the consequences of tests and treatment, to adjust their expectations, and accept their situation.

Be realistic about your chances and keep your feet firmly on the ground, but don't give up if you don't meet with success right away. IVF doesn't work for everyone, but there is a great deal you can do yourself to improve your chances of success.

Write a list of positive affirmations and repeat them to yourself every day:

- my body is healthy and able to grow and sustain a pregnancy
- I accept each stage of this process and believe that it will have the best possible outcome
- everything is working as it should be and going according to plan

Always bear in mind that the IVF process is taking you closer to your goal of having a baby. Don't be overwhelmed by any one stage, test result, or consultation, and constantly keep an eye on what will hopefully be the end result.

It is important to keep communicating with your partner and offering each other mutual support. It is all too easy to allow the stresses of treatment to come between you, particularly if you have different ways of dealing with things. Not all men will share their partner's obsession with researching the finer points of treatment, while others will read the technical manuals in order to avoid dealing with the emotional implications.

I have seen some women grow increasingly frustrated with what they perceive to be their partner's lack of understanding of, and commitment to, the treatment program, while others go overboard trying not to burden their partner with their concerns. Recognize that IVF may be tough for you, but it can be a really difficult time for your partner as well. He may feel frustrated, powerless, even guilty, as he watches you taking medication and undergoing the various procedures. Find out if he wants to become more involved in the process, perhaps by helping you with the injections or accompanying you to scans. If he doesn't want to, try not to take it personally and, whatever you do, don't put him under pressure to do what doesn't come naturally.

CONSIDERING COSTS

● **My husband and I are wondering how we'll pay for IVF. What costs should we budget for?**
Fertility treatment costs vary from clinic to clinic. The cost per live birth can be as much as $55,000. You need to find out exactly what the charges are, what they include, and whether the cost of a treatment cycle (each attempt at achieving a pregnancy) includes items such as drugs, blood tests, scans, or sperm, egg, and embryo storage.

Insurance coverage varies from plan to plan. Many insurance companies will not pay for fertility treatment, but will cover the costs of diagnosis and treatment of an underlying condition, such as endometriosis, polycystic ovarian disease, varicocele, blocked epididymis, or blocked vas deferens. Find out if your insurance plan covers any part of the investigations or treatment. Also, ask whether any of the fee is refundable by the clinic if a treatment cycle has to be abandoned for any reason.

● **What if we can't afford IVF? Is there any way to get around the high costs?**
There are no bargains to be had, and reproductive medicine and your best interests may not always coincide with those of the clinic. So it is important to get as much information as you can on variation in costs and recommended treatments from a nonprofit organization such as RESOLVE or the American Society for Reproductive Medicine (ASRM).

AVOIDING TIME LIMITS

Don't set yourself time limits at the outset: this will make you feel under even more pressure. Take the treatment program one step at a time and keep reviewing the situation, being prepared to change course (even clinic) as circumstances change. Keep focusing on the positive: if at first you don't succeed, your fertility specialist will have gained a great deal of information that will help fine-tune your treatment in any subsequent cycles. Always ensure that you review each failed cycle to see what can be learned and reworked next time.

your body and IVF

IVF is a highly technical procedure, so it is easy to feel that you are merely the object of a scientific process and have little influence on that process or the outcome. There is, however, a great deal you can do physically and mentally to minimize side effects and enhance treatment, and to help your body to recover afterward.

TAKING CONTROL

The procedures and drugs of IVF will place huge demands on your body. To give yourself the best chance of success, start to prepare physically at least four to six weeks before treatment begins.

In my experience, IVF seems to work better in spring and summer, the time for growth and renewal within the natural cycle. In fall and winter, nature is dormant and the body needs rest and sleep rather than action. If time is on your side and you have the choice, opt to begin treatment in spring rather than winter.

There is a great deal that you can do to help the process along and to give yourself a greater sense of control over the course of events. When I assist women about to undergo IVF, I prepare them mentally, physically, and emotionally, offering appropriate help and advice at each stage of the treatment. Some of them have had bad experiences previously, but if you are prepared and focused, you can cope with anything and make the most of every attempt. Much of the fear and anxiety you might have can be alleviated by understanding how IVF makes use of the body's natural

processes, the particular objectives of each stage of the treatment, and the possible results. Use this knowledge to strengthen your natural resources and to help visualize a successful program.

PREPARING THE BODY

Prepare yourself physically for the months of treatment ahead by doing the following:

- if you have already been through one cycle of IVF, you should ideally allow your ovaries to recover for a month or two before embarking on another treatment program
- keep tabs on your weight, because IVF will have a better chance of success if you are not carrying too much weight (see page 29). If you are, improve your eating habits so that you lose weight gradually, without depriving yourself of vital nutrients
- similarly, if you are significantly underweight, reassess your diet so you can gain the weight you need steadily and healthily

Yoga postures help you to relax and promote harmony in mind and body.

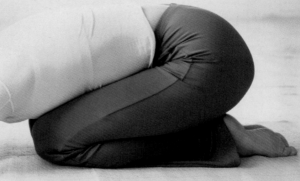

- do not smoke and avoid smoky atmospheres: smoking damages the lining of the uterus
- try to avoid strenuous exercise, such as aerobics. Your body needs rest as your hormonal system shuts down to prepare for IVF. Try gentle forms of exercise instead, such as walking or yoga.

THE IMPORTANCE OF GOOD NUTRITION

Maintaining a healthy diet and following a general detox program can help you to fortify those body systems that are going to come under the most stress during the IVF process. A good dietary practice to start with is to avoid chocolate, sugary and processed foods, salty snacks, coffee, tea, cola and other carbonated drinks, and alcohol. These all counteract the beneficial effects of vital nutrients, and some have a diuretic effect.

TAKING SUPPLEMENTS

If you have already been trying to conceive for a while, you and your partner may already be taking nutritional supplements. If not, invest in the best-quality preconception multivitamins and minerals that you can afford (see pages 59–64). Start taking them at least three or four months before your IVF treatment commences. Be wary of some of the anecdotal advice found on Internet bulletin boards. This has led some women to take excessive amounts of certain vitamins and minerals. It is worth seeking the advice of nutritional experts.

- Vitamin B-complex: will help your body cope with the stress of invasive procedures
- Vitamin C: 500 mg a day will help collagen production and is vital for wound healing following egg retrieval. There is some evidence to suggest that it may help to prevent miscarriage
- Vitamin E: enhances healing
- Zinc: promotes cell formation and wound healing after surgery and is vital for hormone production and implantation. Many women who come to see me because they have fertility problems are deficient in zinc. This is especially likely if they have been taking the Pill for a long time.

ZITA'S TIPS

I believe it is as important to prepare your body in the run-up to a cycle of IVF treatment as it is to prepare it in anticipation of natural conception. There are a number of measures you might like to consider.

- A **7- or 10-day liver detox program** (see pages 50–53) will help to clear out your system and boost the liver's detoxifying capacity so that it is able to cope with the drugs that you will have to take during the treatment. So, if you have a few weeks before beginning an IVF cycle, spend one of them doing a liver detox program.

- **Certain vitamins and other nutrients,** such as vitamin C, vitamin E, selenium, bioflavonoids, and glutathione (an amino acid), also help to optimize liver function and protect it from the effects of toxins by increasing the rate at which it processes them. (See pages 59–63 for good food sources of these key nutrients.)

- **Make sure that you take a good multivitamin and mineral** supplement. It should contain magnesium, selenium, and zinc. Also consider taking a vitamin C supplement (500 mg a day), which will help to replenish the ovaries.

- **Drink** lots of water (see page 58).

- **Consider having a course** of lymphatic drainage (see page 149).

- **Sleep or rest** as much as you can in the weeks leading up to the start of your IVF program, in order to build up your reserves of energy. You are certainly going to need lots of physical and mental energy to keep you going during the months to come.

- **Spend 10 minutes a day** practicing deep breathing techniques (see pages 42–43) and visualization (see pages 43 and 163).

A good supply of essential nutrients is vitally important in preparation for IVF to support your body's ability to:
• develop mature follicles and eggs
• establish the lining of the uterus
• heal after the retrieval of eggs
• implant an embryo following transfer

Egg quality will become one of your overriding concerns during the course of your treatment. Make sure you eat plenty of:
• protein: studies have shown that insufficient protein in the diet can result in a reduced number of eggs. So you should make sure you eat about 2 oz (60 g) of protein a day (see also pages 55–56). The best-quality protein foods, in terms of amino acid balance, include eggs, meat, fish, beans, lentils, and quinoa. Avoid eating too many dairy products (since milk contains artificial hormones) and eat only organic meat
• vitamins and minerals: take a good-quality multivitamin and mineral supplement every day. Various studies have also shown that in women who are on supplementation, the fluid surrounding and nourishing the eggs is rich in vitamins C and E. Zinc, magnesium, selenium, and vitamin A are all vital nutrients for egg production; selenium and magnesium have been shown to improve fertilization rates; and folic acid is also important
• essential fatty acids: these are vitally important (see pages 63–64). I put all my clients on a DHA supplement in the period leading up to the start of their IVF program and increase the dosage once stimulation treatment has begun.

Egg retrieval and other invasive techniques used in the IVF program are regarded as minor surgical procedures, but you need to recover and heal quickly so that you will be ready to receive the embryos shortly afterward.
• Vitamin C and zinc: take vitamin C (500 mg) and zinc (20 mg) daily for at least two weeks before the procedure.
• Arnica: this homeopathic remedy may help prevent damage to internal tissues. Consult a practitioner or take the remedy four times daily (6c potency) from the day before retrieval until after the transfer of embryos into the uterus.

The endometrium needs to be thick enough to receive the embryo and facilitate implantation. The following measures may help to build it up:
• eat foods that are rich in vitamins B1 and B6. The latter is needed for the production of progesterone and hence the development of the uterine lining. You should also have good intakes of iron and coenzyme Q10, which is excellent for improving blood flow generally. These vitamins and minerals will help to support and enrich the endometrium. (For good food sources of these nutrients, see pages 60–63.)
• the use of acupuncture on certain points on the back has been shown to be of benefit to the uterine lining and to improve blood flow through the pelvis
• drink plenty of water every day

- avoid vigorous exercise
- use a hot-water bottle to keep the abdomen warm and assist healing

ACUPUNCTURE AND IVF

You may find acupuncture treatments beneficial as you prepare for IVF and during the procedures themselves. Research suggests that acupuncture on a weekly basis may help to build up the lining of the uterus, develop follicles and, after the transfer of embryos, encourage implantation and the maintenance of pregnancy.

I really believe that, in accordance with traditional Chinese beliefs (see pages 72–73), if your lower abdomen is cold to the touch, you should apply warmth to improve your chances of conception. In addition, the kidneys and the liver are considered to be very important for reproduction. The liver is associated with anger, frustration, and irritability. Women often complain of experiencing these emotions when they are taking IVF drugs, so encouraging a healthy liver may help to improve the way you feel during your treatment cycle. Acupuncture at certain key points on the liver meridian will help to improve the flow of blood and life energy (*qi*) to a woman's reproductive organs. Treatment of acupoints along the kidney meridian may also help to restore energy depleted during IVF treatment.

POSITIVE VISUALIZATION

At each stage of your IVF treatment, I want you to visualize what you want to happen in your body— the eggs maturing, the lining of the uterus thickening, the embryos implanting.

The Chinese believe that if you focus your mind on a particular area in the body, life energy will flow to that spot. Write descriptions of these positive visualizations on cards and place them at points around the house so that you are reminded to repeat them out loud regularly throughout the day. Add other positive affirmations (see page 159) as well as some statements about how well your

body is responding to the drugs and processing them. You may feel a little eccentric doing this, but remember that the mind is an incredibly powerful tool. What you believe shapes what you become. You need to really believe that you are going to have a baby and that in the course of doing so you will remain healthy and not compromise your immune system.

DEEP-BREATHING TECHNIQUES

Breathing slowly, deeply, and smoothly (see pages 42–43) can be of great benefit if your stress levels are high and you are emotionally tightly wound. Relaxing your body, encouraging life energy to flow freely, and calming your mind will equip you well for the ups and downs of IVF treatments.

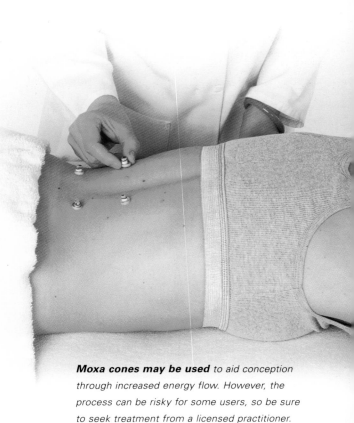

Moxa cones may be used to aid conception through increased energy flow. However, the process can be risky for some users, so be sure to seek treatment from a licensed practitioner.

FSH and IVF

Many women are unable to start IVF treatment because their levels
of follicle-stimulating hormone (FSH) are too high. They feel as if
they have fallen at the first hurdle and are disappointed, faced with
the prospect of putting life on hold as they wait for levels to fall.

THE IMPORTANCE OF FSH

FSH is the hormone released by the pituitary gland that causes eggs to ripen and mature. If your FSH levels are beyond the expected range, your eggs are likely to be of poor quality. They are much less likely to result in a healthy embryo and consequently a pregnancy. There are several reasons why you might have raised levels of follicle-stimulating hormone (see pages 128–29). In some cases, levels may be low enough to embark on an IVF cycle. Some clinics will begin even if your FSH is relatively high, but the success rate for women who have raised levels is not as good as for those whose levels are normal.

To maximize your chances of success with IVF, it is important to wait until conditions are right, with a reading of less than 10 (see box, left) and an estradiol level below 70 (see pages 99–101).

If your FSH levels are raised, it is important not to put yourself under pressure and increase your stress levels. I often suggest to my clients that they take a break from testing in order to relax. Finding out that your levels are high can be devastating. Explore all the options open to you as a result before deciding whether or not to move on to the next step.

LOWERING LEVELS

There is currently no conventional treatment for raised FSH levels. There is some research to suggest that acupuncture may be of benefit, especially using acupoints to help balance the pituitary gland. I treat a number of important points for reproduction

INTERPRETING FSH LEVELS

DAY-3 FSH (PG/ML)	INTERPRETATION
Less than 6	Excellent result. Very reassuring level.
6–8	Normal. Expect a good response to stimulation.
8–10	Fair. Response is likely to be between normal and slightly reduced (though it will vary widely).
10–12	Lower than normal ovarian reserve. Likely to be a reduced response to stimulation and a reduction in egg and embryo quality with IVF. There are also reduced live birth rates.
12–17	Generally indicates a more marked reduction in response to stimulation and further reduction in egg and embryo quality with IVF. Low live birth rates.
More than 17	Very poor or no response to stimulation. No live births. "No go" levels will be determined by the particular laboratory analysis and IVF center.

and hormone regulation, usually during the last two weeks of a woman's cycle.

Other measures that may help bring levels down include:

- putting yourself on a detox program (see pages 50–53), by drinking plenty of bottled or filtered water, reducing salt intake, and avoiding coffee, tea, and sugary, carbonated drinks. Try drinking hot water with lemon juice instead
- getting gentle exercise and, if you are overweight, losing weight
- spending time relaxing by practicing deep breathing or meditating on the color blue
- taking B-complex and zinc supplements (see pages 59–63)
- keeping the lower abdomen warm
- taking a herbal supplement of *Vitex agnus-castus* (chaste-tree berry), an herb that is known to suppress elevated FSH levels, but this must be under the supervision of a qualified herbal practitioner
- taking an essential fatty acid supplement (see pages 63–64)
- including beans, legumes, onions, and garlic in your diet to help the liver break down estrogen, and cabbage to increase the rate at which the liver converts estrogen into its water-soluble form so that it can be excreted. In addition, eating foods that are good sources of phytoestrogens (see page 31), such as alfalfa sprouts and flaxseed, legumes, oats, parsley, broccoli, and Brussels sprouts may also help to correct hormonal imbalance.

AGE AND EGG QUALITY

While an abnormal result (which means high-baseline FSH) tends to be indicative of poor egg quality, a measurement within the expected range does not necessarily mean that the quality of your eggs is good. There are significant numbers of women with normal-baseline FSH values who have poor egg quality that is not reflected in their FSH reading. This is particularly true of women in their 40s.

An infertile 44-year-old woman with normal FSH (for example, 6) still has a very low probability of conceiving as a result of using IVF, or any other assisted reproductive technique for that matter. It is the fact that she is 44 that diminishes her chances. This is, of course, why IVF programs have age limits. These restrictions vary

Spend time relaxing,
using deep-breathing techniques and perhaps meditation or visualization.

from clinic to clinic, but most of them have an age cutoff of between 42 and 45. Older women who have fertility problems will rarely be successful using their own eggs. However, women in their 40s with raised FSH levels may have IVF treatment and consider using donor eggs.

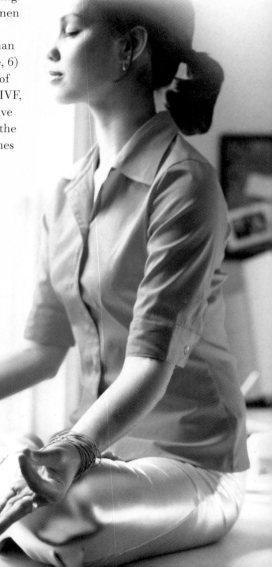

IVF protocols

There are two main procedures, or protocols, but the details differ from one clinic to another. Your circumstances will determine which is for you: your response may deviate from the generalized descriptions below.

WHO FOLLOWS WHICH PROTOCOL?

The long protocol is for women whose hormones are functioning normally and who have regular cycles. The short protocol is for those who have high FSH (follicle-stimulating hormone) levels or who have responded poorly to ovarian stimulation before.

THE LONG PROTOCOL

In this protocol, the body's natural production of FSH and luteinizing hormone (LH) is suppressed, or "down-regulated." The cycle is then carefully controlled with drugs to stimulate the ovaries so that many eggs can be produced and harvested.

LONG AND SHORT IVF PROTOCOLS (GENERALIZED)

Stage	LONG PROTOCOL (LP)		LONG PROTOCOL (LP) AND SHORT	
	Menstruation	Down-regulation	Menstruation/ stimulation	Stimulation continues
Day of cycle	2/3	21–31/33	2–5	6–10
Stage of follicle development				
Treatment and procedures		● Suppression drug	● LP: (days 3, 4 or 5) FSH + suppression drug ● SP: (day 2) suppression drug; (day 3) FSH	● Possible FSH adjustments + suppression drug
Tests and scans	● Blood test to check levels of FSH, LH, and estradiol		● LP: suppression check on day 3. Scan to check for cysts and/or blood test to check estradiol and possibly other hormone levels	● Scans to check progress of follicle development and check thickening of the endometrium ● Blood tests to check estradiol levels

You may be given a blood test on day two or three of your menstrual cycle to check levels of FSH, LH, and estradiol (see pages 99–100). If these hormones are at their optimum levels (see box on page 101), you will be able to start the long protocol on day 21 of your cycle.

Down-regulation

At the beginning of a natural ovarian cycle, gonadotrophin-releasing hormone (GnRH) is released into the blood from the hypothalamus in the brain. It is only active for a few seconds, but this is sufficient to stimulate the pituitary gland to release FSH, which in turn stimulates several follicles that have begun to develop to continue their growth (see page 10). Under the long protocol, you will be given drugs that have an effect similar to GnRH but remain active in your system for longer than would occur naturally, over-stimulating the pituitary gland so that, in effect, it releases all of its FSH and LH. As levels of these hormones fall, the follicles "recruited" for this cycle do not receive enough hormones to enable them to continue their development. This suppression of the reproductive system wipes the slate clean, so to speak, so that it can begin to be manipulated. The suppression drugs are administered either by injection or nasal spray and common brand names include Buserelin, Nafarelin, Synarel, and Zoladex.

PROTOCOL (SP)

Follicles ripe	Eggs mature	Egg retrieval	Fertilization	Transfer of embryos
11	12	13	14	15–18
• Possible HCG, depending on scan + blood-test results		• Vaginal ultrasound probe or laparoscopy to collect eggs	• IVF or ICSI method of fertilization • Grading of embryos	• Embryos loaded into catheter and inserted into uterus through cervix • Progesterone or HCG
• Final scan				

Checking suppression

Suppression takes 10–12 days: your period should arrive 7–9 days later. Your clinic will schedule a suppression check (ultrasound scan to see if there are any follicular cysts and/or blood test to measure estradiol levels) on day three of your period. What is considered a "normal" estradiol level varies from one clinic to another. If the scan detects no cysts and estradiol levels are down, you are ready to move on to the next stage of the procedure.

Ovarian stimulation

In the next stage of the long protocol treatment, the recruited follicles (see page 10) are stimulated to grow by means of injections of FSH (follicle-stimulating hormone) or FSH and LH (luteinizing hormone) combined. In a natural cycle, the release of FSH is controlled by the pituitary gland so that there is only enough to stimulate the largest follicle to ripen fully. In a stimulated cycle, almost all the recruited follicles get that chance.

Q&A

○ How do I know if the drugs are working?

You only find out when you have a blood test to check your hormone levels after suppression.

○ How do I know if I am using a nasal spray properly?

You will receive instructions from the clinic on the use of a spray. Most women don't have any problems, although it may feel different each time you inhale. Check with your clinic if you are in doubt.

○ What side effects can I expect from the suppression drugs?

Different women respond in different ways: some are very sensitive to the medication, while others hardly feel any effects at all. If you are concerned, contact your doctor. Common side effects include:

● mood swings/emotional fragility
● irritability and bad temper
● tiredness
● hot flashes and sweats
● breast tenderness
● vaginal dryness

● flulike aches or headaches
● changes in sex drive
● irregular bleeding

○ Should I get my period while on the suppression drugs?

Yes, your period will usually arrive 7–9 days after you start taking the drugs. Most clinics will wait until your period starts before commencing stimulation drugs.

○ What if a period doesn't come?

Either your system has not shut down yet or you were pregnant before treatment began. Some women do become pregnant by chance while taking the down-regulation drugs, and your clinic will test to rule out this possibility.

○ What if my system has not shut down?

Usually when this happens, a follicle is left over from a previous cycle, or hormone levels are not what your doctor wants them to be. You will have to re-bleed and a drug will be given to start this process. Such a

delay will be discouraging. I have found acupuncture may help to start the bleed.

○ What can go wrong at this stage?

Not everybody responds to the suppression drugs. Sometimes estradiol levels remain high. The most common problem is an ovarian cyst revealed on an ultrasound scan.

○ What if I have a cyst?

Some women are prone to cysts, or they may be exacerbated by the drugs. Instead of bursting, as they do in normal ovulation, follicles fill with fluid and estrogen is produced, interfering with FSH and estradiol levels. Cysts are not dangerous, although they may be painful.

○ How will the cysts be treated?

Some clinics allow you to stay on the suppression medication for a while to see if the cyst disappears on its own. Some clinics will want to remove or drain the cyst before continuing, while others will keep you on the cycle to see if estradiol levels fall.

You will have injections at timed intervals during the day, starting on days 3–5 of your period. The drugs used will depend on your particular body chemistry: common brand names include Menogon, Menopure, Puragon, Metrodin High Purity, and Gonal-F. Some are pure FSH: others are a combination of FSH and LH. Your doctor will decide which is the most suitable for you. Every woman responds differently to the drugs; some only need a low dosage, while others need more to achieve the same effect.

You will also continue to take suppression drugs in order to maintain a delicate hormonal balance that will allow eggs to ripen, but prevent ovulation from occurring before the clinic has a chance to retrieve your eggs. You will continue to take both stimulation and suppression drugs, with possible dosage adjustments, until the eggs are ready to be retrieved (see page 173).

MONITORING YOUR PROGRESS

Your progress should be closely monitored. Ultrasound scans of the ovaries and blood tests to measure hormone levels will determine how the follicles are developing. Your doctor will also measure the thickness of the endometrium (by means of ultrasound scanning): 8–10 mm is the optimum. Depending on how your body is responding, drug dosage will be adjusted (within a range of 150–450 mg). Some clinics recommend higher dosages for older women.

If possible, take your partner along with you when you go for a scan, or at least make sure you talk to him on the phone. You may feel the need to discuss the results and their implications with him there and then. Alternatively, you might like to take a friend with you for support in case you hear slightly less-than-positive results from your doctor.

EGG MATURATION

Around day nine of your cycle, a final scan will check the number and size of follicles and a blood test will check hormone levels, determining when

ZITA'S TIPS

- **Most women cannot** realistically take the whole time off work during suppression, but be aware of what is happening to your hormonal system and take things as easy as you possibly can. Go with the flow of your body and relax as much as possible.

- **Avoid all aerobic exercise.** I advise all my clients to avoid strenuous exercise. While the reproductive system is shutting down during suppression, they should follow suit. During stimulation while the body is growing eggs, aerobic exercise will take away from this by redirecting blood flow away from the follicles.

- **Sleep is very important:** get plenty of early nights.

- **Keep the lower abdomen warm** to improve the flow of blood in the pelvis.

- **Drink plenty of water**—filtered or bottled.

- **Spend time alone** if you feel like it: being a bit self-indulgent can do no harm.

- **Acupuncture may help** during the stimulation process.

- **Make sure your diet** includes lots of protein and oily fish such as salmon. I recommend a supplement of evening primrose oil plus DHA. Amino acids are also important. Vitamin C will help to replenish the ovaries. Vitamin E is necessary for the maintenance of cell membranes. (For good food sources of these essential nutrients, see pages 59–64.)

- **If you suffer from headaches,** gently rub lavender oil into your temples.

- **Meditation and visualization** will help you to relax (see page 43). Surround yourself with the colors indigo and blue. Burn lavender oil and focus on the middle of your forehead (the site of the pituitary gland). Visualize your ovaries shutting down.

you should have an injection of human chorionic gonadotrophin (HCG—common brand names are Pregnyl or Profasi). The injection will be timed to coincide with the natural surge of luteinizing hormone (LH) that triggers the final maturation of the eggs and ovulation (see page 10). With IVF, the eggs are retrieved (see page 173) 36 hours after the HCG injection, after the final maturation, but just before ovulation.

At the end of stimulation, most of the follicles should vary in size from 18–23 mm in diameter, but at this stage it is impossible to tell whether or not there is an egg that can be collected from every follicle. Sometimes the follicle develops at a faster rate than the egg, so when it comes to egg collection, the egg is so immature it cannot be removed. And it is quality, of course, not quantity, that counts when it comes to eggs. About 90 percent of visible follicles of the right size

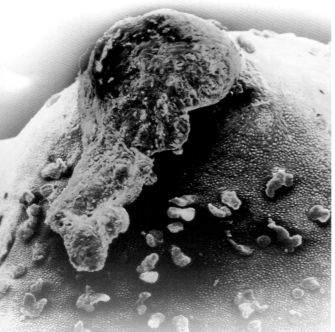

Follicular fluid *(blue) is expelled as a mature follicle, lying beneath the swollen surface of the ovary, ruptures at ovulation. The ovum is in the follicle, ready to be ejected into the fallopian tube.*

produce a collectible egg, but a substantial number of eggs does not necessarily mean that they will all be of good quality. On average, about 7–12 eggs are collected from among the 10–20 follicles that started to ripen at the beginning of the cycle.

THE SHORT PROTOCOL

This protocol is also known as the boost or flare regime. The short protocol takes advantage of the natural flare in FSH and LH levels around day two or three of your cycle, which stimulates follicles to develop. A suppression drug that has the same effect as gonadotrophin-releasing hormone (GnRH)—see page 167—is given on day two of the cycle to prevent premature ovulation.

In contrast to the long protocol, which waits 10–12 days for you to be down-regulated before starting stimulation drugs, the short protocol prescribes FSH injections the next day (day 3). From here on, the two protocols are the same (see under Monitoring your progress, page 169).

MANAGING INJECTIONS

You will be expected to administer the injections yourself: the clinic will give you clear instructions. If you doubt you will be able to manage this, talk to your clinic about arranging a way of having it done under medical supervision. For most women, self-injection becomes easier with practice: a few times is usually enough for them to become confident. You might find the following useful:

- allow plenty of time for your first few injections. If you are working, prioritize this time and make sure nothing infringes upon it
- get your partner involved, as long as he's not too squeamish. Many partners overcome their initial nervousness to become experts at giving injections
- sometimes the site of the injection can feel hot. A dab of aloe vera is soothing and cooling
- apply arnica cream if bruises start to form
- warm up the area to be injected first by rubbing the skin or applying a hot-water bottle. This will make it easier to get the needle in.

FEELING THE EFFECTS

Every woman responds differently to the drugs. Mood swings, tearfulness, general emotional fragility, and abdominal bloating are all common symptoms. Remember that this stage does not last for long. Most symptoms will disappear when you have finished the injections. If you have serious concerns, contact your fertility consultant.

I see a lot of anxiety in women, especially around the time of their scans, as they discover how their bodies have responded to treatment.

You are at the mercy of your hormones and for a few days will be riding an emotional roller coaster. You may be difficult to live with and your partner may find it impossible to say or do the right thing. Accept the fact that you will have good days and bad. You each need to observe these mood swings objectively and rationally for what they are instead of falling prey to them. Bear in mind that at any point, the treatment may not go according to plan. And if the response is poor, it may mean that the cycle has to be abandoned.

Q&A

○ **What if I have a poor response?**

About 10 percent of women do not respond to stimulation, which means estrogen levels are low and follicles are not growing. The definition of "poor response" varies from clinic to clinic. It is important to check follicle-stimulating hormone (FSH) levels at the beginning of a cycle before treatment to get an indication of how you will respond. Careful monitoring will allow the drug dosage to be increased or reduced as necessary. If you respond poorly, don't give up hope. A first IVF cycle is very much a case of trial and error, finding out how you will respond and what combinations of drugs suit you best. It isn't always possible to get it right the first time. Talk to your doctor about varying the drugs next time or, if necessary, try another clinic.

○ **What happens if my ovaries are stimulated too much?**

Some degree of overstimulation occurs in all women going through this procedure because the drugs are making the ovaries ripen as many eggs at one time as occurs in more than a year of normal ovulation. If more than 30 follicles are stimulated, you may have ovarian hyperstimulation syndrome (OHSS)—see below.

If your doctor is concerned that too many follicles have grown and your estradiol level is high, you may be left to "coast." The HCG injection will be withheld, the stimulation drugs stopped, and suppression continued. You will be closely monitored. Get plenty of bed rest and drink lots of water at this time.

Occasionally, the ovaries become massively enlarged and fluid starts to build up in the abdomen and thorax. This is ovarian hyperstimulation syndrome (OHSS). Symptoms include:
● severe pain in the lower abdomen and bloating
● breathing difficulties
● nausea and vomiting
● faintness
● reduced urination

In extreme cases, OHSS can result in thrombosis, heart attack, or stroke. The condition can develop quickly, which is why regular monitoring at this stage of the IVF procedure is so important. Familiarize yourself with the symptoms of OHSS and contact a hospital immediately if you experience any of them.

○ **What happens if the lining of the uterus does not thicken enough?**

By the time of egg collection, your uterine lining should be about 9–10 mm thick (about a third of an inch)—see page 12. Poor uterine lining may be the result of a previous infection in the uterus (see pages 108–11), fibroids (see pages 117–19), or the repeated use of clomiphene (see page 151). If the endometrium does not thicken adequately during the stimulation program, it will be very difficult for an embryo to embed. I often use acupuncture at this time to improve blood flow to the endometrium.

ZITA'S TIPS

Your main aim is to grow eggs, so concentrate all your efforts and visualization on this. Try to stay relaxed and take each day as it comes. Getting overanxious about the results of scans and tests will release adrenaline into your bloodstream, which may counter the effects of the drugs you take.

Go to bed early. Never underestimate the power of sleep and rest to enable the body to adapt, repair, and grow.

Rest is vitally important. Lie down and put your feet up whenever you can. Exercise and activity directs blood to your extremities, but you want it to feed your uterus and the eggs. Even just sitting at a desk or driving a car restricts the flow of energy to the abdomen.

Grapefruit, lemon, or lime essential oil in a warm bath will relax you and lift your spirits.

Make a conscious decision to get rid of negative thoughts as they arise. Repeat positive affirmations out loud, even if it makes you feel as though you are a bit eccentric: "My eggs are growing and ripening and maturing; my eggs are of good quality; my womb lining is growing thick."

Use visualization to try and bring about what you are trying to achieve (see page 43). Imagine that you are directing the delivery of oxygen to the lining of your uterus, helping it to develop. Try to visualize the eggs growing. Focus on how you want your body to respond and use these positive images to help you banish fear. This technique also helps you to sit quietly and relax, and it improves the flow of blood and therefore the supply of energy around the body.

Avoid stressful situations. Spend some time each day sitting quietly and breathing slowly and deeply. Use breathing techniques (see pages 42–43) to encourage blood flow through the uterus.

Make sure your diet includes lots of protein (see pages 55–56), which will improve egg quality.

Take a daily supplement of evening primrose oil or DHA (see pages 63–64) to encourage the development of cell membranes.

Take a good general vitamin and mineral supplement, one containing vitamin E and coenzyme Q10 (see pages 61 and 63).

Drink plenty of water. Two to three quarts (liters) a day helps the follicles develop. Avoid alcohol, coffee, tea, and other stimulants.

Try regular acupuncture treatment with an experienced practitioner (see pages 72–73). There is research to suggest that acupuncture may stimulate the follicles to grow.

Keep your lower abdomen warm, using a hot-water bottle, for example. In Chinese medicine, warmth is considered necessary for the development of a baby.

Surround yourself with orange-colored things. This color is considered to be good for fertility.

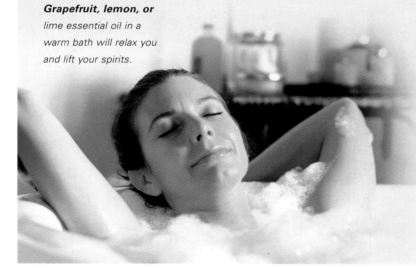

egg collection and transfer

The egg retrieval procedure varies from one clinic to another, but you are most likely to be either heavily sedated or given a general anesthetic. This stage may be a source of anxiety for you.

WHAT IS THE PROCEDURE?

Retrieval of the eggs from the follicles is generally done using a vaginal ultrasound probe, which guides a needle to aspirate each follicle. Most clinics will give you a sedative. Sometimes a laparoscopic procedure (see page 102) is used, but this requires a general anesthetic.

The length of time egg retrieval takes depends on the number of follicles, but it is not a lengthy procedure. Once the egg has been aspirated from the follicle, it is carefully inspected under a microscope and given a grading (see page 175). You will be anxious to know how many eggs have been obtained, but it is quality, not quantity, that matters. Not all the eggs will be fertilized, so the number retrieved is no indication of how many embryos there might be in the end.

On the evening after retrieval (or on the day of the transfer, depending on the clinic) you will start taking progesterone, either by vaginal or anal suppository or by injection. This prepares the uterine lining to receive the embryo. If your pregnancy is positive, you will take it for up to 12 weeks, depending on the clinic. Side effects include nausea, constipation, and fluid retention.

SPERM COLLECTION

Your partner will now have to produce sperm ready to fertilize the eggs, having abstained from sexual intercourse for two days. Providing a sperm sample at the clinic can be a stressful experience for a man (see page 133). It may be possible to produce a sample at home, but you must be able to get the sample to the clinic immediately for preparation for the next stage of the procedure.

FERTILIZATION

Fertilization protocols also vary from clinic to clinic, but a decision will already have been made about the best fertilization option for you. This will mean one of the following:

- **IVF** (in vitro fertilization) Sperm are prepared, washed, and counted and then combined with the eggs in a culture medium in a shallow dish or test tube in the laboratory and incubated at 98.6°F (37°C). After 18 hours, they are examined. If fertilization has occurred, there will be two pro-nuclei—one from the egg and one from the sperm. Within 48 hours, cell division will have begun and the embryo will be ready for transfer.

Q&A

○ **How will I feel after retrieval?**
You will feel a little groggy from the sedative and your abdomen may be swollen and sore. You might also experience some cramping, but this will pass within 24 hours. There is a slight risk of hyperstimulation if a large number of follicles have been emptied and they fill up with fluid (see OHSS in the box on page 171). Contact a doctor immediately if you start to develop symptoms.

○ **Is it normal to have spotting after retrieval?**
You may experience bright red vaginal spotting for 24–48 hours, caused by puncture wounds in the vagina. If bleeding develops, call the clinic immediately.

○ **What can go wrong at this stage?**
The biggest problem at this stage of the procedure will be the failure of the sperm to fertilize the eggs.

ZITA'S TIPS

Before retrieval

● **Take the homeopathic remedy** Arnica (6c potency) four times a day starting the day before the procedure, to help prevent soreness and bruising. Continue until after transfer.

● **Take supplements of DHA** (see pages 63–64 and 162) and vitamins C and E (see pages 61 and 162), and eat plenty of foods rich in iron (see page 61).

● **Acupuncture** (see pages 72–73) can help to prepare the endometrium to receive the embryos and assist the healing process.

● **Practise breathing techniques** to help you to relax during the retrieval process. As you inhale, imagine the breath going to your solar plexus. As you exhale, imagine all the stress and worry that you are experiencing, as well as any physical discomfort you have, being expelled from the body.

● **Spend 20 minutes** each morning and evening repeating positive affirmations, telling yourself that everything is going according to plan. Refuse to dwell on "what if..." speculation or possible negative outcomes.

Following retrieval

● **Rest as much as you can** in preparation for the placing of the embryos in the uterus. Rest will aid recovery and healing.

● **Take a coenzyme Q10 supplement** (see page 63), which will help to improve blood flow after retrieval.

● **Visualize** the healing of the ruptured follicles following egg collection and the thickening of the endometrium to receive an embryo.

● **Practice deep breathing** and relaxation techniques (see pages 42–43) to encourage a good flow of blood and energy around the body.

● **ICSI** (intracytoplasmic sperm injection) A single sperm is injected into the egg under a microscope using a fine glass needle. This is the technique generally used when:

  • the sperm have poor motility and cannot penetrate the egg; the sperm count is too low for IVF; there is a very high proportion of abnormal sperm; or there are very high levels of antibodies in the semen

  • the sperm has to be surgically obtained

  • there has been a poor rate of fertilization, or none at all, with previous IVF attempts

You can normally expect a fertilization rate of 60–70 percent. Some eggs will not be successfully fertilized because they are too immature, too ripe, or of poor quality generally; some eggs might be fertilized by defective sperm; and not all eggs that are fertilized will go on to divide. Fertilization may, of course, fail to occur at all.

EMBRYO GRADING

You will, at this stage of the IVF procedure, be very interested in the quality and development of your embryos, and you will probably want regular progress reports. Remember that the grading of the embryos does not correspond directly to your chances of becoming pregnant. High-grade embryos show a tendency to higher pregnancy rates, but they are not a guarantee. I have treated couples whose grading was high-quality but who

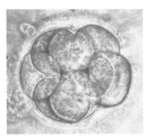

Grade 1 embryo: *even cell division, an appropriate number of cells for the culture time, and no fragmentation.*

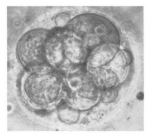

Grade 2 embryo: *even cell division and a small amount of fragmentation (extracellular debris) between cells.*

failed to achieve a successful pregnancy, and I have known couples who were dependent on one frozen embryo and went on to have a baby.

Grading helps to determine how many embryos should be transferred, but it is not an exact science. Try to be positive about your embryos, regardless of their grading, and have faith in the decisions of your medical team. Multicell embryos are usually graded from one to four (see below), where grade one is best. Sometimes, however, four is best. Your embryos are likely to be of different grades.

TESTING FOR GENETIC DISORDERS

Preimplantation genetic diagnosis (PGD) is used to test embryos for genetic disorders: only embryos without abnormalities can be transferred in an IVF cycle. Half of miscarriages following IVF are believed to be the result of abnormal embryos, so PGD may increase the chances of a successful pregnancy. It also allows people who have a genetic disorder to minimize the risks of passing it on.

PGD is very expensive and is used for a relatively small number of couples at high risk for producing children with genetic disorders. The number of centers offering PGD, though, is growing.

On day three of the embryo's development (see box, right), an embryologist carefully extracts, using microscopic instruments, one cell from each embryo. These cells are then analyzed for genetic abnormalities. Currently, PGD investigates

indications for more than 20 diseases, including cystic fibrosis, Huntington's disease, Duchenne muscular dystrophy, Tay-Sachs disease, sickle-cell disease, Marfan syndrome, retinitis pigmentosa, hemophilia A, and fragile X syndrome. It can also reveal chromosomal abnormalities, such as that associated with Down syndrome, although it does not eliminate the need for prenatal testing such as amniocentesis.

You will be referred to a genetic counselor to identify specific risks of genetic diseases. You may be given carrier testing to see if you are carrying a disease that you do not have.

EMBRYO DEVELOPMENT

To help you visualize what is happening to your embryos in an attempt to encourage the process to be successful, it might help to know how an embryo develops.

- **Day 1** The first cell division, or cleavage, takes place 33–36 hours after insemination. The eggs are checked to see if fertilization has occurred, identified by the presence of two pro-nuclei. The fused egg and sperm nuclei are known as a zygote, or early embryo.

- **Day 2** At this stage the embryo usually consists of between two and four cells. The second cell division takes place 45–46 hours after insemination.

- **Day 3** The third cell division takes place about 54–56 hours after insemination. By this stage, the embryo has 6–8 cells. The individual cells that make up an embryo are known as blastomeres.

- **Day 4** Compaction (when cells start to merge together) occurs and the embryo is known as a morula.

- **Day 5** The embryo now has many cells and develops a fluid-filled cavity. Now it is a blastocyst.

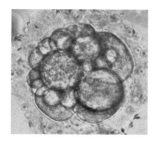

Grade 3 embryo: *slightly uneven cell division with much fragmentation between cells.*

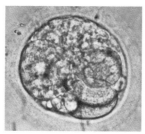

Grade 4 embryo: *uneven cell division and excessive amounts of fragmentation between cells.*

Q&A

○ **Which drugs accompany this stage?**

Most clinics will prescribe progesterone or HCG (human chorionic gonadotrophin)—the hormone that is produced once the placenta attaches—to prepare the uterine lining to accept a fertilized egg and provide support for a developing embryo. Heparin, ritalin, or aspirin are also prescribed by some clinics to help blood flow.

○ **How many embryos should I transfer?**

You will not be allowed to transfer more than two embryos at a time, since the danger of complications rises significantly with a multiple pregnancy. Talk to the clinic about this early on, so that you feel comfortable with the decision before it is time to transfer.

○ **What happens to embryos that are not transferred?**

Most clinics can freeze embryos and store them for about five years to use in other IVF cycles. The live birth rate per cycle from frozen embryos, however, is usually lower than from fresh embryo transfers.

○ **Is bed-rest recommended after transfer?**

Complete bed-rest, for a minimum of three days, is very important. It will not guarantee a pregnancy, but gives the embryos a better chance of implanting. Activity diverts blood to your extremities and vital organs, while lying down allows blood to flow to the endometrium. Do not feel guilty about taking time off work or staying in bed.

○ **When does implantation occur?**

An embryo reaches the blastocyst stage five days after fertilization and starts to break out of its outer shell during the following 48 hours. Only then can it implant. How soon this happens after transfer depends on the the stage of the embryo.

○ **Which factors affect implantation?**

The embryos must be of good quality, the endometrium needs to have thickened, and your body must not have an immunological reaction to the embryos.

TRANSFERRING EMBRYOS

This procedure happens between 48 hours and five days after fertilization, depending on what you and your fertility specialist have decided. It is quite an achievement to have gotten this far, so think positively and try to ignore your anxiety as you progress to the next stage. Always keep in mind that nothing is certain, and it is possible to beat the odds. I have seen successful pregnancies result from low-grade embryos, from frozen embryos, and from poor-quality sperm.

Your embryos will be loaded into a small, flexible catheter that will be inserted through the vagina and cervix into the uterus. Ideally, you should have an empty bladder, so avoid drinking very much liquid on the morning of the transfer. Some clinics map out your uterus in advance: others use an abdominal ultrasound to guide embryos into place, in which case your bladder needs to be full. When the catheter is in the optimum position near the top of the uterus, the embryos are expelled and the catheter slowly removed. It is then checked back at the lab to make sure that there are no embryos sticking to it.

KEEPING CALM

The smoother the transfer, the greater the chance of success. Lying on your back for a clinical procedure may contribute to your anxiety. The adrenaline released by the body in response to the stress you are experiencing may cause the uterus to contract, which will not be helpful to the procedure. So use relaxation techniques such as deep breathing, visualization, or meditation (see pages 42–43) to calm yourself down. If you are able to watch what is taking place on a screen, it will give you a better idea of what is happening to your embryos and make visualization easier.

It may be reassuring to have your partner along with you for the transfer, but don't insist upon it if he is reluctant. You need someone to help you reduce stress levels during the procedure, not contribute to them.

the two-week wait

Remember that to have come this far is fantastic, considering all of the other hurdles you have had to negotiate. I believe that women have forgotten how to convalesce—you have been through a lot, so give yourself time!

THE WAITING GAME

There will be good days and bad days over the next two weeks as, full of anxiety, hope, and a desperate longing to know if you're pregnant or not, you ride yet another emotional roller coaster. Allow yourself to be optimistic. Even if this is not your first IVF cycle, you are bound to feel a sense of anticipation. Try to banish negative thoughts and repeat to yourself—"I *am* pregnant. This *is* working."

DAYS 1 TO 4

After all the regular scans and tests, you may feel a bit lost and cut off. You should call the clinic at any time if you are concerned. A friend can be a great support, especially if your partner is adopting a pragmatic "either it's worked or it hasn't" attitude. You could use an IVF website or chatroom to "talk" to other women who are going through the same experience.

Rest and relaxation "Carry your embryos with pride," one woman once said to me. Don't feel guilty about taking time off work and lying in bed. You will want to be very careful with yourself. Rest and sleep will give your body the best chance to repair and take the course you want it to. At the very least, lie on the sofa with your feet up as often as possible. Watch videos back-to-back; read books.

Your body prepares for the implantation of an embryo with a cycle of hormonal stimulation. The ovary continues to produce progesterone, the cells of the blastocyst start to release HCG (human chorionic gonadotrophin), the endometrium thickens, and the site of implantation becomes swollen with a supply of new blood capillaries.

The Chinese believe that if you focus your mind on a particular area in your body, *qi* or life energy will flow to that spot. So spend 15–20 minutes every morning and evening visualizing what is going on inside your uterus: the embryos are floating safely and are ready to embed in the endometrium, which is thick and well prepared.

In traditional Chinese medicine, the kidneys play an important role in reproduction. They may quickly become depleted of energy during an IVF cycle. The kidneys are particularly active from 5 PM to 7 PM, so make sure you rest quietly then. Deep breathing will help you relax and enhance the supply of oxygen reaching your uterus.

Other measures Certain essential oils used in burners or candles can help to lift your mood or soothe and calm you. Try lavender for relaxation; lemon, lime, or grapefruit to raise your spirits; or jasmine if you are feeling low. Alternatively, the flower remedy (see page 147) mimulus may help if you are feeling overly anxious about the

---

WHAT NOT TO DO

During the two-week wait, you must avoid:

- caffeine, tobacco, alcohol, drugs
- heavy lifting
- strenuous exercise, including housework
- bouncing activities, such as horseback riding or aerobics
- sun bathing, saunas, hot tubs, jacuzzis, hot baths
- swimming
- sexual intercourse

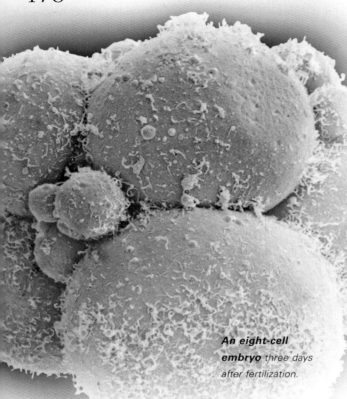

An eight-cell embryo three days after fertilization.

outcome of your egg transfer. If you are finding it difficult to relax, try white chestnut flower remedy. If you are haunted by past failures, take walnut.

Keep the lower abdomen warm—I cannot stress this enough—but stop using a hot-water bottle. Remember that you cannot "grow" a baby if this part of the body is cold. Eat warm, nourishing food.

Finally, make sure your diet is rich in protein, zinc, and essential fatty acids (see pages 55–56 and 59–64). Take a good multivitamin and mineral supplement and DHA. Eat foods that are rich in selenium (see page 63), and remember to drink a minimum of two quarts (liters) of water a day.

DAYS 5 TO 7

You may be starting to get restless, obsessively thinking about the implantation, looking for signs that things are going according to plan, and possibly misinterpreting every symptom. Sore breasts, mild shooting pains, and bloating are all indications, in fact, that things are going well.

It's very important to keep yourself occupied. Go for a leisurely walk or do some gentle yoga. Focus on the color blue if you feel yourself starting to panic. Practice deep breathing and meditation (see pages 42–43) to help you relax. Talk your worries through with a friend or your partner but focus on the positive.

You might like to consider acupuncture (see pages 72–73) seven days following transfer, when the embryo will be starting to implant. Try to imagine the embryo embedding in the thickened endometrium. Ideally, it will implant on the back wall of the uterus. New blood capillaries then start to develop and the placenta begins to form. The cells in the embryo continue to divide rapidly, forming a two-layered disk, the top layer of which will become the embryo and the amniotic cavity, and the lower of which will be the yolk sac.

DAYS 8 TO 14

The waiting game seems to be going on forever. Even if you have gone back to work, you must still try to take things easy and avoid any stressful situations. Only do light tasks, and rest as much as you possibly can. Spend your free time seeing friends or plan a long weekend away, rather than doing lots of things around the house.

Acupuncture may be beneficial at this stage to boost your kidneys. Make sure you see an acupuncturist who has experience of treating women who are pregnant as a result of IVF treatment. Interestingly, one of the relevant acupoints treated on the kidney meridian is called the Gate of Life (see page 73).

There are a number of other complementary treatments you might like to try at this point. Have an aromatherapy massage, but make sure you visit a qualified practitioner and tell them about the treatment you have been having. Meditate for at least 20 minutes every day.
Do lots of positive visualization.

By all means, exercise, but keep it low-key, such as leisurely walking, gentle yoga postures, tai chi, or qigong. Avoid all forms of aerobic exercise.

PREGNANCY TESTING

The only way you can be sure whether or not you are pregnant is to have a blood test—an HCG (human chorionic gonadotrophin) or beta blood test—at your fertility clinic. It really is best not to use a home testing kit, which might give you an agonizingly misleading result, but of course I know that in reality many women will just not be able to resist doing so.

HCG is the hormone that starts being produced as soon as the embryo attaches to the endometrium (see page 12). The level doubles every 48 hours in the first six weeks of pregnancy and then every 72 hours for the next 2–4 weeks after that. The level peaks at about 8–10 weeks, then declines and remains at a lower level until term.

Even the most sensitive blood test cannot detect HCG until about ten days after ovulation, and there is huge variation in what is regarded as the "normal" level. Pregnancies that eventually miscarry or that are ectopic often show normal HCG levels initially, while low levels may still produce a healthy pregnancy.

If you were given an HCG injection as part of your fertility treatment, it might distort readings for 14 days. Doing two tests on different days usually solves this problem: if the level increases on the second, the likelihood is that you are pregnant. So try not to resort to using the "evil pee sticks"—wait until your clinic can give you a definite and accurate result that will not be accompanied by any nagging doubts.

GETTING THE RESULTS

If the result of your pregnancy test is positive, many congratulations! Your longed-for goal has been realized at last. Take a moment to absorb the information, relax, and then celebrate. Be prepared, however, for conflicting emotions as you think about what lies ahead. Many women feel lost when they suddenly have no medication to take or doctors to visit. Nurture yourself, especially if you have been anxious.

CASE HISTORY

Elizabeth, aged 26, was diagnosed with polycystic ovary syndrome (PCOS) after her periods stopped. She took the contraceptive pill until she got married, but then found her periods stopped again. After a year she sought help and was prescribed clomiphene. The next three months she describes as "absolutely horrific. I couldn't sleep, I was tearful; it was like having bad PMS all the time."

It became clear that Elizabeth was still not ovulating. She felt very discouraged and "ready to give up" the idea of having a baby altogether. A friend of hers recommended that she come to me for acupuncture treatment. I referred her on for further fertility testing. Following a hysteroscopy and laparoscopy, which confirmed that Elizabeth was not ovulating, she decided to opt for IVF. "I felt bloated and hormonal when I started the treatment, but I just had to get on with it."

Elizabeth's first cycle of IVF was successful but, sadly, she lost her baby at seven weeks. Four months later she began a second cycle and is now pregnant again. "The whole experience has brought my husband and I much closer together and has made this pregnancy even more special."

DEALING WITH A NEGATIVE RESULT

If the result of your pregnancy test is negative, do not despair. Don't try to put on a brave face: accept the fact that you feel devastated. Many of my clients who have received a negative test result report that a failed IVF cycle resembles a mini-miscarriage, with exactly the same feelings of loss and grief. Allow yourself time to mourn the collapse of your dream of a baby this month. Take a few days off work if necessary. Be antisocial if you want to be. It will be hard to imagine at the time, but you will feel stronger after a few weeks.

Although you may feel at your lowest ebb right now, the experience you have just been through has by no means been a waste of time. Your clinic will have learned a great deal about you and your physiology that will enable them to make adjustments to the treatment program if there is going to be another attempt. If you are anxious to try again, arrange a meeting with your fertility consultant and talk about what has been learned and what could be done differently next time.

I have seen very many women go on to conceive at their next attempt at IVF, after they have taken three months off for rest and recuperation, physical as well as mental. If, however, you feel you have reached the end of the road and you cannot put yourself through it again, talk to your doctor about other options, but always try to keep an open mind. You might change it.

ZITA'S TIPS

● **The second week is the worst** One minute you will be fairly sure that the treatment has worked and you have conceived a baby, but the next minute you will be plunged into despair, convinced that it hasn't worked and your period is imminent.

● **You will feel very hormonal** Emotional fragility may make you feel very vulnerable and as if you have no control over your fate.

● **Reading the signs** Remember that every woman's experience is different. There is no standard set of symptoms that you get as side effects of all the drugs you have been taking, or as you recover from the IVF cycle, or during the early stages of pregnancy (see opposite), for that matter. Whatever the "signs" are, you will probably be just as able to translate them negatively as positively, depending on the mood you are in at the time. You may have no symptoms at all, but you might have bloating and fluid retention, breast tenderness, drowsiness and exhaustion, slight cramping, PMS symptoms, night sweats, aversions to certain foods, nausea, and slight bleeding or a brownish discharge. If you are not pregnant, you may start to bleed before two weeks after transfer.

● **Stay focused on your goal** Continue to practice relaxation techniques, meditate, and visualize positive outcomes. Don't look too far ahead; stay in the present and take each day as it comes. Banish negative thoughts as they arise and only listen to stories and read statistics if you can deal with them, whatever they are, without overreacting.

● **Seeing babies** You may find there is a recurrence of the phenomenon you experienced as you set out down the road to conception— seeing pregnant women or people with babies everywhere you look!

● **After a negative result** Don't make any rash decisions. If you want to try again with IVF, your initial instinct may be to make a fresh start at another clinic. Listen to what your consultant has to say about the recent attempt, however, before you make up your mind, and don't forget how many factors you had to weigh up carefully before you made a choice in the beginning. Take time out before you decide.

pregnancy following IVF

Receiving the longed-for "positive" result of a pregnancy test may have seemed like an end in itself. Finding out that you are expecting a baby, however, may just be the start of a whole new wave of anxieties—about how best to prevent a miscarriage and maintain the pregnancy—as well as a source of deep joy.

THINKING PREGNANT

It can be really difficult to let go of what has gone before and think of yourself with confidence as a pregnant woman. Take each day at a time, and remember that the odds of your pregnancy being successful improve with every week that goes by. Anxiety tends to be a much more common feature of pregnancy following IVF. Every twinge or ache or pain can be a source of worry.

Getting to the 12th week is the first big hurdle. The fetal heartbeat has usually been detected by this point. Your doctor will listen for it using an ultrasound device as part of a routine prenatal check. Ninety-four percent of pregnancies carry through to a positive conclusion once the fetal heartbeat has been picked up.

A transvaginal scan will ensure that your pregnancy is not ectopic. There is a higher risk of an ectopic pregnancy following IVF because the embryos float around for longer before implanting. Try to limit the number of transvaginal scans you have and opt for abdominal scans instead.

TAKING CARE

Many women who have been through IVF feel terribly sick in early pregnancy. Welcome this as a good sign and expect to feel exhausted: in other words, feel good about feeling bad. But if you don't feel bad, don't worry! Bear in mind the following:

- spotting or a slight brownish discharge are normal and nothing to worry about. If bleeding gets heavier, call your clinic immediately.

- avoid caffeine, alcohol, tobacco, strenuous exercise, and hot baths, just as you did during the post-transfer period (see page 177), and drink two to three quarts (liters) of water a day.

- I advise couples not to have sex for the first 12 weeks of pregnancy if they can avoid it.

- get plenty of rest and early nights. Take time off work if you need to. Right now, maintaining your pregnancy is more important than anything.

- consider a course of acupuncture to replenish and build up energy in the kidneys. Acupuncture has also been shown to be effective in helping to relieve nausea and sickness.

ZITA'S TIPS

To relieve nausea and sickness in early pregnancy:

- **eat small, frequent meals**, avoiding spicy or fatty foods. Take a good multivitamin and mineral supplement to ensure that you are not deficient in vitamin B6, magnesium, or zinc.

- **be sure to get as much rest** as you can during the day and as much sleep as possible at night, since fatigue and severe sickness seem to be linked.

- **stimulate the Pericardium 6 acupoint** on your forearm, three finger-widths above the wrist crease between the two tendons. Apply gentle presssure for ten minutes, four times a day.

looking at other options

If diagnosis and treatment have ruled out the possibility
of having your own child, you need to ask yourselves some
important questions. Can you accept that only one partner
is a biological parent? Should you consider adoption?

SPERM DONATION

If your partner is producing no sperm at all, or if
he is at risk of passing on a genetic disorder, donor
insemination (DI) may be the only way that you as
a couple can have a child. Sperm banks vary in
methods of screening anonymous donors' sperm.
Seek out banks that follow guidelines such as
those of the American Association of Tissue Banks.
DI is being used less with the success of micro-
manipulation techniques such as ICSI (see page
174), which enable men who have low sperm
counts to fertilize their partners' eggs.

Donors can be matched to your partner for race,
build, coloring, and blood group. "Quarantining"
procedures also ensure safety. Check that the
donated sperm has been thoroughly tested for HIV
and a variety of infections before being frozen and
quarantined for six months. It should be thawed
immediately before use.

Your cycle will be monitored by body temperature,
an ovulation prediction kit, or ultrasound scans
and, if necessary, you will be given fertility drugs
to ensure ovulation. Insemination occurs at
ovulation, when sperm are placed in the vagina,
cervix, or uterus. If several cycles do not produce
a result, DI may be combined with IVF.

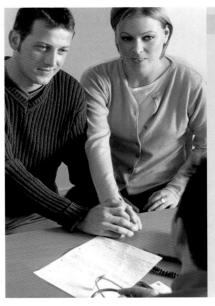

WHAT YOU NEED TO KNOW ABOUT DI

Although donor insemination may be the next logical step, it has psychological and
emotional implications, particularly for your partner, who will be fathering a child
that is not genetically his. Consider the following before you make a final decision.

- **You must both take the time to talk** about all the issues involved. Don't
  pressure your partner if he isn't willing—DI must be right for both of you.

- **Counseling is essential** because of potential ethical, legal, and social
  repercussions. Your partner should consent, in writing, to become the legal
  father of any child born as a result of donor insemination.

- **Many states allow donors to relinquish parental rights** so they have no
  legal claim to children conceived and born using their sperm.

- **Your decision to opt for donor insemination remains private**. You don't
  have to tell anybody, and nobody else ever needs to know.

EGG DONATION

Egg donation is becoming an increasingly common option and may be one you should consider. If you are not producing eggs, perhaps because of an inherited condition, surgery, chemotherapy, ovarian disease, or early menopause, the only way you may be able to conceive and carry a child yourself is by using donated eggs. This is also an option for women over 40 whose egg quality is declining and for women who are at risk of passing on a genetic disorder to their offspring. If you use a donated egg, you and your partner will still be able to bond with the baby throughout your pregnancy and the birth. Half your baby's genes will belong to your partner and you will both be the baby's parents. As with sperm donation, however, you do as a couple need to think long and hard about all the issues involved.

Both you and the donor should get counseling to help you consider the emotional, social, medical, legal, and ethical issues surrounding egg donation. You need to consider, for example, how and when you will tell your child about his or her genetic origins. As with donor insemination, your decision to use donor eggs can remain private.

WHAT IS INVOLVED?

The donor has to go through the IVF cycle as far as egg collection. The donated eggs are then fertilized by your partner's sperm and the resulting embryo is frozen until you are ready for it to be transferred. This may occur immediately if your cycle has been manipulated to match that of the donor.

IVF success rates with egg donation cycles tend to be higher than with routine IVF because the eggs are almost always from women under the age of 35, and you (the recipient) have not gone through super-ovulation drug treatment. This means that your endometrium is in a more natural state of receptivity, although you may be given estrogen to encourage implantation. On the other hand, egg donation can be emotionally stressful and you will have to deal with the uncertainty about whether or not the donor will produce enough eggs.

In the US, egg donors can be compensated for their time and trouble. Organizations like the American Society for Reproductive Medicine (ASRM) can tell you where treatment is available and offer guidelines on screening for viral conditions and genetic disorders. Although a relative can be a donor, you are more likely to use an anonymous donor, who will be matched as closely as possible with you for race and blood type, among other characteristics.

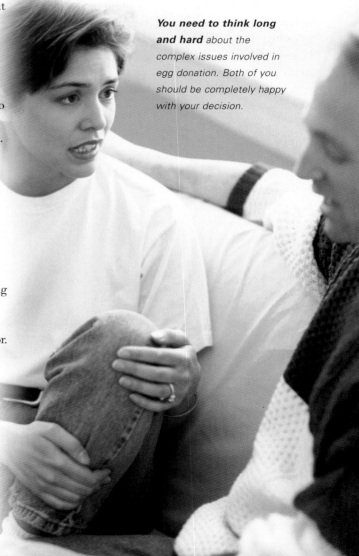

You need to think long and hard about the complex issues involved in egg donation. Both of you should be completely happy with your decision.

moving on

"How will I know when it's time to give up and move on?" That's the million-dollar question I get asked time and time again. The answer is, of course, different for every couple.

COMING TO A CONCLUSION

The decision that you are ready to give up the fight to have your own biological child is possibly the one stage in the process of planning for a baby that is the least predictable. If you have fertility problems and have been undergoing treatment, you will keep moving the goalposts until you reach the point at which you realize that enough is enough and you have gone as far as you are prepared to go. It is possible for almost every couple to have a baby if they really want one. It is a question of how far they are prepared to push the limits as they deal with their fertility problems and, perhaps at the end of a long treatment road, they consider options such as egg donation, surrogacy, or the adoption of a child.

You won't know exactly when this realization is going to dawn until it occurs. The factors conspiring to bring about the decision might include:

• whether or not you think your relationship can withstand any more of the pressures of trying to have a baby of your own
• whether or not you have the financial resources to pursue any more options
• whether or not you have the emotional strength to keep going
• whether or not you feel as if your body has been through enough
• the advice of your doctors and the predicted odds for success of any further treatment or option
• your age at your next birthday

There is usually a doctor somewhere who, with the best possible intentions, will offer "just one more thing you could try," and it is tempting to hang on to yet another last thread of hope. Don't, however, become so fixed on an endless pursuit that you lose all sense of perspective. Be careful not to become so wound up with the quest to become a parent that a sense of failure overshadows all the positive aspects of life, destroying your self-esteem.

Some women wake up one day knowing they have reached the end of the road, and are ready to reclaim their life and their body. They want to stop defining themselves in terms of their fertility and regain a sense of normality. Others realize this gradually. If you and your partner do not get to this point at the same time, you will need to give each other time and support, and you may need counseling to help you do this.

NO REGRETS

It is important, as far as possible, to move on from fertility treatment knowing that "you've given it your best shot," and to be able to look back in five years and view the whole experience without any regrets. That means knowing that you:

• adopted all the necessary nutritional and lifestyle changes that were recommended to you to enhance your fertility
• received the best medical attention that you could afford at the time
• followed the recommendations of your doctors and specialists
• pursued all the treatment options that were appropriate for you and that had a reasonable chance of success
• gave each option your best effort, thinking positively about it and believing in it

MIXED EMOTIONS

You may have made a monumental decision, but the emotional roller coaster of the last few months or years may not be over just yet. Expect to feel some, if not all, of the following:

- **relief** that there are no more tests, scans, injections, or other procedures that you will have to endure
- **liberation** from what felt like a never-ending cycle of hope and despair
- **anger** because "this wasn't the way it was all supposed to end"
- **betrayal** because the medical profession has failed, despite all the resources and latest technology at its disposal, to give you the right answers or solutions
- **grief** and a huge sense of loss as you mourn the child you will never have
- **exhaustion**, both physical and emotional
- **strength,** because you've not only survived intact but have grown in the process
- **freedom** to take back your life and return to some kind of normality
- **hope** as you plan for a new future

Give yourself as much time as you need to work through each of these emotions. Complete emotional healing and recovery may take years, but it is important to come to terms with some of these feelings as soon as possible. Talking them through with a friend or therapist and reviewing the road you've traveled since you first started to think about having a baby can be a very constructive part of the healing process.

WHAT ABOUT THE FUTURE?

You will then be ready to move on and investigate the options of surrogate parenting, adopting, fostering, or, of course, child-free living. It is now time to think very carefully about these issues:

- how important to you and to your partner is the experience of raising a child?
- how important is the necessity for one of you to have a biological/genetic link to that child?

Make sure that you and your partner understand each other's needs so that the solution you choose suits both of you equally. The more clearly you can identify and fully appreciate your reasons for wanting to be a parent in the first place, the more clearly you will be able to identify the right path forward in the future. As many couples will tell you, there are more ways to create a happy family than by giving birth to a baby.

CASE HISTORY

Having suffered seven miscarriages over five years and tried four IVF cycles, all of them unsuccessful, Sarah started to think about surrogacy. "I first heard about surrogacy in the 1980s when it was making the news. I never thought I'd be in a situation where I had to consider it. But soon the idea of conceiving a child of our own, carried by a surrogate, started looking better and better to me." *Sarah decided to pursue a surrogacy program and started to learn about the laws in her state regarding surrogacy.* "It has proved to be yet another emotional roller coaster. I had slight misgivings about the first surrogate, so I decided not to go ahead. I didn't want to act out of desperation but to keep looking until I found someone with whom I felt totally comfortable. The second attempt has gone well so far. It's still early, but I'm optimistic it will work out."

further information

REFERENCES

Page 20
Journal of Family Planning and
Reproductive Health Care, 2001, 27 (2),
103–10

Page 30
Longscope C G, Orbach S, Goldin B et
al, 1987, *Effect of low-fat diet on
oestrogen metabolism*, J Clin Endocrinol
Metab, 64 (6), 1246–49

Page 31
Arnold S E, Klotz D M, Collins B M et al,
1996, *Synergistic activation of oestrogen
receptor with combination of environmental
chemicals*, Science, 272, 1489–92; Baird
D, *Smokers face higher infertility*, J Am
Med Assoc, 1985, 253, 2979–83;
Bopp B and Shoupe D, 1993, *Luteal Phase
Defects*, J Repro Med, May, 38 (5), 348–56;
Tuormaa T E, *Adverse effects of alcohol
on reproduction: literary review*,
International Journal of Biosocial and
Medical Research, 14 (2), In press, 1994

Page 33
Wilcox A et al, *Caffeinated beverages
and decreased fertility*, The Lancet, Vol
2 (1998), 1453–55

Page 34
Baird D, *Smokers face higher infertility*,
J Am Med Assoc, 1985, 253, 2979–83;
Tuormaa T E, *Adverse effects of alcohol
on reproduction: literary review*,
International Journal of Biosocial and
Medical Research, 14 (2), In press, 1994;
Ward N et al, *The placental element
levels in relation to foetal development
of obstetrically normal births. A study of
37 elements. Evidence of the effects of
cadmium, lead and zinc on fetal growth,
and smoking as a cause of cadmium*,
International Journal of Biosocial
Research, Vol 9 (1), 1987, 6308;
Wyn M and Wyn A, *The case for pre-
conception for men and women*, AB
Academic Publishers (1991)

Page 36
Batzinger R P, Ou S Y L, and Bueding
E, *Saccharin and other sweeteners:
mutagenic properties*, Science, 1977, 198,
944–46;
Fertility and Sterility, vol 71, no 3,
March 1999;
Goyer R A, *Lead toxicity: a problem in
the environment*, Am J Pathol, 1971, 64,
167–79;
Ondrizek R R, Chan P J, Patton W C,
and King A, Department of Gynecology
and Obstetrics, Loma Linda University
School of Medicine, California, USA,
*Inhibition of human sperm motility by
specific herbs used in alternative
medicine*, J Assist Reprod Genet, 16,
87–91, Feb 1999;
Reif-Lehrer L, *Possible significance of
adverse reactions to glutamate in
humans*, Federation Proceedings, 1976,
35, 2205–11, 1976
Schroeder H A and Tipton I H,
The human body burden of lead,
Arch Environ Health, 1968, 18,
965–78;

Page 41
Fertility and Sterility, 2001, 76:3, 10–16.
©2001 by American Society for
Reproductive Medicine.

Page 46
Grant Ellen, *Sexual Chemistry*, Cedar
Press, 1994

Page 47
Farrow A, Hull MGR et al, *Prolonged
use of oral contraception before a
planned pregnancy is associated with a
decreased risk of delayed conception*,
Human Reproduction (ALSPAC study),
Vol 17, 2002, 10, 2754–61
Gnoth C, Frank-Herrmann P, Schmoll
A et al, *Cycle characteristics after
discontinuation of oral contraceptives*,
Gynecol Endocrinol, 2002, Aug 16 (4):
307–17

Vessey M P, Smith M A, Yeates D,
Oxford, FPA study, *Return of fertility
after discontinuation of oral
contraceptives – influence of age and
parity*, British Journal of Family
Planning, 1986, Vol II, 120–40

Page 59
Crawford M A, *The role of dietary fatty
acids in biology: their place in the
evolution of the human brain*,
Nutritional Reviews (1992), 50, 3–11;
Czeizel A E et al, Dept of Human
Genetics and Teratology, WHO
Collaborating Centre for the
Community Control of Hereditary
Disease, Budapest, Hungary, *The effect
of pre-conceptional multivitamin
supplementation on fertility*,
International Journal for Vitamin and
Nutrition Research, 1996, 66 (1) 55–58;
Shrimpton Derek, *A scientific evaluation
of the range of intakes*, commissioned
by the European Federation of Health
Product Manufacturers' Association and
published by the Council for
Responsible Nutrition, October 1997;
Olsen F F, *Does fish consumption during
pregnancy increase fetal size? A study of
the size of newborn, placental weight,
gestational age & fish intake*,
International Journal of Epidemiology
(1990), 19, 971–77

Pages 68–75
Journal of Family Planning and
Reproductive Health Care, 2001, 27 (2),
103–10

Page 69
Rex K M et al, *Nocturnal light effects on
menstrual cycle length*, Journal of
Complementary Medicine, 1997, 3,
387–90;
Roennburg T and Aschoff J, *Annual
rhythm of human reproduction: 11
environmental correlations*, Journal of
Biological Rhythms, 1990, 5, 217–39

Pages 72–73

Chen B Y, *Acupuncture normalises dyfunction of hypothalamic-pituitary-ovarian axis*, Acupunct Electrother Res, 1997, 22, 97–108;

Steer C V, Campbell S, Tan S L, Crayford T, Mills C, Mason B A et al, *The use of transvaginal colour flow imaging after in vitro fertilization to identify optimum uterine conditions before embryo transfer*, Fertil Steril, 1992, 57, 372–76;

Stener-Victorin E, Waldenström U, Andersson S A, and Wikland M, *Reduction of blood flow impedance in the uterine arteries of infertile women with electro-acupuncture*, Hum Reprod, 1996, 11 (6), 1314–17;

Stener-Victorin E, Waldenström U, Nilsson L, Wikland M, and Janson P O, *A prospective randomized study of electro-acupuncture versus alfentanil as anaesthesia during oocyte aspiration in in-vitro fertilization*, Hum Reprod, 1999, 14 (10), 2480–84;

Stener-Victorin E, Waldenström U, Tagnfors U, Lundeberg T, Lindstedt G, and Janson P O, *Effects of electro-acupuncture on anovulation in women with polycystic ovary syndrome*, Acta Obstet Gynecol Scand, 2000, 79 (3), 180–88

Page 74

Costa M, Canale D, Filicori M et al, *L-carnitine in idiopathic asthenozoospermia: a multicenter study*, Andrologia, 1994, 26, 155–59;

Dawson E B, Harris W A, Teter M C, and Powell L C, *Effect of ascorbic acid supplementation on the sperm quality of smokers*, Fertil Steril, 1992, 58, 1034–39;

de Aloysio D, Mantuano R, Mauloni M, and Nicoletti G, *The clinical use of arginine aspartate in male infertility*, Acta Eur Fertil, 1982, 13, 133–67;

Fraga C G, Motchnik P A, Shigenaga M K et al, *Ascorbic acid protects against endogenous oxidative DNA damage in human sperm*, Proc Natl Acad Sci, 1991, 88, 11003–06;

Schacter A et al, *Treatment of oligospermia with the amino acid arginine*, Int J Gynaecol Obstet, 1973, 11, 206–09;

Tanimura J, *Studies on arginine in human semen. Part III. The influences of several drugs on male infertility*, Bull Osaka Med School, 1967, 13, 90–100.

Page 109

Morton R F, *Candidal vaginitis natural history predisposing factors and prevention*, Proceedings from the Royal Society of Medicine, Vol 70 (4), 1997, 3–6;

Sutton G, *Genital infections*, Midwife and Health Visitor and Community Nurse, 18 (2), 1982, 42–45;

Weidner W, *Ureaplasmal infections of the male urogenital tract in particular prostatitis and semen quality*, Urology International, Vol 40, 1982, 42–45

Page 113

RS *Microbiology of the female genital tract*, Am Obstet and Gynae, 1987, 156, 491–95

Page 120

Yu J, Zheng M, and Ping S M, *Changes in serum FSH, LH and ovarian follicular growth during electro-acupuncture for induction of ovulation*, Chung Hsi I Cheih Ho Tsa Chih, 1989, 9, 199–202

Page 131

Sliutz G, Speiser P, Schultz A M et al, *Agnus Castus extracts inhibit prolactin secretion of rat pituitary cells*, Horm Metab Re, 1993, 25, 253–55

Page 149

Gravitz M A, *Hypnosis in the treatment of functional infertility*, Am J Clin Hypno, 1995, 38, 22–26;

Hernandez-Reif M, Martinez A, Field T, Quintero O, Hart S, and Burman I, Touch Research Institute, University of Miami School of Medicine, Florida, USA, *Premenstrual symptoms are relieved by massage therapy*, J Psychosom Obstet Gynaecol, Mar 2000, 21 (1), 9–15.

USEFUL WEBSITES

UNITED STATES

American Society for Reproductive Medicine (ASRM)
www.asrm.com

Society for Assisted Reproductive Technology (SART)
www.sart.org

RESOLVE
www.resolve.org

American Infertility Association
www.americaninfertility.org

American College of Obstetricians and Gynecologists Resource Center
www.acog.org

American Urological Association, Inc.
www.auanet.org

American Association of Tissue Banks
www.aatb.org

Fertilitext
1-900-PREGNANT

Polycystic Ovarian Syndrome Association
www.pcosupport.org

Compassionate Friends
www.compassionatefriends.org

SHARE—Pregnancy and Infant Loss Support, Inc.
www.nationalshareoffice.com

SIDS Alliance
www.sidsalliance.org

MEND (Mommies Enduring Neonatal Death)
www.mend.org

Child Welfare League of America
www.cwla.org

Organization of Parents through Surrogacy
www.opts.com

The Triplet Connection
www.inreach.com/triplets

Mothers of Supertwins
www.mostonline.org

CANADA

Infertility Awareness Association of Canada
www.iaac.ca

Multiple Births Families Association
www.mbfa.ca

index

acknowledgments

Zita West would especially like to thank Sharon Baylis for helping her to collate the raw material for this book and to write it. She would also like to thank: Jude Garlick for her help and enthusiasm over the last six months; her family—husband Rob, Sofie and Jack; Vicki McIvor; Anna Davidson, Anne Esden, Salima Hirani, and Corinne Roberts at DK; Dr. Sheryl Homer for her input on male fertility and IVF; Melanie Brown and Jane Knight; Emma Cannon, Sally-Anne Caplin, Hilary Haines, Jane Knight, Chew yeen Lawes, Clare Mellon, Joanne Miller and Karen Taylor at her clinic; Paul Armstrong (Consultant in Obstetrics and Gynaecology), Gerad Kite, Julia Leonard, Karl Olah, Pandora, Bernadette Kelly Rivers, Ian Spiers, Titiana Wait, and Martin Watt.

DK Publishing would like to thank Dr. Mary Jane Minkin for U.S. medical advice and Dr. Chris D. Meletis for his help with herbs and botanicals. Dorling Kindersley would like to thank Lucas Mansell for proofreading, Sue Bosanko for the index, and picture librarians Hayley Smith and Romaine Werblow. They also thank the following for their kind permission to reproduce their photographs: (Abbreviations key: t=top, b=bottom, r=right, l=left, c=center)

1: Getty Images/Paul Vozdic (c); 3: Getty Images/Sarah Jones (Debut Art); 4-5: Science Photo Library/Dr. Yorgos Nikas; 6-7: Getty Images/Deborah Jaffe; 8-9: Getty Images/Roz Woodward;

10: Science Photo Library/Alfred Pasieka (bl), Professor P. M. Motta et al. (br); 11: Science Photo Library (bl), Dr. Yorgos Nikas (br); 12: Science Photo Library/Pascal Goetgheluck (b); 13: Science Photo Library/D. Phillips (cll), Dr. Yorgos Nikas (cl), (crr), Professor P. M. Motta & J. Van Blerkom (cr); 15: Science Photo Library (br); 18: Corbis/Rick Gomez; 21: Getty Images/Joe Polillio; 23: Getty Images/Color Day Production; 25: Getty Images/Paul Viant; 34: Getty Images/Romilly Lockyer; 36: Getty Images/Eric Larrayadieu; 39: Getty Images/David Seed Photography; 44: Getty Images/V.C.L.; 46: Getty Images/HOM; 48: Getty Images/Stephanie Rausser; 50: Science Photo Library; 54: Getty Images/Chris Cole; 60: Getty Images/Jed & Kaoru Share; 62: Getty Images/Dennis O'Clair; 65: Science Photo Library/Martin Dohrn; 69: Getty Images/David Sacks; 74: Getty Images/Lori Adamski Peek; 77: Science Photo Library/Innerspace Imaging; 80: Getty Images/Ghislain & Marie David de Lossy; 82: Getty Images/Anthony Marsland; 83: Getty Images/Ghislain & Marie David de Lossy; 84: Getty Images/Alexander Walter (tl), Yorgos Nikas (bc); 85: Getty Images/Ron Chapple; 86: Getty Images/Sarah Jones (Debut Art) (br), Werner Bokelberg (tl); 89: The Wellcome Institute Library, London; 90: Getty Images/Jerome Tisne (tl); 91: Corbis/Donna Day (b); 92: Corbis/Roy Mchon; 94: Getty

Images/Antonio Mo; 97: Getty Images/Rob Van Petten; 99: Mother & Baby Picture Library/emap esprit; 100: Science Photo Library/Professors P. M. Motta & S. Makabe; 103: Science Photo Library/Nancy Kedersha; 110: Science Photo Library; 111: Getty Images/Romilly Lockyer; 115: Science Photo Library/Chris Priest; 123: Getty Images/Zigy Kaluzny; 127: Getty Images/Ghislain & Marie David de Lossy; 129: Getty Images/Frederic Tousche; 138: Getty Images/Color Day Production; 140: Getty Images/Romilly Lockyer; 142: Getty Images/Derek Berwin; 146: Getty Images/Michelangelo Gratton (t); 147: Getty Images/Jim Franco; 148: Science Photo Library/Cordelia Molloy; 151: Science Photo Library/Edelman (br); 154: Getty Images/Oliver Strewe (bl); 157: Getty Images/Paul Vozdic; 160: Getty Images/Peter LaMastro; 165: Getty Images/Gary Buss; 170: Science Photo Library/Prof. P. Motta/Dept. of Anatomy; 172: Getty Images/Daniel Bosler; 174: The Wellcome Institute Library, London/K. Hardy (bc), (br); 175: The Wellcome Institute Library, London/K. Hardy (bl), (br); 178: Science Photo Library/Dr. Yorgos Nikas; 182: Mother & Baby Picture Library/emap esprit (bl); 183: Getty Images/David Harry Stewart.

All other images © Dorling Kindersley. For further information see: www.dkimages.com

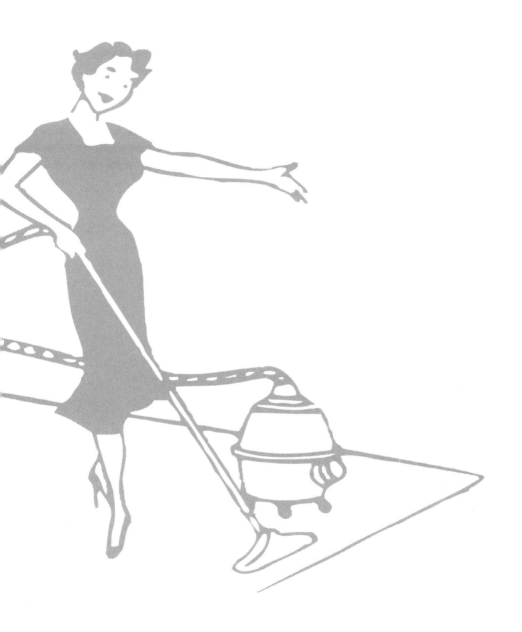

mediaworks

nancy paterson

surrey art gallery

ISBN 0-920181-52-x

Canadian Cataloguing in Publication Data
Paterson, Nancy, 1957 –
Media works, Nancy Paterson

Catalogue of an exhibition held at the
Surrey Art Gallery, Feb. 6 – May 14, 2000.
Includes bibliographic references.

1. Paterson, Nancy, 1957 – – Exhibitions. I.
Davison, Liane, 1960 – II. Gigliotti, Carol.
III. Cutler, Randy Lee. IV. Surrey Art Gallery
(B.C.) III. Title.
N6549.P39A4 2001   709.2   COO-911526-9

This publication was produced to accompany
the exhibition "Second Nature:
Autobiographies in New Media by Nancy
Paterson" held at the Surrey Art Gallery
February 5 - May 14, 2000.

Cyberfeminism was first published online
on the echo gopher server (NYC) in 1992.
First hard copy publication in *Fireweed, A
Feminist Quarterly of Writing, Politics, Art
& Culture*, issue #54 (summer 1996).

Technology ≠ Art was first published in
Fuse, Vol. 20, #5, (Fall 1997)

Curly, Larry & PoMo was first published in
Astrolabe: Online Journal, 1998.

The artist would like to thank the Canada
Council for the Arts, the Ontario Arts
Council and the Toronto Arts Council. She
would also like to acknowledge donations
from the following companies: Pioneer,
Casio, Polaroid, GVC Canada, Toronto Stock
Exchange, Biolink Computer R & D, Protec
Microsystems, Platinum, Apple Canada, ATI
Technologies, SGI, Leeson Motors and
Globe Motors.

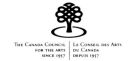

Surrey Art Gallery
13750-88th Avenue, Surrey, B.C. Canada V3W 3L1

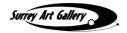

BRITISH
COLUMBIA
ARTS COUNCIL

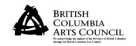

THE CANADA COUNCIL | LE CONSEIL DES ARTS
FOR THE ARTS | DU CANADA
SINCE 1957 | DEPUIS 1957

SURREY
CITY OF PARKS

designed by the Rädish design studio
printed at Kromar Printers, Canada

contents

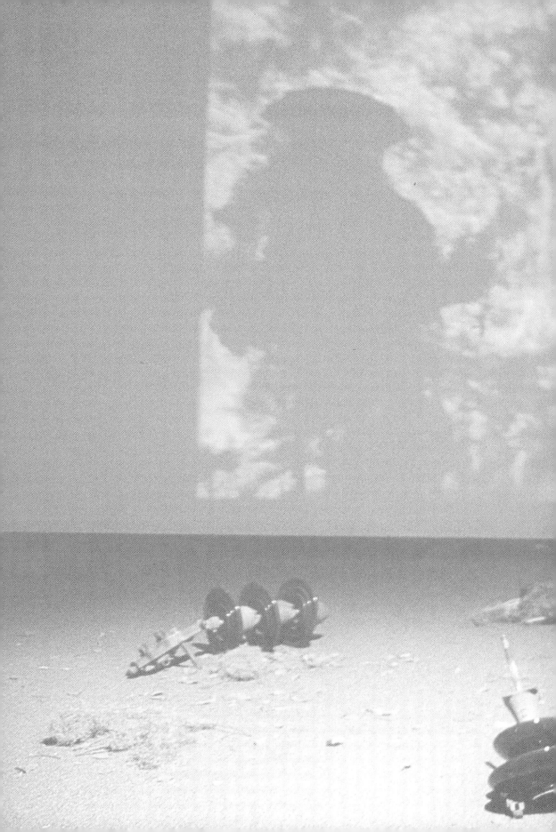

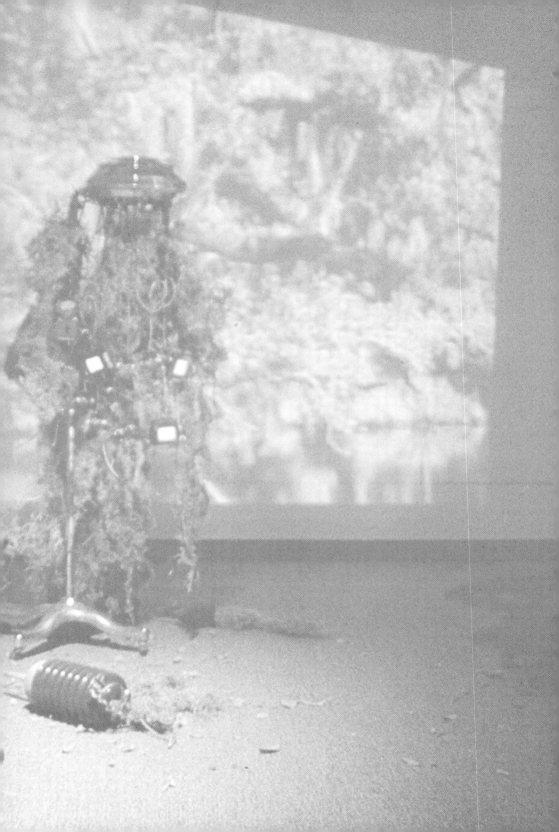

introduction   liane davison

Electronic technology represents for us the development of an external central nervous

system. And inevitably, our hearts will truly beat within the machine.[1]

New electronic technologies are like a jar of marbles that has slipped off the edge of a table

and crashed, shattering, scattering marbles in a million different directions. Inconsolable, you

are <u>never</u> going to gather up all those marbles again, and it's slightly dangerous to try.[2]

Just as artists have helped envision and even create the future with their experimentation and exploration of new technologies, they also have the skills to open our eyes to the present. Nancy Paterson is one such artist, versed in new media, who doesn't hesitate to poke at our complacency and with her humour chide us to remain conscious of our assumptions about the world. She twists media into forms that reveal the mechanisms and means of our seduction, exposing the powers that are manipulating us. Paterson provides a perspective as a Canadian, as a woman, and as a citizen of the world concerned about the future.

Our culture has become dependent on computer technology, as the recent Y2K paranoia, clearly indicated. On December 31, 1999, at New Year's Eve parties around the world, people were carrying pagers or cell phones – just in case. Meanwhile, their less fortunate friends were bunkered in at work as members of "first response" teams for possible Y2K disasters. Globally, billions of dollars were spent to ensure technology's continued momentum. In the end, nothing much went wrong. But as we entered 2000 it was as if the toboggan of our culture had been pulled over a precipice and there was no turning back. Are we sliding down a thrilling, slippery slope to be totally engulfed by a techno-wonderland? Nicholas Negroponte, originator of the Media Lab at MIT, recognized the force of techno-progress when he said, "Once a new technology rolls over you, if you're not part of the steamroller, you're part of the road."[3] Generally, we're dazzled and delighted by technology. We want it to be faster, smaller, lighter, more convenient, cheaper, and even invisible. What is the implication of this for our society – a utopic cyberspace or something less optimistic? Artists like Nancy Paterson ask themselves these kinds of questions, and their work illustrates their thinking.

Named by *Shift* magazine as one of the 10 "digerati to know" in 1995,[4] Nancy Paterson continues to be hailed as one of Canada's foremost cyberfeminists and techno-media artists. She has lectured and exhibited her media works around the world. Her projects consistently maximize whatever technology she can get her hands on. In the mid-1980s, she designed video matrixes with complex switching systems to control the logic and presentation of imagery. In the early 1990s, she used laser discs to create immersive, interactive video environments. Her recent computer work has resulted in one of the first telerobotic sculptures totally interfaced with the Internet. And at the turn of the millennium she employed computer graphics and VMRL to produce one of the most complex and detailed 3D environments available on-line. Although her use of technology is impressive, it is her ideas, and the forms that they take, that make her work significant and original.

Paterson's art not only looks towards the future but also holds hands with the past, particularly with the 1950s, when technology still held forth the promise of building a utopia by the year 2000. When you think of art using the latest in digital technology, you probably wouldn't expect to see wringer washers, electric hair-curling machines, or old bicycles in a gallery. But a hallmark of Nancy Paterson's art has been the combination of '50s "automations" with today's technology. Old machines, particularly the ones designed by men for women (to "help" women with their domestic work, or to make them more beautiful) fascinate her. Paterson's media works often juxtapose the promise of these machines (reduced work, increased pleasure) with the socio-political reality. The optimism of a machine's "space age" industrial design is revealed to be ironic, and issues such as women's oppression and environmental decay are shown to be unresolved. Paterson challenges the viewer to recognize that even though technology and machines have come a long way, other aspects of our culture have not progressed as quickly.

Paterson didn't originally plan to become a media artist. Her education began at the Victoria College of the University of Toronto. In first year, she was accepted into a third-year course taught by Northrop Frye. This class, along with others in literature and philosophy, gave her a solid grounding in the classics and trained her to be articulate and clear in her thinking. In late 1982, she went across campus to the engineering department, and secured her first Internet account. Although she eventually completed an honours degree at the Victoria College in 1985, she interrupted her academic studies at one point to follow a radical impulse and applied to the Ontario College of Art. There she became embroiled in student politics while she learned the basics of visual art practice. During OCA's four-year program, she joined up with fellow artists Derek Dowden, David Andrews, Graham Smith, and Ed Mowbray to launch Toronto's first media gallery, the Artculture Resource Centre (ARC) in 1979.

At ARC, Paterson became familiar with early new media works that employed the still-novel personal computers, fax machines, and Telidon.[5] The exhibitions she organized at ARC by artists such as Vera Frenkel, David Rokeby, and Brian Eno inspired her to pursue her interest in cultural theory and feminist politics through her own video installations. Her skills in mechanics and electronics, honed since childhood, encouraged her to experiment with the splitters and relays for video signals. She began work on her first video installation project, *HairSalon TV*, in 1984. The feminist content evident in this early work recurs throughout Paterson's *oeuvre*. Curator Daina Augaitus commented on the significance of the video clips in a 1987 essay: "As compulsive consumers of hygiene and home products, women are depicted in a master/slave involvement with technology. . . . These videos also recall the oppressive factors of the ongoing technological revolution, especially its high toll on the growing number of workers who are in servitude to increasingly exploitative technocratic developments in the worksite. . . . Paterson's chosen clips also portray the rare instances where women's participation on the upper rungs of the hierarchical ladder has been significant."[6]

After ARC folded in 1985, Paterson began working at another artist-run centre in Toronto, Charles Street Video. There she played a role in the unionization of that facility, while continuing to create more video sculptures, including *Wringer/Washer TV* completed in 1989. By the late 1980s, Paterson was experimenting with new technology to create interactive video experiences. Her *Bicycle TV*, an interactive installation produced in 1990, and one of the first of its kind internationally, provides a viewer/bicycle-controlled tour through Bracebridge, a small town in Ontario. Continuing to experiment with interfaces for interaction, Paterson eventually replaced the bicycle with a joystick for *Expo92*, so named after its exhibition at the Canadian pavilion at the world's fair in Seville, Spain. The video tour is in fact a video maze wherein viewer "virtually travels down interconnected paths that eventually lead back onto themselves." Paterson comments that she mapped the video sequences so that the viewer wouldn't "slip off the edge of the disc." For its time, the creation of this parallel world — where one may imagine one has control — represented a very sophisticated use of laserdisc technology. *Bicycle TV* presents an alternative to the computer graphics-dominated industry of virtual reality, actualizing the techno-worlds imagined for *Star Trek's* holodeck, or the 1998 movie *The Truman Show*.

Paterson continued to investigate technology that would allow her to create immersive video environments responsive to a person's presence and activity within a gallery venue. For *The Meadow*, produced in 1996, she videotaped the surrounding of a selected site in rural Ontario from four different perspectives (to the north, south, east, and west) over the course of a year. These views are projected onto the gallery's four walls to simulate a wraparound landscape in different seasons. Paterson utilizes ultrasonic transducers to read visitor position and movement within a fixed area, triggering changes in the seasons depicted, from winter to spring and so on, forwards and backwards in time. The movement of visitors also controls and composes the sequence and selection of sounds in the environment, as though technology is rewarding their actions. This viewer-manipulated virtual-reality landscape, like *Bicycle TV*, appears to give participants some measure of control over nature. In fact, in these works nature is fully mediated.

Meanwhile, Paterson was also engaged in the theoretical discourse surrounding the use of technology. She began work towards a master's degree in education which she completed in 1997, split between Brock University and the Ontario Institute for Studies in Education. While, working on her thesis on the topic of cyberfeminism, she created what can be considered a self-portrait: *The Medusa Project (Autobiography)*. For the artist, this work brings together several concerns: her interest in feminism and technology, the relationship between nature and culture, and her own personal history. The work presents a contemplative non-interactive environment featuring a figurative form created from a six foot tall, 1920s electric hair-curling machine, draped with Spanish moss, and several small LCD screens that shed blue-green light (and sometimes captured ambient TV signals). Projected across the sculpture onto a length of wall is video footage of a tangled swamp environment, shot near a small town in Florida where the artist spent time as a child. The installation is strange, with this quiet "monster" centrally present in the landscape. But it is also peaceful, with the sounds of water, rustling foliage, and birdsong filling the gallery.

The *Medusa Project* is a response to the rhetoric that nature and culture are not compatible, arguing against the cultural assumption that women are more "natural" and therefore do not have a significant place in the world of high technology. This work invites the viewer into a very techno-mediated environment from a woman's perspective. Paterson's use of the name Medusa is also revisionist. We popularly know Medusa as a murderous monster with hair of snakes so frightening that those who looked upon her turned to stone. But the ancient version of the myth is quite different. Medusa was one of the Gorgons, a trinity of three goddess sisters, along with Stheno and Euryale. Together they represented Wisdom, Strength, and Universality. Born of the gods of the Earth and the Ocean, Medusa was the only mortal.[7] The power to turn men to stone was the power to protect secrets and mysteries.[8] Also believed to be the goddess of the Libyan Amazons, Medusa, by being the guardian of divine female wisdom, was also thought to possess knowledge of the future and to protect it with her fearful powers.[9] Paterson's Medusa, constructed of equal parts machine, technology, and nature, presents the symbolic intertwining of the past, present and future. She is bathed in mediated nature, a figure that is both in and of technology.

Unlike artists working in traditional media, who are able to maintain a private studio and be fairly self-sufficient in the use of their tools and the production of their art, Paterson eventually required partnerships and support that, for many, stretches the concept of who artists are, what they can do, and how they work. In 1997, Paterson was invited to become an Artist in Residence at the new Bell Centre for Creative Communications (Centennial College) in Toronto. [10] BCCC provided Paterson with not only a studio space but also access to tools and resources essential for an artist working on the cutting edge of new media — constantly upgraded, state-of-the-art computer equipment, technical specialists, information and computer networks, media facilities, and exceptional bandwidth — to help her visions become reality. In return, Paterson was asked to be available as a lecturer and mentor to students, to conduct research, and to participate in information sharing. This arrangement at BCCC, and increasingly at other institutions, recognizes artists as intellectuals who, with their imagination and creativity, are contributing to the envisioning and realization of the future of computer technology.

One of the projects enabled by Paterson's BCCC residency was the *Stock Market Skirt*, her first work involving the Internet. "I wanted to make an artwork that dealt with the Internet as an emerging intelligent thing itself, because it is. Granted, it's a mile wide and an inch deep. It's a lot like watching [the game show] *Jeopardy!* There's a thin veneer of information with not a lot of depth or context to it."[11] Running on the open-source Linux operating system, *Stock Market Skirt* uses a specialized program developed to continuously check the value of a composite index or a selected stock. These values, retrieved from various financial Web Sites on the Internet, activate the sculpture every second. When no real-time stock prices can be obtained (such as when the markets are closed) the system defaults to other foreign exchanges or uses archived data. The changing stock prices trigger a stepper motor, which mechanically lifts or lowers the hemline of a blue taffeta and black velvet party dress made by Paterson, exhibited on a dressmaker's mannequin called a "Judy."

Arguably one of the first pieces to not only comment on the Internet but also to rely on it for interactivity, this telerobotic work responds to the global flow of information and a capitalist culture. Accessible both on-line via a Web cam and in a gallery setting, the work expresses a relationship between the stock market and the length of women's hemlines, echoing the Desmond Morris theory that fashion responds to the economy. Described by Paterson as a cyberfeminist fashion statement, *Stock Market Skirt* has been featured in fashion and business magazines as well as in art journals such as *Flash Art*[12] and *Tema Celeste*.[13] Paterson laughs when she talks about the microprocessor controlled Singer sewing machine used to make the dress. The mostly male computer technologists were puzzled because they weren't familiar with that particular "computer," she says.

For *Stock Market Skirt* and other recent works, bandwidth has become the broad brush with which Paterson has learned to "paint." She is often quoted as saying that "bandwidth is political" and is quick to point out that "very few cultural facilities in Canada have any bandwidth to speak of"[14] and are therefore unable to exhibit many kinds of new media work. *Stock Market Skirt*, like e-mail, "slurps" very little bandwidth; but at the same time, connectivity is integral to the project. For exhibition, this work, *Stock Market Skirt* requires constant and reliable connectivity to enable perl[15] scripts to continuously request and retrieve the stock data that control this installation.

At the other end of the spectrum, but still focusing on bandwidth, Paterson developed a 3D project titled *The Library*.[16] Initially produced as an on-line VRML environment at the Bell Centre, this project was supported in part by the Canada Council's Millennium Arts Fund. The design of this 3D virtual environment is based on an extraordinary building, the beautiful rotunda of the Canadian Library of Parliament in Ottawa.[17] *The Library* contains interactive objects and sculptures distributed throughout the environment. These objects, including a globe and a telescope, represent different creative interpretations of the themes of the project: navigation and wayfinding, as they relate to the millennium. The first phase of this project, which premiered in at BCCC in early 2000, uses a broad bandwidth of 200 Mbps. "I've always wanted to build a library," says Paterson of both her personal and professional motivations behind the project. "They represent the important core repositories of science, language, culture, and heritage within a society. But the library of the 21st century must move beyond the physical limitations of shelf space and two-dimensional cross-referencing. I see information as a living entity, and a creative work that's always in progress."[18]

In 2000, Paterson became the Coordinator of the artist-in-residence program at BCCC, opening up the opportunities offered by this facility to other artists, after she was invited to be a visiting artist at Seneca@York University,[19] also in Toronto. At this institution, Paterson had the opportunity to further develop *The Library*, when she was given access to ORAD Virtual Studio technology. This technology allowed her to "composite" people into her computer graphic environment, enabling them to walk around and behind virtual objects. The new version of the project was titled *The Library²*. *The Library³* is under development.

As her relationship with Seneca@York continues, Paterson has embarked on a project that has interested her for years: the retelling of *Coppelia*, from the robot's point of view. *Coppelia*, considered the first feminist ballet, premiered in Paris in 1870. It is a comedy about a pair of lovers who overcome a problem in their love affair. Franz blows one too many kisses at Coppelia, thinking the life-size creation of Dr. Coppelius is really alive. To create this work, Paterson has begun working with dancers and a life-size custom-constructed robot. The ORAD is being used for the production of video sequences, which will appear in both an installation and a performance. Paterson says: "Working with dancers, the robot, and the ORAD has opened up a whole new area of experimentation and improvisation for me."[20]

The marketing of technology and its products promises that we will be better connected, more efficient, more beautiful, or richer with them in our lives. We're entertained and seduced, no differently than those who saw the first electric appliances 60 years ago. Paterson quipped in one interview that the centrefolds of *Wired* magazine were airbrushed computers, that they were the pornographers of digital culture, selling increasing desire for more technology. But she doesn't want our response as consumers of technology to be complacency or awe. Paterson is more demanding of those who view her works: "*Working with video and electronic technology, I am interested in engaging the viewer in an active and introspective analysis of the role of electronic media in contemporary culture . . .I am interested in the development of virtual reality systems and the sociological implications of this new technology.*"[21]

Whether it is her innovative work with the Internet and dynamic 3D environments or her deconstruction and hybridization of machines from the 1950s, Paterson offers insight into our desires and our humanity. When she says, "In the future, everyone will be famous for 15 megabytes,"[22] she is commenting on the Internet and the issues regarding copyright and creativity. And, anticipating the day when "our hearts will truly beat within the machine," she refers to biotechnology and the ethical dilemmas inspired by technology's physical and medical interventions. Nancy Paterson, through her media works and her writing, challenges us to explore our power to design the future while recognizing technology's impact on every aspect of our culture.

notes

1   Nancy Paterson, "Lust & Wanderlust: Sex & Tourism in a Virtual World," *Media Information Australia, Art & CyberCulture*, No. 69, 1993.

2   Quoted from a presentation by Nancy Paterson at the Kunst und Ausstellungshalle der Bundesrepublik Deutschland, in Bonn, Germany.

3   Nicholas Negroponte, quoted in *The Media Lab: Inventing the Future at MIT*, by Stewart Brand (New York: Viking, 1987).

4   Rodney Palmer, "Who to Know: The Digerati," *Shift*, November 1995: p. 30.

5   Telidon, a graphics system that offered the possibility of two-way television, was a Canadian invention developed by the Communications Research Centre in the late 1970s.

6   Daina Augaitus, in a catalogue essay for *Siting Technology*, Walter J. Phillips Gallery, Banff, 1987.

7   *The New Larousse Encyclopedia of Mythology* (Prometheus Press, 1968), p. 183.

8   Barbara G. Walker, *The Women's Encyclopaedia of Myths and Secrets* (New York: Harper & Row, 1983) p. 349.

9   Ibid: p. 629.

10   Focusing on education in communications media, the Bell Centre has the world's largest single educational installation of Silicon Graphics workstations and one of Canada's most advanced fibre-optic networks. Web site: <www.bccc.com>.

11   Quoted in a review in *Cybertimes*, by Matt Mirapaul , New York Times, February 5, 1998.

12   David Pescovitz, "Be There Now: Telepresence Art Online," *Flash Art*, March/April 1999, p. 51.

13   Daniele Perra, "Navigando in Rete con Gli Artisti," *Tema Celeste* (Milan) May/June, 1999.

14   E-mail from the artist to the author.

15   Perl is a programming language commonly used for writing interactive applications for the Internet.

16   This project incorporates the work and input of a team of people, including Ann Medina, Beryl Fox, Al Razutis, and modellers/programmers Paul Dobson and Peter Robbinson. The Banff Centre for the Arts was also a supporting partner. Paterson also acknowledges the support of companies including Platinum, Apple Canada, and SGI, and organizations including Human Resources Development Canada through Youth Employment Services and the Information Technology Association of Canada (IRAP).

17   The Library of Parliament in Ottawa, Ontario, was built between 1859 and 1876, to plans drawn up by the architectural partnership of Thomas Fuller and Chilion Jones. Modelled on the Reading Room of the British Museum, this distinctive circular structure features a ring of 16 flying buttresses, pinnacles, decorative windows, and beautiful ornamental ironwork. It is the only part of the original Parliament Buildings to survive the 1916 fire.

18   "Virtual Library Project: Waiting for the Future," *New Media Pro*, May 1999, p. 14-16.

19   Seneca@York is a partnership between Seneca College of Applied Arts and Technology and York University. It is housed in a new facility that provides state-of-the-art learning opportunities using the newest electronic communications and network technology. Web site: <www.senecac.on.ca>.

20   E-mail from the artist to the author.

21   As quoted in the exhibition catalogue for *TechnoArt: An Interactive Media Exhibition*, Ontario Science Centre, 1994.

22   Nancy Paterson, quoted from a presentation at the Surrey Art Gallery, February 2000.

the perogative to change our minds :

The environment in which we find ourselves is familiar but incongruously strange. We immediately recognize items: televisions, mannequins, a bicycle, a satellite dish. After that first
recognition, however, the item's individual place among other items and our surroundings
betrays wisps of unfamiliarity, like puffs of gas from a canister ready to explode. Suddenly, the
explosion of disorientation overcomes us. For that minute, all meaning disappears. The smoke
blinds our eyes, as they burn and water. Sight leaves us, and with it goes understanding.
Soon, though, the smoke begins to clear. Now, each object seen previously brings with it several descriptions. It's a satellite dish, yes, but it's also a weapon, or maybe a religious symbol.
And that is a TV set, but it only has one image on its screen. What is that teepee doing there?

That disenchanted, disconnected feeling is now, more than ever, not unusual to us. We of the
twenty-first century are here, now, forever, and in the future. It is no longer a fantasy, but a
reality of time. Unable to go back, doomed to move forward, we can never go home again.
Wherever that was.

Calmed by this realization, since the feeling of unfamiliarity has become a familiar one, we
can turn our attention to the direct inspection of these objects and this place in which we
find ourselves. It occurs to us that perhaps they have something important to say. I go
through something like this every time I see an installation by Nancy Paterson. Paterson's
work always sneaks up on me, knocks me out for a time, and then leaves me room to breathe
and think. Sort of a pugilistic Zen experience. Having followed Paterson's work for the last
seven years or so, I continue to have that experience upon seeing each new piece. I believe it
has as much to do with Paterson's understanding of the technologically human present as it
has to do with her take on the cyborgian future. And curiously enough, like a Zen experience,
her environments clear a space for me to consider both the possibilities and the dead-ends
each of these phases of the future- present provide for the practice of the spiritual.

Many other contemporary artists are hard at work translating, reconfiguring, re-shaping, and
re-interpreting our relationship with technology. Just as the familiar objects in Paterson's
pieces belie the deeper meaning of their situations, so do surface familiarities with
Paterson's work belie the wider influences with which that work is interconnected.
International artists such as Char Davies, Eduardo Kac, Brenda Laurel, Victoria Vesna, Jill
Scott, Christa Sommerer and Laurent Migonneau, and Thecla Schiphorst, among many others, are attempting to look beyond the acceptance of assumptions upon which the development of current technology is based. Their work offers alternatives to the acquiescence usually
offered in the face of scientific activity.

the work of nancy paterson carol gigliotti

Underlying the misgivings fostered by our hard-driving commitments to computer technology is a deep-seated concern about our spirit. A central tenet of this concern is the constraint technology places upon our ability to define and communicate that spirit. Artists involved with computer technology are simultaneously questioning, supporting, repudiating, subverting, altering, and sustaining particular processes integral to computer technology as a communication medium and as an aesthetic process.

The design and development of contemporary interactive computer technologies innately involve aesthetic choices. Aesthetic choices have the capacity for mediating sensory perception and affect judgment. In affecting judgment those choices convey both value and meaning, and in that capacity become ethical choices as well.[1] For those working to develop these technologies, both artists and other kind of developers, the aesthetic, the ethical, and the spiritual are inextricably mingled with the functional, the expedient, and the materialistic.

In *Beyond the Postmodern Mind*,[2] religious historian Huston Smith, outlines what he considers to be the four major phases of religious activity throughout the world thus far. His description of these phases, which exhibit similarities across cultures, revolves around an understanding of personal, social, and environmental ethics. For Smith,

"An ethic is an assemblage of guidelines for effecting the self-transformation that enables the world to be experienced in a new way."[3]

According to Smith, the first phase, Archaic age, lasted until the beginning of the first millennium and did not focus on humanity. People in the Archaic age focused instead on the beyond, seeing it as a bearer of meaning and timelessness in sharp contrast to the finite and confusing quality of life itself. Humans living in small familiar groups saw the rituals and myths that grew out of these concerns as more immediately integral to their lives than interpersonal matters. The second phase, the Axial age, saw prophets, seers, and mystics in Israel, Persia, India, and China preaching similar messages of interpersonal ethics. In this phase, the goals of conscience, compassion, self-knowledge, and forgiveness were nurtured. The third phase, the Modern age, added a sense of collective responsibility to the religious agendas of the Archaic and Axial ages. The rise of modern science in the seventeenth century and the age of enlightenment in the eighteenth led people to see that social structures are changeable. As Smith points out,

"if society can be changed, it often should be changed, in which case its members are responsible for seeing to it that it is changed."[4]

The earlier religious agendas of timelessness, interpersonal matters, and social ethics are being extended during the current and fourth phase, the present age, by concerns for and feelings of connection with other species and the environment. Smith insists, however, that religion in its many forms can only remain relevant and useful, if both the spirituality of the Archaic and Axial ages and the social and environmental interests of the Modern and present ages remain vital.

I quote Smith at length because his wide-ranging view of religion and spirituality is helpful to any discussion of the spiritual dimensions of artistic work within the electronic medium. This focus, I think, comes not only from past spiritual traditions in the arts, but from spiritual concerns of the Modern and present ages. These concerns are most clearly implicated in electronic culture's discernible impact on an emerging worldview of a global market and culture. Despite many hyperbolically positive descriptions of this impact, it needs to be stated that negative outcomes are just as possible.

I propose here that Paterson's work is better understood and appreciated in a wider context of current art-making as offering contemporary environments for debating, investigating, and formulating alternative perspectives to current and future problems. These aesthetic environments are similar to spiritual organizations in their search for alternative ethical solutions.

The ubiquitous and wide-ranging possibilities of current interactive technologies raise many such ethical questions, including a fundamental one involving technology as the epitome of rational thinking, specifically of logic. This, in turn, raises the question of whether we are able to comprehend the logic of a system by that same logical method. The incompleteness theorem, also known as Godel's proof, has allowed scientists to perceive many forms of rationality as well as the possibility that among these forms no rational thought processes can be used to comprehend why multiple rational methods might work.[5]

Many artists involved with the electronic medium have found the polarization of rational thought and creativity to be counter/productive. They have found, instead, the need to access as many cognitive processes as possible to grapple with this medium in what they perceive to be an ethical and spiritual way. Scientific thinking makes every effort to banish mysticism, just as mystical thinking attempts to banish rationality. Each type of cognition attains its peak performance if it can achieve its goals completely. Yet both kinds of cognition are possible in everyone. Human thinking is composed of the mixed strategy of these two radically opposing methods of cognition. Humanity itself cannot exist without these two methods. They exist in individuals in varying proportions, but all of us use both of them.[6]

This approach, helpfully outlined by game theorist Mero, is reiterated by a number of contemporary ethical theorists. One is Mark Johnson, whose philosophical theory of "moral imagination"[7] is based on current research in cognitive science. Others, such as the feminist ethicists Noddings, Gilligan, and Ruddick,[8] see ethics as a process of growth and change. The point on which these ethicists agree is an embodied understanding of ethics based on metaphor, imagination, and reflection. Artists such as Paterson are concerned with the fact that we practise ethical decision making through daily actions, many of which today are mediated by technology.

"The crux of this view, moral criticism as fundamentally imaginative is that moral objectivity consists not in having an absolute, God's-eye point of view, but rather, a specific kind of reflective, exploratory, and critical process of evaluation carried out through communal discourse and practice."[9]

In her aesthetic decisions, Paterson practises multiple strategies, both rational and mystical, to enhance our experience of technologically mediated ethical questioning. Her work aggressively asks us to question our normal reactions to technology by simultaneously using distancing methodologies of rationality and logic, morally imaginative methodologies of ethics and aesthetics, and intuitive methodologies of mysticism. The interactive punch in Paterson's work, aside from the participation it requires, is the engagement it demands.

Paterson uses technology itself in her work to highlight several consistent and interrelated themes. These themes, simply put, are the consequences of technology for women, for nature, and for notions of destiny and chance. Paterson constantly throws us up against a difficult issue that at first seems to have only one solution. What we find, however, after our initial shock, anger, irritation, amusement, or resignation at being cornered, is encouragement to disagree. Paterson's skilful use of layered metaphors often allows for hilarity at that first solution, and so makes a space within that solution to imagine other alternatives.

In *The Machine in the Garden*, the casino slot machine appears to control the video monitors and the images they display. The passiveness of the woman covering her eyes, ears, and mouth on both the LCDs and the monitors bookends the images of war, game show hosts, religious figures, children's programming, and TV commercials. The cause and the effect seem evident and inevitable. We have been silenced by our own greed. We have listened to the charlatans of contemporary market culture and even though the consequences of acquiescence have been disastrous, we continue to listen.

Pulling the lever a second time, however, allows us a second chance to question the cause and the effect. Are the images from the slot machine or the video monitors? On second glance this woman doesn't look like a passive victim, instead she looks like the proverbial mischievous monkey. Is she offering, in the Zen Buddhist sense, a koan on which to meditate? Are negative consequences merely the luck of the draw or can we make different choices? The text that Paterson usually uses to accompany this piece quotes Stephen Hawking's response to Einstein's famous edict, "God does not play dice." Hawking's response, "Not only does God play dice, but sometimes he throws them where they can't be found," explains the post-Godel outlook. This acceptance of non-rational understanding is a central motif in Paterson's branch of cyberfeminism.

Paterson's construction of a feminist technological and ethical program for action – one on which a spiritual approach to technology can develop – includes hard-driving rational action combined with mystical amusement and humility. Her work demonstrates Huston Smith's wide-ranging view of religion as a combination of multiple strategies of ethics and mystical understanding. As well, it may be seen in contemporary quantum physics' to demonstrate the same use of multiple strategies for understanding cosmology.

The Meadow explores this cosmological space through metaphors of nature and of technology, helping us to place ourselves in a world that is both real and simulated. In *The Meadow*, the physical space between the video displays is an ambiguous one. It is neither nature simulated for us on the monitors and through the sound system nor technology that both constructs and mediates our experience. This space has been fabricated by another set of technologies, that of architecture, and, perhaps, the cultural space of the gallery. This "real" space, of seeming emptiness and yet, full of its own set of metaphors, offers a place to imagine other possibilities. Johnson's description of moral criticism as "a specific kind of reflective, exploratory, and critical process of evaluation carried out through communal discourse and practice,"[10] works well in generating these possibilities. This kind of moral imagination is nothing new to feminists, nor for that matter to any sincere practitioners of spiritual traditions.

Paterson's *Stock Market Skirt* also generates possibilities. Here our immediate response is, "Oh yes, Paterson is right. The stock market, fashion, the fashionably fascinating fashion of the internet are only just as meaningless as each other." But then, look again and you may see Paterson's *Stock Market Skirt* as a spiritual icon for cyberfeminists. The image of the leaping heroine, with her transparent levels of skirt gaily holding aloft the laptop, and all the literature accompanying the piece certainly push my thinking in that direction. Joan of Arc, Shiva, the Virgin Mother, and the Black Madonna are all rolled into one powerful symbol of the prerogative of each woman to change her mind. And then to change all our minds.

This capacity for the spiritual, and the ethical is not a new one for art. The capacity art has for wisdom and change, however, is currently being tested by artists such as Paterson through their involvement with a medium belonging not only to the sphere of the arts, but to the wider world of human, and perhaps other, forms of communication.

notes

1 C. Gigliotti, "Aesthetics of a Virtual World: Ethical Issues in Interactive Technological Design," (Ph. D. diss. Ohio State University, 1993), abstract in *Dissertation Abstracts International*.

2 H. Smith. *Beyond the Postmodern Mind*, 2nd ed. (Wheaton, Illinois: Quest Books, 1989).

3 Smith, 72

4 Smith, 187

5 L. Mero, *Moral Calculations: Game theory, Logic and Human Frailty*, (New York: Springer-Verlag, 1998, 252.

6 Mero, 254

7 M. Johnson, *Moral Imagination: Implications of Cognitive Science for Ethics*, (Chicago: University of Chicago Press., 1993).

8 See especially, C. Gilligan, *In a Different Voice*, (Cambridge, Mass.: Harvard University Press, 1982), N. Noddings, *Caring*, (Berkeley: University of California Press, 1984), and S. Ruddick, "Maternal Thinking." *Mothering: Essays in Feminist Theory*. J. Treblicat (Totowa, N.J.: Romand and Allenheld, 1983).

9 Johnson, 217.

10 Johnson, 217.

The human artifice of the world separates human existence from all mere animal environments, but life itself is outside this artificial world, and through life man[sic] remains related to all other living organisms. For some time now, a great many scientific endeavors have been directed toward making life also "artificial," toward cutting the last tie through which man[sic] belongs among the children of nature . . .

— Hannah Arendt [1]

new beginnings: nature is not the opposite of culture In 1958, Hannah Arendt wrote about technology and how it leads to a split between culture and nature. In the 1950s things were a bit more cut and dry. Even so, Arendt was a female philosopher writing about the narrow direction that humanity was moving towards. In her vision, culture and nature were in opposition and never the twain shall meet. Forty years after Arendt's warning, at the dawning of a new millennium, we understand that 'nature' is not a pure entity but often overlaps with artifice.[2] Nature has become a construct, an idea for advertisers to hawk or an unstable commodity in the hands of corporate greed. And yes, this too was part of Arendt's message. The confusion around nature's corporate image can result in a relinquishment of agency. "What can I do?," we ask ourselves. Back in 1958, Arendt engaged with the thinking of the day by polarizing the issues. Today, we see more clearly that by relegating the world into binaries, nature/culture, woman/man, mind/body, we lose control of our images, then our bodies and finally our natural environment.

While technology itself is not the enemy, our attitude is. We need to reinvest meaning into the world and the stories we tell. The blurring of nature and artifice need not lead only toward cutting the last tie through which we belong among nature. The fusion of boundaries and points of view can also produce promising alternatives to traditional scientific objectivity. Lived reality is a lot more complicated and the picture more blurred than we are prepared to admit. The ties through which we belong and connect with the world can also come from science and technology. Artifice can be reframed and given new meaning. There are many Canadian media artists who explore these issues by engaging with the creation, manipulation and images of technology. In so doing they challenge the simplistic thinking of binary logic. Nature is both inside and outside our bodies. In particular, work by Canadian media artists like Nancy Paterson, Catherine Richards, Nel Tenhaaf and Thecla Schiphorst offer provocative, metaphorical readings of nature by problematizing the boundaries between nature and culture. By nature, I am thinking of the landscapes, bodies and forces that have become a recurring subject of contemporary media practice. These artists offer imaginative contexts and fascinating interfaces that engage the embodied viewer, making awareness a priority. In this essay I will explore the production of awareness and engagement with regard to artificial constructions in the art of Nancy Paterson.

remapping the terrain randy lee cutler

responsive awareness Awareness of the interconnections between technology and affect is central to any thoughtful consideration of new media art practice. Embedded within the structures of at least some of these 'artificial worlds' (as Arendt put it) is a deep ecology of nature, gender and empowerment. Affect is the emotional and mental influence of a given phenomenon or set of ideas; it has the power to inform, alter and change all those who experience it. Where effect is the (passive) *result*, affect is the (active) *response*. Arendt's caution toward the destructive power of scientific endeavors does more than sound an alarm. It can mobilize and redirect energies. Current practices in new media, particularly those by women, have visualized invisible forces and investigated the pervading paradigms of technoculture which inform our everyday lived realities.

In *Understanding Media: the Extensions of Man* (1964), Mcluhan reminds us of the effects that technology can have on our relationship with the world. "It is a necessary approach in understanding media and technology to realize that when the spell of the gimmick or an extension of our bodies is new, there comes narcosis or numbing to the newly amplified area."[3] Narcosis insinuates itself on one's body, mind and spirit. It is the *result* of passively accepting the limited information that crosses our paths. Nancy Paterson's artwork is an intelligent, cyberfeminist response to the numbing effect that images can have by inserting novel forms of interface. Her work allows the viewer to engage with ideas and appreciate more exciting interventionist strategies; tools and visions that circumnavigate the negative effects often induced by technology.

cyberfeminism or bust! Since the early eighties, Nancy Paterson has been working with and addressing the evolution of technologies and their impact on our everyday lives. As a self described cyberfeminist, Paterson engages with the implications of new media on women and how marginalized groups might wrestled control from the dominant techno-narratives. Her work embraces a range of issues, too numerous to be considered here. I will therefore contextualize the themes of nature, irony and interface in Nancy Paterson's work within the discourse of cyberfeminism. Cyberfeminism provides the ground on which affective relations might occur; Cyberfeminism retells the techno-myths of the past and rewrites the codes for the future. Images from nature are often used in electronic culture to signify a utopian nostalgia for the untainted and free experience.[4] What else can 'nature' signify? What can its representations teach us about how we live? Paterson's use of 50s techno-icons and new technologies investigates this. Equipped with irony she revisits the nostalgia for the 'natural' and introduces engaged readings of culture.

In 1990, Nancy wrote a timely essay entitled *Cyberfeminism*. In it she showcased the evolution of a new movement in feminist history and called attention to women's role in the future of technology. What underlies this attitude is that cyberfeminists are fully engaged in resignifying women's relationship to technology. "Multimedia, interactive video, virtual reality; for women these new technologies present opportunities to break out of prescribed roles and away from scripted dialogues."[5] In fact the short history of cyberfeminism is an ongoing call to arms, so to speak, to find alternatives "left for women who are not satisfied with the roles which patriarchal culture has designated."[6] This is especially true when the dominant images of technology have been industrial and disembodied in their epistemology. Paterson situates her art within the larger, complex and often contradictory network of cyberfeminism.

Many contributions have been made to cyberfeminist discourse, among them Sadie Plant's book *Zeros+Ones: digital women + the new technoculture* (1997). Plant traces the contributions of women to the evolution of the digital culture through the filter of feminine mythological constructs. Weaving is the metaphor used to describe the female relationship between computing and telecommunications. *Zeros+Ones* takes as its starting point the 19th century mathematical contributions of Ada Lovelace to the first cybernetic machines. There is another history, seldom told which catalogues a longstanding involvement between women and the design of technology. Ada's calculations heralded further engagements and history making.[7] In the diverse examples of cyberfeminism, the rewriting of myth and history as well as the use of metaphor has been a recurring strategy to break away from received and patriarchal history. Plant has also worked closely with the women's art collective *VNS Matrix* [http://sysx.org/vns/] who rewrite the logic of gaming and insert a decidedly cyberfeminist attitude that takes no prisoners. In the electronic magazine *Switch—electronic gender: art at the Interstice*, Anne-Marie Schleiner offers a gender analysis of the 1st person shooter/-adventure game with female heroine entitled; Does Lara Croft wear fake polygons?[8]

Cyberfeminism has taken much of its inspiration from Donna Haraway's important essay *A Cyborg Manifesto; Science, Technology and Socialist-Feminism in the Late Twentieth Century*.[9] Written in 1984, this text addressed the relationship between women, race and technology. By calling her work an ironic political myth, Haraway offered future cyberfeminists the tools for subverting the traditional, patriarchal trajectory of technoculture. According to Haraway, "Irony is about contradictions that do not resolve into larger wholes, even dialectically, about the tension of holding incompatible things together because both are necessary and true."[10] This irony is central to Paterson's media work and our present investigation of the imaging of nature.

making irony today through technologies of tomorrow Nancy Paterson makes techno-cultural hybrids; a fusion of information and communication technologies with simulated 50s nostalgia thrown into the potent mixture. She recycles broadcast imagery and retells stories and myths with a cyberfeminist slant. Paterson's use of irony resonates throughout her media work where 'ultramodern' postwar visions are factored into the realities of an increasingly unwieldy future. 50s icons of feminine domains including a beach cruiser bicycle, a wringer washer, a hair salon style dryer and a vibrating exercise-belt machine symbolize the utopian dreams that were offered to women in the cold war era. These icons which represent the kinds of engagement women have conventionally had with technology are reimagined in Paterson's media installations. Here interactions and interfaces are orchestrated between new technologies, e.g., the Internet, micro-controller for laserdisc, LCD monitors, PERL scripts, webcams, ultrasonic transducers and centralized micro processor units, complicating our understanding of women's relationships to technology and electronic culture. The domestic machines of the 1950's have given way to technologies that are reconfigured by women themselves. It is in this transition that irony resides.[11]

On the subject of irony Paterson has this to say: *Postmodern culture thrives on irony – in courtrooms, in politics, in science, in art. Irony is a means for addressing the tensions created by rapidly increasing diversity and the blurring of distinctions based on both sex and gender. Irony delineates an expression of technological realism, an epistemological grounding of one-self and a way of responding to the accelerating pace of communications. Through irony we represent what is otherwise unstated or unstateable - what is meant or implicated, but never quite articulated. Irony is a key component of millennial theory. Both symptom and remedy for postmodern culture, irony represents a possible path up and out of a pessimistic quagmire of simulacra and meaninglessness.*[12]

This ironic aesthetic gets your attention and demands a response, an interaction. The contradiction, which ricochets across your brain, demands reconciliation, though simplistic resolution is impossible. Irony exposes irrationality that may be subtle and unrecognized. It contests the strength of those dominant cultural forces of history and memory. Irony is ambiguous though its effectiveness works when the contradiction is made obvious. Through adroit elaboration, it is often used to make a false conception conspicuous. A cyberfeminist take on this strategy inserts a voluptuous and tough understanding of gender and power. Irony also highlights the space between two antithetical vantage points and creates a new realm out of the remains. This is a space for reflection as opposed to narcosis; a space for affective response.

weaving tales of nature *Stock Market Skirt* (1998) is a sophisticated example of how irony weaves its way into a cyberfeminist critique of the representations of women, market economics and information technologies. The piece is a telerobotic response to the Wall Street lore that the Dow affects the lengths of women's hemlines. "The better the market, the more leg shown." Paterson made this apocrypha tangible by wiring continually updated equities markets to the hem of a dress on dressmaker's mannequin, visualizing the willing connection between profit and desire. The piece, which was first shown at the Bell Centre for Creative Communications in Toronto, is also visible via a Webcam. Rather than an individual, it is the Internet, the posthuman flow of information that drives *Stock Market Skirt*. Women's bodies are often used as a sign of technology and desire. *Stock Market Skirt* makes manifest the libidinal economy of technology, money and gender. The irony is in the ambiguity of the source material that is dislocated from human agency. *Stock Market Skirt* is driven by the collective unconscious of human greed and illuminated through an appetite for fashion. What we learn is the 'emerging intelligence' of the Internet to alter information and direct meaning. More than a sophisticated technology, Paterson illustrates the power of collective desires, digitally.

Irony is in full force in Paterson's work when it is applied to the electronic visualization of natural forms. The fullness of nature, redolent with aromas and breezes are captured to hyper real effect. In works like *Bicycle TV* (1991), *The Medusa Project* (1997) and *The Meadow* (1996), Paterson reconfigures nature in the space of the virtual. Nature becomes a construct, an organic, wet, realm reduced to the zeros + ones of digital language. Always within reach, images from the natural environment seduce the viewer into having an intimate experience. This of course is limited by what the artist has allowed into the interface: what we the user actually experiences.

With *Bicycle TV*, we enter this 'artificial world' via a 1950s woman's bicycle. The act of steering and pedaling creates the experience both in terms of direction and speed. The user winds their way down country roads experiencing the freedom signified by the rural landscape. The images are calibrated as a relatively seamless experience of each transition, each new road taken. Ironically though, "the cyclist is . . . contained within the defined 'world' of the laserdisc."[13] The experience is reminiscent of the final scene of Ridley Scott's *Blade Runner* (1984), where Deckard and the replicant Rachel drive off into the American sunset. Allegedly they are escaping the dystopian world of the Tyrell Corporation for greener pastures. As the credits roll though one wonders whether even the benign ending is not another illusion, another artificial world.

The Meadow also explores the ambiguous space between the 'simulated' and the 'real'. Paterson suggests that "it is here that new mythologies and realities may be imagined." The work simultaneously asks what sort of images do we want to engage with virtually and short-circuits this openness by the limits of the configured space. In *The Meadow* four large video displays simulating the change of seasons in what appears to be a random fashion surround the viewer. The sound of birds, mosquitoes and children intermittently enter the metaphorical space. The installation gives the illusion of spontaneity and challenges the viewer's assumptions of scripted programming possibilities. This is especially true when chance elements seem to enter the experience. Certainly we can use these virtual landscapes to interject new fictions, but only within the confines of the program. Nature is not free but has been seduced into the ambiguous and artificial space of 'the virtual'. The question though is what do these images of nature signify?

The Medusa Project (Autobiography) (1997) takes an interesting trajectory by reflecting upon the interconnections between technology, communication and autobiography. As Paterson states: "This mediawork is in keeping with my series of installations combining video with technological icons from the 1950s." The 6' high chrome hair-curling machine is covered in Spanish moss, LCD monitors hanging down from the clamps, glow in various shades of blue, green and white; projected video of a semi-tropical landscape bring the viewer into a liminal space between imagination and memory. The mythological figure of Medusa is empowered by the screen of digital images projected onto her monstrous body. The Medusa figure is unruly and assertive as she conflates the mythic past with the mythic future. This work considers how women incorporate new electronic media into our lives without handing over control. Can we rewrite the past using the trope of nature? What kinds of responsibilities are there in representing 'the Real'?

Each successive work by Paterson develops the configuration of natural spaces as well as natural stereotypes. Images of femininity are inverted to expose the proscriptions of gender assigned by dominant broadcasting signals. Works like *Hair Salon TV* (1987), *Wringer/Washer TV* (1989), *The Machine in the Garden* (1993) and *Ex(or)ciser* (1994) sample the dustbin of history, reconfiguring images of the past. With playful irreverence, these works redefine 'reality' and 'the Real' by showing alternate routes for electronic communications. Rewriting code has numerous and contradictory implications for the cyberfeminist.

the thinking body A strong sense of subjective knowledge informs all of Paterson's media practice. Subjective knowledge is embodied, related to and informed by the body. This is also known as feminist epistemology because it takes context and the status of the knower into account. "Feminist epistemology as we use the term, marks the uneasy alliance of feminism and philosophy, an alliance made uneasy by this contradictory pull between the concrete and the universal."[14] Paterson's deconstruction of nature and gender bring lived experience into the design of interfaces and configuration of the techno-apparatus. Particularly in her most recent work, she grafts personal history and cultural influences onto the objective protocols of scientific method. The power of affect blurs the boundaries between subject and object, truth and fiction, nature and artifice; it demystifies technology, and encourages access to these tools.

Perhaps the most exciting aspect of Paterson's work as well as that of her contemporaries are the imaginative interfaces employed. Rather than a phallic joystick, 'ergonomic' control pad or text based environments, much Canadian media art proposes modes of communication beyond the exclusively ocular. Paterson's recent project, *The Library*, is a 3D environment containing numerous interactive and animated objects designed to be explored via the Internet. In this media work Paterson pushes the boundaries of our perception of the 'interface' creating a strong case for the transformation of the web by 3D technologies. In *Charged Hearts* (1997), Catherine Richards invites the 'user' to lift a bell jar holding a glass heart. The action charges electrons that glow and pulse in time with one's own heart. Thecla Schiphorst's *Bodymaps: artifacts of touch* (1997) highlights responsive spaces by inviting the viewer to touch an activated surface. What kinds of knowledge are afforded by touch? What forces can be materialized in the proprioceptive sense?[15] Nel Tenhaaf's *Fit* (1995) is also activated through a touch interface. An animated image of DNA strands accompanied by evocative narration challenges the proscriptions of biological determinism. The tactile interface complicates science's ability to represent the self.

Interactivity can work on many levels. Key to this is the materialization of forces often undetectable to the human eye. The result in the work of Paterson is that meaning is available, and narcosis next to impossible. Analysis of one's own experience is framed and the viewer is afforded an opportunity to consider their relationship to video images, representations of nature, gender construction and nostalgia for the 50s. Room is always left for affective response and thoughtful interaction should the user wish to move forward in the game. Pull the slot machine arm, ride the bicycle or strap on the vibrating belt.

I began this essay with a consideration of nature as more than a discursive construct. I would like to conclude by suggesting that within media art, nature is not only landscape but also how the body interacts with organic and artificial worlds. Just as the constructs are unstable, so too is the experience. Embodied experience, as a form of knowledge, shifts ones own relations to technology, its myths and representations. Our bodies are also our knowledge centers. While cyberfeminism is multiple, its strategies usually produce further awareness of complexity. An imaginative interface and a critical sense of irony can inform our experience, producing affective responses as we move through natural and artificial worlds. [16]

notes

1 Hannah Arendt, *The Human Condition*, Chicago: University of Chicago Press, 1958, p. 2. The date of publication frames this discussion, a period when the world appeared more straightforward and man was the symbol for universality. This will be made explicit in the discussion of Nancy Paterson's reworking the fifties icons of domestic technology.

2 "On one level 'nature' is like all concepts, a product of discourse, but its referent is also the subject of politics." Jon Bird et al, *FutureNatural, nature/science/culture*, Routledge, 1996, p.1.

3 Marshall McLuhan, 'Clocks; The Scent of Time' in *Understanding Media: the extensions of Man*, New York: McGraw-Hill, 1964, p. 149.

4 In both its editorials and advertising *Wired* magazine has trafficked in nature as a trope for freedom, open spaces and mobility.

5 Nancy Paterson, *Cyberfeminism*, http://internetfrauen.w4w.net/archiv/cyberfem.txt

6 Ibid.

7 The contributions to technological innovation by women are impressive. Ida R. Forbes invented the electric water heater in 1917. In 1919 Alice H. Parker received a patent for an improved home-heating furnace. Lise Meitner became the first person to split an atom in 1938. Erna Schneider Hoover created a computerized system in 1954 that monitored incoming telephone calls. Stephanie Louise Kwolek discovered one of the key components of Kevlar in 1965. Marie Brittan Brown created the first home-security system in 1969. Cisco Systems was founded in 1984 to market Sandy Lerner's router that linked university computer networks for e-mail communication. M. Katherine Holloway and Chen Zhao invented protease inhibitors in 1990. See *Ms.* magazine, December1999/January2000, pp. 52-57.

8 http://switch.sjsu.edu/web/v4n1/toc.html

9 Donna Haraway, Simians, *Cyborgs and Women: the reinvention of nature*, London:Free Association Books,1991.

10 Ibid. p, 149.

11 While some critics see irony as a stance of the cynical and mean spirited, it can also be understood as an enabling strategy.

12 Nancy Paterson in *Curly, Larry & PoMo* (c) 1998 Astrolabe online Journal
[http://www.cgrg.ohio-state.edu/Astrolabe/journal/inaugural/paterson.html]

13 Nancy Paterson, www.vacuumwoman.com

14 Linda Alcoff and Elizabeth Potter in *Feminist Epistemologies*, New York: Routledge,1993, p. 1.

15 This is the awareness of living in a physical body.

mediaworks

the library This project began as a 3D environment modeled on the Library of Parliament in Ottawa, available online. Accessing this environment using a VRML-enabled browser, viewers explore interactive and animated objects created in collaboration with selected Canadian artists and programmers. These objects are metaphors for the new millennium, referring to the emerging themes for this project: navigation and wayfinding. Included are an aurory which spins inside the dome of the Library, and a world globe, the texture a constantly updating satellite image retrieved (every 5 minutes) from the NASA website and wrapped around a rotating sphere. Clicking on various reference points on this globe triggers images of selected cities to be displayed, rotating suspended in the air around the globe. Navigating to the second floor of the Library, the viewer may choose to enter an opaque sphere which contains a model of the Giza plateau, comparing the course of the Nile and position of the pyramids/sphinx to an overlaid chart of the Milky Way. Throughout the 3D environment viewers may encounter literary characters who act as guides; these characters also point towards future educational applications, as books are transformed from linear stories into narrative experiences. At the turn of the millennium, *The Library* represents one of the most complex 3D environments on the net, designed for the future of bandwidth. *The Library* can also be exhibited as an installation, with a large screen projection and 3D trackball for user participation. ● Fully optimized for online access, this mediawork was futher developed for use with the ORAD Virtual Studio (CyberSet M), while Visiting Artist at the School of Communication Arts, Seneca@York. Titled *The Library* [2], this 3D environment was ported to the ORAD virtual set, allowing for the seamless integration of people and computer-generated imagery. A system of infrared transmitters makes it possible for the viewer to not only see themselves in the *Library* environment (on a wall size screen opposite the blue screen CyberSet) but also to move around and behind 3D objects such as the world globe. In *Stock Market Skirt*, perl (under Linux) was utilized to extract a value from various internet pages. This value controlled a stepper motor located under the dress, raising or lowering the skirt hemline as the tracked stock price rose or fell. Conceptually similar to this and to the retrieval of the NASA satellite image for the world globe, I am pursuing the development of *The Library*[3], retrieving data and multimedia elements from the internet (using perl, javascript, java) and incorporating them into the LIBRARY environment along with live people. In *The Library*[3] (under development) utilizing an upgrade for the CyberSet M, this environment will be sent out live over high speed networks, interactive via a browser.

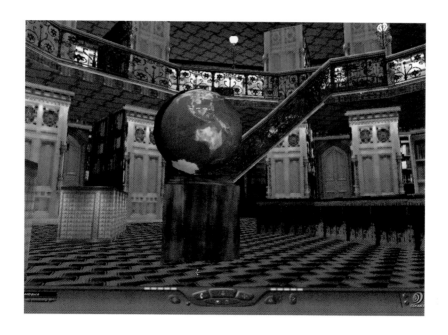

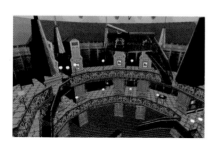
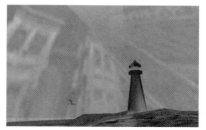

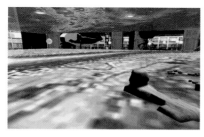
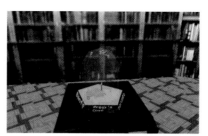

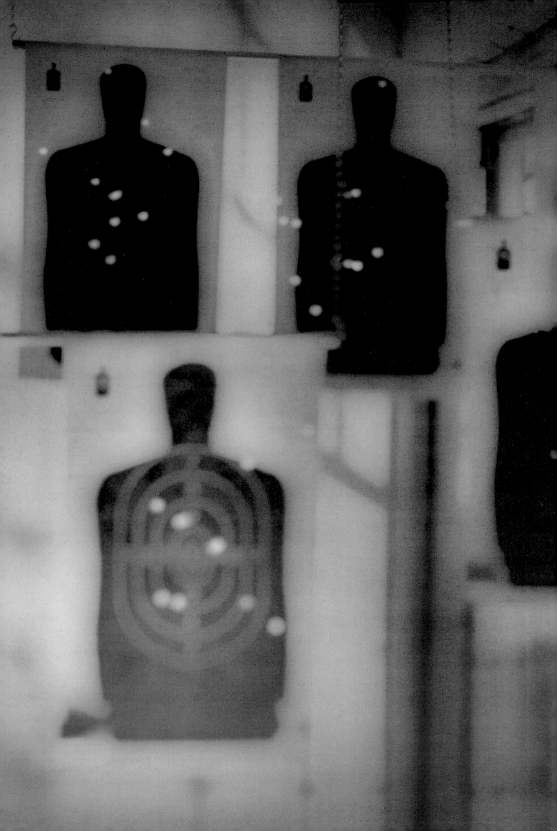

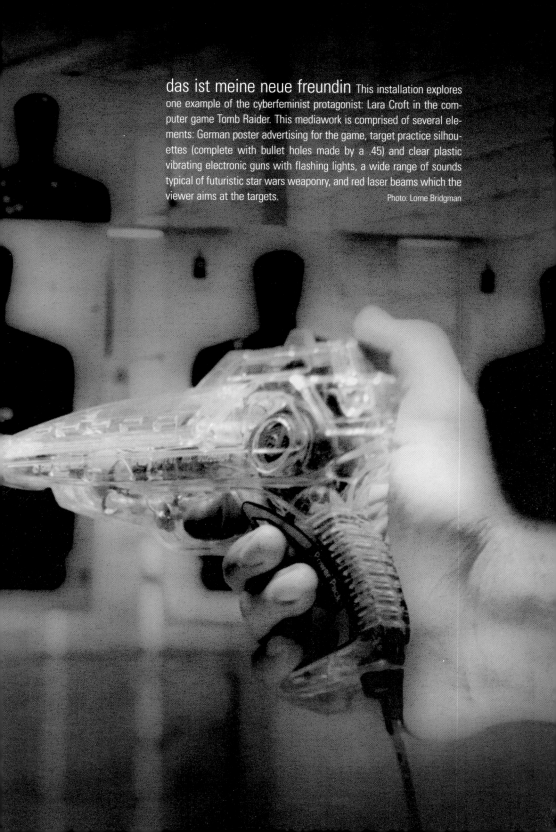

das ist meine neue freundin This installation explores one example of the cyberfeminist protagonist: Lara Croft in the computer game Tomb Raider. This mediawork is comprised of several elements: German poster advertising for the game, target practice silhouettes (complete with bullet holes made by a .45) and clear plastic vibrating electronic guns with flashing lights, a wide range of sounds typical of futuristic star wars weaponry, and red laser beams which the viewer aims at the targets. Photo: Lorne Bridgman

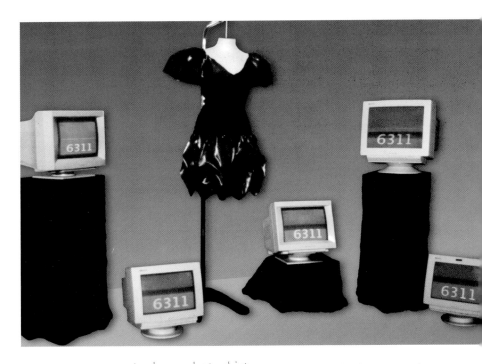

stock market skirt This 'cyberfeminist fashion statement' was created to challenge traditional, patriarchal values and new media applications. *Stock Market Skirt* was conceived long before the technology was available to make it a reality. When this work was first undertaken, online stock quotes were available only to brokers by subscription through expensive services such as Bloomberg. A blue taffeta and black velvet party dress is displayed on a dressmaker's mannequin or 'Judy,' located in the Gallery next to a computer and several monitors of varying sizes. In large white type against a blue background (tastefully matching the blue of the taffeta skirt), the stock ticker symbol and constantly updated price scroll in simulation of the pixel board displays used to track stock values on traditional exchange room floors. Stock quotes are retrieved at least once per second (depending on the speed of connection) from stock quote pages online, with the hemline moving in unison. Custom-designed PERL running under Linux, retrieves and parses HTML code. This data is conveyed to a custom-designed controller which accordingly sends positive or negative pulses to a stepper motor mounted up and under the skirt. A complex system of cables, loops and weights sewn to the interior of the skirt ensure that the hemline length changes smoothly. When the

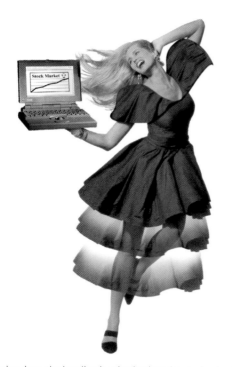

stock price rises, the hemline is raised; when the stock price falls, the hemline is lowered. ⬩ Unlike the majority of tele-robotic works, *Stock Market Skirt* is interactive with the flow of data within the internet itself (rather than being interactive through the internet as a pipeline or conduit). Written into the program is a script which sets the skirt's range of movement based on the selected stock's previous day's performance. This range is monitored throughout the day, and is automatically adjusted if necessary. ⬩ *Stock Market Skirt* is capable of being configured to track the price of any stock on any exchange which provides online updates: North American, European, Asian, etc. At the end of the trading day, *Stock Market Skirt* is programmed to switch to the next time zone to continue tracking a select stock in real time. When all exchanges are closed, it switches to historical data. ⬩ This mediawork utilizes a webcam to capture and display real-time images of the hemline as it fluctuates. A website simultaneously displays these images as well as the stock market quotes which are controlling the length of the hemline. This site is made available in conjunction with the exhibition of this installation. ⬩ *Stock Market Skirt* addresses issues such as the convergence between technology, feminism and art, as well as the emerging intelligence of the internet.

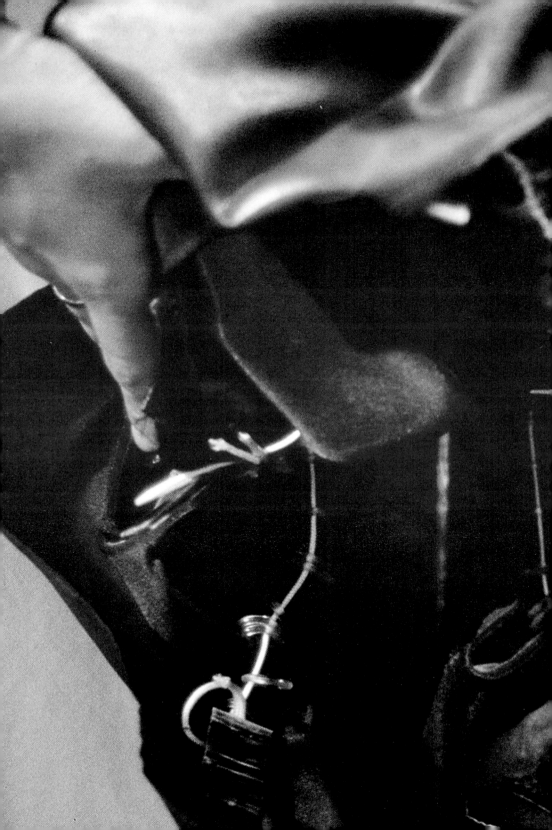

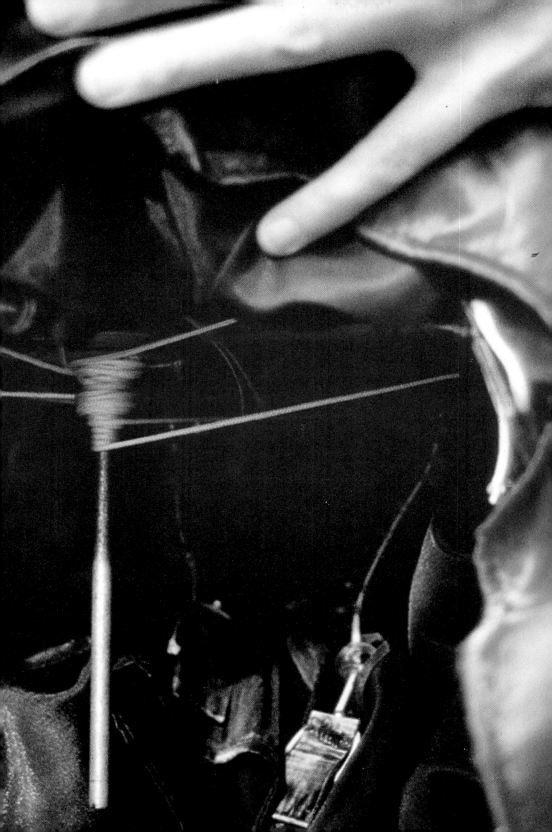

the medusa project (autobiography)

This media-work represents an attempt to directly merge personal history and influences in an installation which addresses my interest in the relationships emerging between feminism, technology and art. Two major influences on my early development were time spent in the southern USA visiting family who had lived in South Miami since the early 1900s, and time spent at my family's cottage near Bracebridge, Ontario (in the heart of the Muskoka region). In Florida I was introduced to the writing of Marjorie Rawlings and Zora Neale Hurston. Through their ideas and my own experiences I fell in love with the buzz of insects and the tangle of tropical growth. The maze of springs, river systems and caves underlying most of the terrain also presented a certain allure. Many summers were also spent at my family's cottage near Bracebridge, on property owned and operated by the Spiritualist Church of Canada – Springdale Park. My interest in seances, telepathy and intuition as well as the creative potential of conditions such as synesthesia, was sparked as I was exposed to their beliefs and attended many of their services. The convergence of these experiences taught me the importance of subtle shifts of perspective, and personal powers of communication. This mediawork is in keeping with my series of installations combining video with technological icons from the 1950s. A central component of this installation is a 6' high chrome hair-curling machine, typical of those found in North American beauty salons from the 1920s to 1950s. The machine stands several feet out from a wall on which video is projected. A looped videotape collage of images and sound locates the machine and the viewer in a semi-tropical landscape. Spanish moss hangs down from tree branches which reach out over clear, blue/green water. The colours of the water in the video projection produce a hyper-real effect. Stunning, sudden transitions of light; a breeze filtering through the trees; the bubbling and churning of the water's surface at the source of a huge natural underground spring - constitute the only movement. Woven in among the wires and cables of the hair-curling machine, are delicate strands of spanish moss. LCD monitors hanging down from the clamps, glow in various shades of blue, green and white, throwing pools of light amongst scattered large high-voltage ceramic coil insulators.

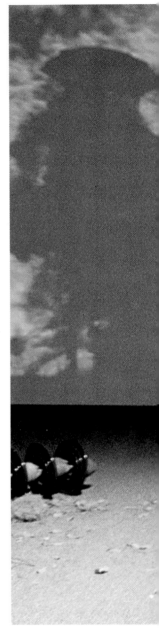

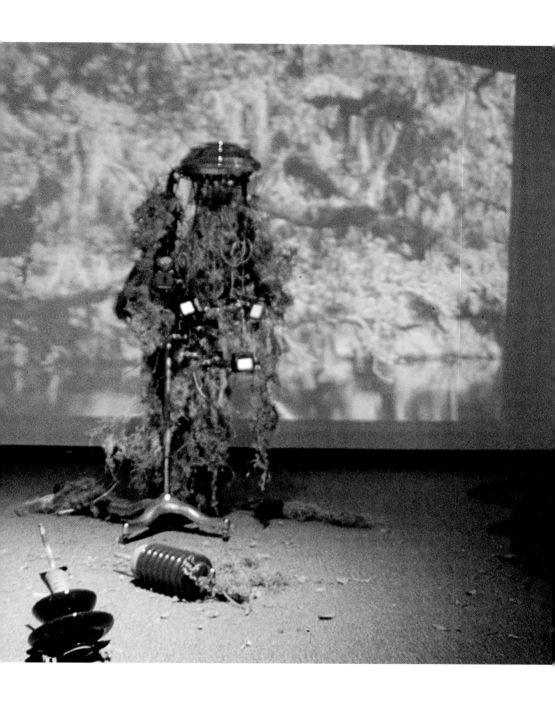

how the rest was won This collaborative project with Shelley Niro arose out of discussions about the impact of new electronic technologies and the often tenuous relationship between the nature of Native cultures and the new technological ethos. It offers a unique opportunity to consider the impact of advanced communications technology on a specific culture with a different perspective of the densely colonized information highway. A canvas tipi, floor mounted satellite dish and imitation Remington 'Bucking Bronco' statue are situated in the installation space. The statue sits on top of a television on which is displayed an Indian Head TV test pattern as a freeze-framed image.   In isolating a popular media stereotype, we raise questions about the perpetuation of systematic barriers and assumptions, the illusion of progress, and the disjunctive relationships between technology and culture.

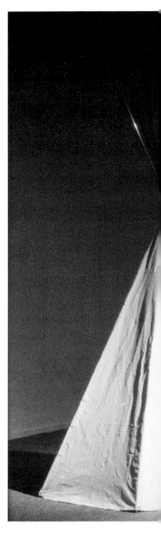

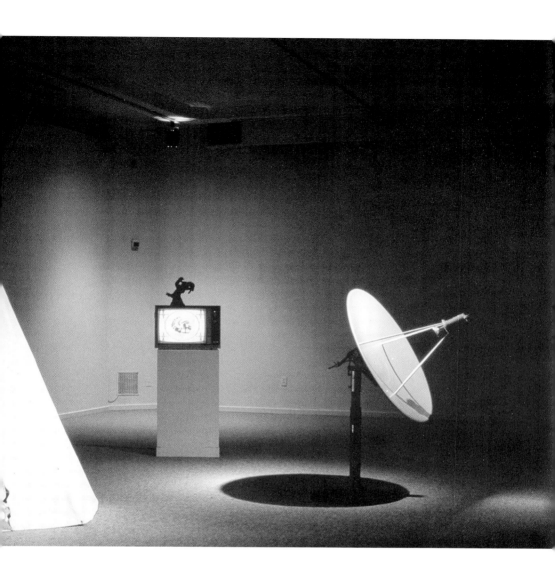

the meadow *The Meadow* explores and manifests the metaphorical space which lies between the 'simulated' and the 'real' – a space to which artists are inevitably drawn. Ambiguity and irony also share this space, and it is here that new mythologies and realities may be imagined. This space is particularly appropriate to artists working with new electronic technologies to bridge the gap between science and fiction. This interactive installation is comprised of ultrasonic transducers, a centralized microprocessor unit and custom-designed micro-controller for four laserdisc players. This system performs two functions: the detection of viewer location/movement and multiple laserdisc control. Stepping into the installation space, the viewer is surrounded by four large video displays. The artificial space created by the video displays is divided into quadrants, each monitored by an ultrasonic transducer. These four transducers cycle to sweep the entire installation space once per second. As viewers enter the installation space, move between quadrants and linger in various positions, their presence and movements are tracked and timed. Displayed on each video display is real-time, full motion video of a different view: the four edges or corners of a meadow as seen from a central vantage point.

As the viewer enters the space, it is winter in the meadow (each video display shows a different scene, blanketed in snow). Taking a clockwise path within the installation space, the viewer's location triggers the four transducers, signalling the controller to change the season on each of the video displays. These seasonal transitions are manifested as slow dissolves and take place on all four video displays simultaneously. The 'season' of the installation space is viewer controlled; the viewer discovers how to manipulate these seasonal changes, and finds it possible to move backwards in time (from winter to fall) or across seasons (from fall to spring) as well. Through further experimentation the viewer discovers that they may also trigger a wide range of audio effects within the installation space: the sound of a flock of geese which suddenly materializes, flies overhead and disappears; the persistent and annoying buzz of a mosquito; children who are suddenly heard laughing or playing just out of sight; a child whispers on your left and is answered by another child whispering, on your right. As in real life, the relationships between cause and effect and the extent to which control is grasped and maintained, is not always clear.

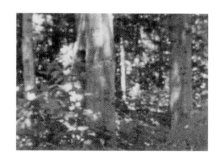

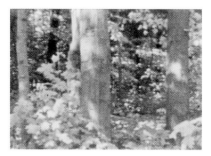

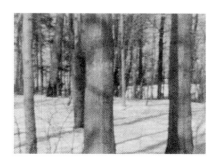

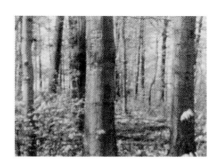

ex(or)ciser This interactive installation addresses issues of mass media and manipulation. In *Ex(or)ciser* individualism and narcissism are revealed as inextricably linked to new electronic technologies and capitalist consumerism. The interface for this installation is a 1950s style vibrating belt massager representative of a tradition of products promising health and beauty with a minimum of energy/effort/sacrifice. The exerciser is placed in front of a colour monitor which is elevated to eye level. A microprocessor controls the playback of video in the installation. When the viewer approaches, they hear audio of rumba music and recorded verbal instructions for learning the footwork for this particular dance. The video screen remains blank until the installation is activated by the viewer turning on the vibrating belt massager. They may choose to step into the exerciser and strap the belt around their hips in the process, or they may simply switch it on, leaving the belt to twist and vibrate seductively in the air. When the exerciser is switched off, the video playback stops while the audio continues. The video program is a montage of short clips including footage of people doing the rumba, imagery of people performing personal hygiene or admiring themselves in mirrors, and images of nuclear power generating stations. The video clips have been edited to be synchronous with the timing sequence involved in dancing the rumba. The vibration of the exerciser is soothing and hypnotic; the juxtaposition of video and audio in this context hints at underlying tactics.

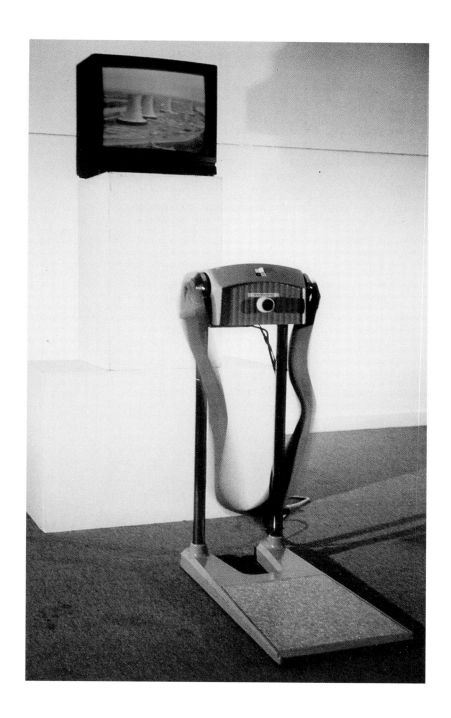

the machine in the garden

Modeled on the design of a casino slot machine, *The Machine In The Garden* incorporates the Buddhist motif of See no evil, Hear no evil, Speak no evil. The viewer sees (on three LCDs mounted on the faceplate of the slot machine and three large video monitors mounted above and behind the slot machine), the same woman's face with hands covering her eyes, ears, or mouth. Viewers activate the installation by either pulling the arm of the slot machine, or pressing the button on the front of the one armed bandit. A contact switch inside the slot machine signals the controller to 'randomly' select three video segments of approx. 13-15 seconds each, to play on the video displays. ■ There are three distinct themes represented in this work: talking heads; images of war; and childrens' television programming. The same theme is always addressed on any particular video display. Each video segment is comprised of dozens of video clips edited as 'wipes' from above, gradually increasing in speed, reaching a peak and then suddenly stopping in staggered sequence, to simulate the 'action' of a real slot machine. Each video segment both begins and ends with one of the three Buddhist images. There are 27 different combination of images on which the video displays may come to rest: 3 images x 3 displays = (3^3). Video/audio from three laserdisc players is routed through a custom-designed A/V controller to the video displays. Juxtaposition of video/audio is available in 729 possible combinations. ■ The *Machine In The Garden* deals with the issues of gambling and spirituality, twin distillates of our obsession with luck and fortune, weighing the apparently random outcome of phenomenon against a possible underlying order. Einstein's Theory of Relativity eliminated Newton's illusion of absolute space and time, and the combined research of quantum mechanics and chaos theory have shown the flaws in the belief that reality is predictable. As inevitably as we turn to organized religion for reassurance in the face of our mortality, and countless other systems of spiritual belief for their promises of miracles, we are just as surely drawn to games of risk and chance. Reconciling spirituality with our apparently reckless attitude towards technology becomes less problematic when we acknowledge that they are opposite sides of the same coin. Playing the odds and betting to win is a decidedly postmodern response to a failing faith in technological utopianism.

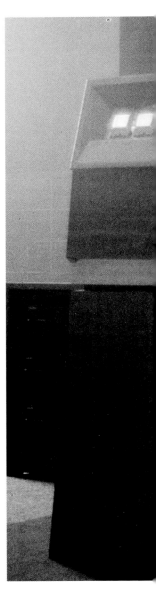

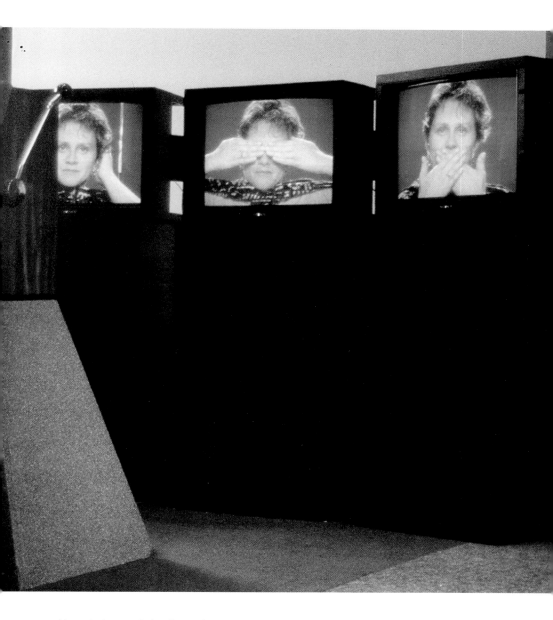

Not only does god play dice . . . but he sometimes throws them where they can't be seen

Stephen Hawking

EXPO '92 For this installation I adapted my interactive mediawork *Bicycle TV*, to work with a joystick interface rather than the bicycle. I recreated the environment of Bracebridge, a small Muskoka town in Ontario, in programming and video. Two channels of Digital Video Effects (DVE) were used extensively in post-production of the *EXPO 92* installation, to produce special effects highlighting scenes of special interest via display of a 'picture within a picture' in one or more corners of the video screen.

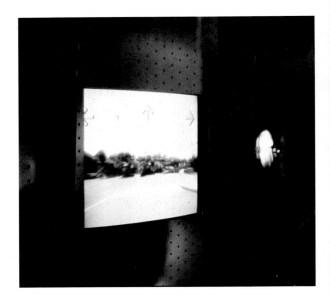

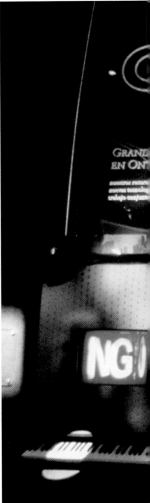

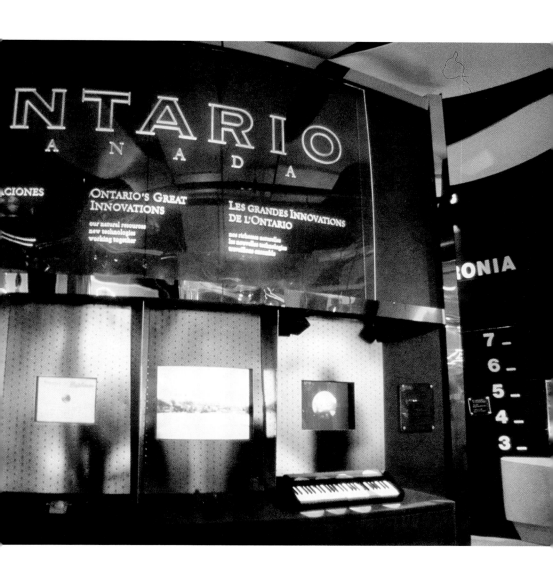

bicycle tv: some interactive excercise

One of the earliest works of its kind, *Bicycle TV* is a rider controlled real-time video tour of a scenic landscape in the Canadian countryside. This interactive installation consists of a 1950s style bicycle, a video display (either a videowall or a 50" colour monitor) mounted in front of the bicycle facing the rider, a laserdisc and player, front wheel direction sensing device and rear wheel motion detector assembly. These devices are linked to the laserdisc player through a programmable controller.   This mediawork presents a contemporary interpretation of ancient designs (mazes and labyrinths) with possible hidden meaning and spiritual significance. It also utilizes the camera as a tool to explore space, a theme similarly addressed in other works such as *The Meadow*. Mounting and pedalling the bicycle activates the video which consists of scenic, winding country roads (shot to simulate the perspective of a cyclist). At all intersections and crossroads the viewer/cyclist has the option of choosing a new path or continuing along the same route. The direction of the video is controlled by the turning of the handlebars where a choice of direction is indicated by arrows superimposed on the video. The opto-electronic front-wheel direction-sensing device sends data to the controller, which is programmed to select and play the appropriate video.   The speed of the video playback is continuously adjusted to reflect the speed at which the bicycle is pedalled. The speed is controlled by the rear wheel motion-detector assembly and is directly determined by the cyclist's pedalling speed. Use of a multispeed laserdisc player allows video that was shot at approximately 17 miles per hour to be slowed by the rider to less than 10 mph, or increased to 35 mph. The rear wheel optical sensor counts pulses via black markings on the rear wheel of the bike. Both the front-wheel and rear-wheel sensors are linked to the laserdisc player through a custom-designed controller.   It is possible for the cyclist to explore many different roads and paths; there is no real beginning or end to the video program. The computer controller is programmed based on a branching system developed in the pre-production stage and the cyclist is thus contained within the defined 'world' of the laserdisc.

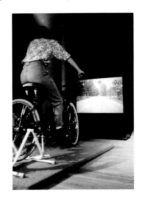

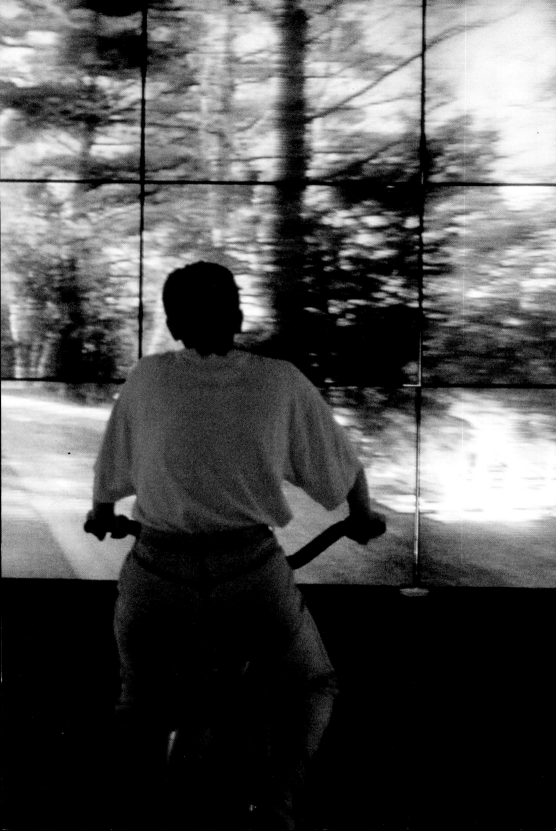

wringer/washer tv This mediawork is a pink, white and chrome wringer washer which has a colour monitor fitted in the bottom of the wash tub facing up. This monitor displays imagery dealing with the issue of abortion in Canada, interspersing opinions and arguments with video footage of a load of laundry going through the wash and rinse cycle. From a distance the viewer sees a variety of poster advertisements for laundry detergent, mounted on the Gallery walls around the wringer/washer. They hear the audio which accompanies the video program, but see only the wringer/washer machine, and the light emanating from its interior (the video playback on the monitor recessed in the wash tub). Upon approaching and looking down into the wash tub they can view the video, and also see it reflected in the polished chrome sides of the tub.

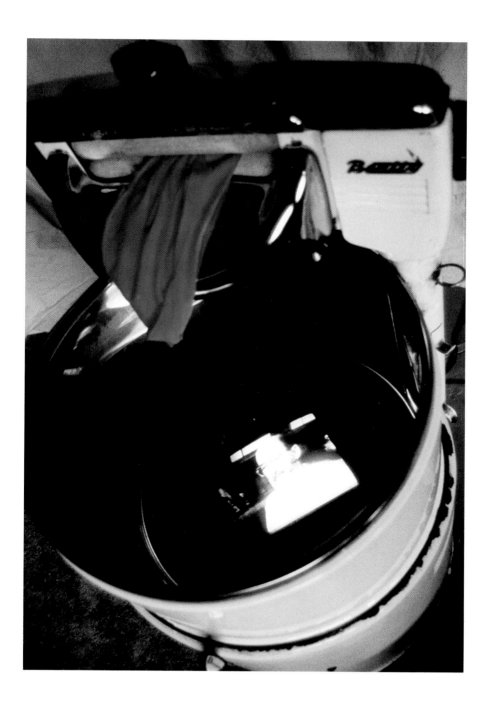

hair salon tv   n *Hair Salon TV* the chrome helmets of three womens' hairstyling chairs are fitted with small colour monitors which display imagery of: 1/ women and domestic technology; 2/ women in the workplace; and 3/ women and scientific discovery/technological innovation. Video imagery on these three themes is routed from three VHS decks to the monitors and this imagery switches randomly.   This early mediawork was produced shortly after I left Art School in the mid 80s. Rather than using a micro-controller to control the switching of the video clips between the three monitors (which would have been expensive at the time), I utilized a bank of relays; a relay is what you would find used in the turn signal indicator of a car.   This was the first mediawork in which I utilized recycled broadcast imagery to demonstrate how our perception and interpretation of issues is shaped and distorted by electronic communications technologies and media. *Hair Salon TV* was also the first in a series of works dealing with themes relating to women and technology and incorporating gender specific technological icons identifiable with the 1950's.

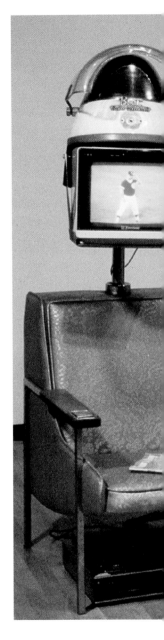

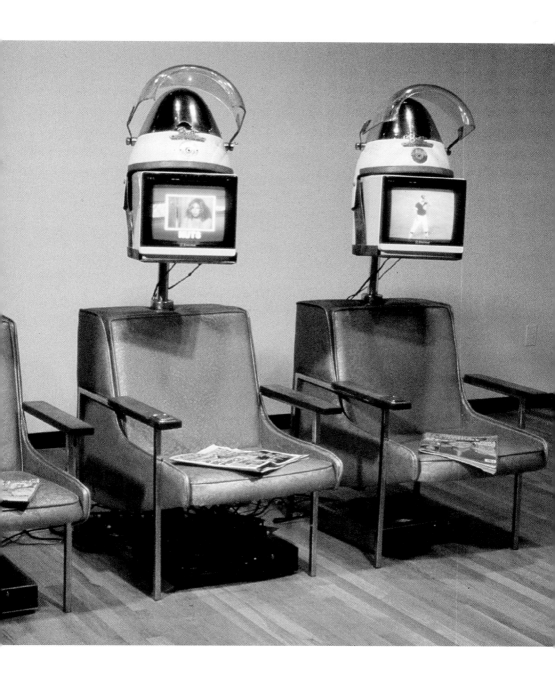

cyberfeminism nancy paterson

In her latest incarnation she is exceedingly voluptuous. The scalpel blades beneath her carefully manicured nails are discreetly retractable. The arm twisted up behind her back is, at first
glance, barely noticeable. Meet Molly in William Gibson's novel *Neuromancer*, or Melanie
Griffith in the film *Cherry 2000* – sexy, tough, aloof, and ultimately a fantasy.[1]

The power which these women wield is evil, technological and, of course, seductive. Any
influence or control which they exert is clearly misguided or accidental. The powerful woman,
bitch/goddess, ice queen, android, is represented in popular culture as a 21st century
Pandora. And the box which she hold this time is electronic and very definitely plugged in.

Linking the erotic representation of women with the often terrible cultural impact of new
electronic technologies is not a new concept. Cinema addressed the desire to anthropomor-
phize machines and vilify women in the process as early as 1927 in Fritz Lang's cult classic
Metropolis. Sex, danger, women and machines: the plot of virtually every futuristic, sci-fi
movie in which women play any role at all. Cyberfemmes are everywhere, but cyberfeminists
are few and far between.

The deconstruction of feminism, the division of women according to geography and sexual or
other politics, is as often self-inflicted as it is due to the acceleration of technology and history. Our lives are careening very nearly out of our control. With the pieces and parts scattered
at our feet, what can be salvaged from 20th century feminism? Through examining the relationship between women and technology, perhaps where science and fiction converge (in the
new technological ethos of new electronic media and art) there may be an opportunity to
reconstruct feminism. Post-gender, trans-gender – the possible parameters of a new philosophy.

Ubiquitous and omniscient, the significance of new electronic technologies, their development, design, implementation and dissemination, cannot be ignored and must not be under-
estimated. Whether directly or indirectly, issues of economics, class, race, nationality, personality and gender, are driven and defined by new electronic technologies. Immersed as we are
in the popular applications of these new technologies and media, their long-term and more
profound impact become invisible.

In *The Media Lab: Inventing the Future at MIT*, Nicholas Negroponte is quoted as saying:
'Once a new technology rolls over you, if you're not part of the steamroller, you're part of the
road.'[2] Without celebrating the military-industrial complex responsible for the origin and
development of these new technologies, what alternatives are left for women who are not
satisfied with the roles which patriarchal culture has designated? Certainly not the association of the feminine with 'nature' advocated by eco-feminists and theorists such as Camille

Paglia. It is no longer possible or desirable for women to capitulate and retreat to this position. The progress of new electronic technologies will leave them in the dust.

There is a school within a school of thought – hard core information processing, as it is known among developmental psychologists – which shares many characteristics and beliefs with a similarly situated "school within a school" – in this case in the field of computer science – artificial intelligence. Tracing the essence of human characteristics back to the intricate twists and turns of the double helix - the DNA - they propose to simulate human thought and behaviour through computer programming. The DNA as a code for the biological and psychological human information processor. With which they relinquish all knowledge and interest in humanity beyond this model and turn their attention to the machinations of computer simulation. A thankless task. For all its merits, the DNA model does not and cannot explain a number of significant aspects of human behaviour and thought. A disappointing but not surprising number of artists are still grappling with this gap between reality and representation. And mainstream media has been wrapped up with this flawed interpretation for some time. The sooner that we grasp the concept that unpredictable random acts, whether of violence or kindness, are almost all that we can expect, the sooner we will gain some insight into the relationship between nature and technology. And yet, we must not perpetuate the myth that technology can or should be developed independently of ethical or humanistic considerations.

The resurgence of determinism, whether biological or technological, is bound to have nasty repercussions for women. The patriarchal system which controls the development and applications of new technologies implies that both the applications and the technology itself are inevitable. Technological utopianism at least encouraged optimism. Technological determinism has a death wish.

Women are not alone in the need to understand how, why and by whom our criteria and confidence for understanding ourselves, each other and our relation to the world, has been stripped away. The dissolution of conventional concepts of time and space through new electronic media has contributed to the acceptance and success of PoMo punk nihilism, pluralism, diversity and the disappearance of dominant history. Simultaneously, we are witnessing a crisis of both individual and cultural identity as we are faced the interminable task of incorporating new electronic media into our lives without handing over control.

Cyberfeminism as a philosophy has the potential to create a poetic, passionate, political identity and unity without relying on a logic and language of exclusion or appropriation. It offers a route for reconstructing feminist politics through theory and practice with a focus on the implications of new technology rather than on factors which are divisive. Cyberfeminism does not accept as inevitable any current applications of new technologies which impose and maintain specific cultural, political and sexual stereotypes. Empowerment of women in the field of new electronic media can only result from the demystification of technology, and the appropriation of access to these tools. Cyberfeminism is essentially subversive.

Vancouver-based author William Gibson is credited with having introduced the word 'cyberspace' into popular culture, in his novel *Neuromancer*, defining it as a 'consensual hallucination.'[3] In fact, this word may be used to describe electronic space in all of its manifestations, ranging from virtual reality to the telecommunications infrastructure or internet. As illustrated by the recent U.S. Clinton/Gore initiative to regulate the internet or Information Superhighway, governments are beginning to recognize in public policy the commercial potential of media which have been under development for several decades. Predictably, the involvement of feminists and other marginalized groups in this process of development and design has not been solicited or encouraged, either in public or in private initiatives.

In the very near future, lines of cultural influence will be drawn based on computer access and literacy. It is becoming the new political divide – those who have access to computers or are computer literate vs. those who are not. The North American Free Trade Agreement, workplace automation, and legislation regarding the 'Information Superhighway,' are generally supported by those individuals, organizations and corporations which have and promote access. Those who have access and/or are computer literate but do not share enthusiasm for these types of policies and initiatives, are severely isolated as they have no one to unite with in their quest for well thought out socio-economic reforms. Those who do not have access, are not computer literate, and are in fact, often technophobic, are critical, but not necessarily constructive in their analysis of new electronic technologies.

New electronic technologies represent a magic circle from which women have been traditionally excluded. It is true that there are tangible barriers to our participation in the discourse shaping the tools and the applications of new electronic media. Women are largely absent from the institutions, networks and structures which determine where and when new technological applications will be developed, and how the potential of these new media will be described. However, lack of initiative, aggression, or determination should no longer be utilized to justify our continued exclusion.

One factor contributing to the discouragement of women in this field may be traced to the historical foundations of these media. The internet, a worldwide computer network, was originally a small military network of four computers known as ARPANET. This computer network was designed to research the feasibility of creating a decentralized system of communication which could survive a nuclear war. Similarly, VR (virtual reality) also had militaristic origins, having been initially envisioned as a tool for battlefield simulations. These origins are clearly acknowledged in every description of current and potential applications of these systems. However, this candor is deceptive, as no links are made between the origins of these media and the future towards which they are being driven. It is obvious that underlying assumptions are manifest in current popular applications of these media. The evidence is in the arcades, where video games such as the Sega Genesis 'Night Trap' challenges players to save scantily clad sorority sisters from a gang of hooded killers.

Margaret Benston, a Canadian activist with a background in engineering and an interest in the social and political dimensions of science and technology, in a chapter of Kramarae's book *Technology & Women's Voices* titled 'Women's Voices/Men's Voices: Technology as Language,' describes technology as a language for action and self expression.[4] Access to machinery and technology has been culturally sex-typed as masculine. In maintaining control over new technologies and by promoting and adhering to a technological world view, men have attempted to silence us. Whether or not we agree whether this world view is appropriate, it is clear that womens' absence from this forum is a problem.

Despite these obstacles, women are increasingly successful in breaking through and stepping inside the circle. Particularly in philosophy and cultural theory, an uneasy realization is dawning that mans' haphazard mastery of nature has not provided an adequate foundation for a vision worthy of leading us into the next century. Across this bleak and plundered landscape cyberfeminist theorists are emerging, speaking and gathering. A new chain of beings and being in the world is constructed; they reshape each other, they redefine themselves, and they reclaim new electronic technologies for women.

Virtual reality and cyberspace – the technologies for living vicariously. Virtual reality describes a wide range of experiences, including the transformation of two-dimensional objects and spaces through media such as holography; installations which use multiple video monitors or projections to surround the viewer; and the 'Hollywood' definition with which we are becoming increasingly familiar – head mounted display, touch sensitive gloves and/or full body suit. Telepresencing and cyberspace, where telecommunications networks enable instantaneous interaction from remote locations, have also been commonly described as virtual spaces.

The body/mind split which has governed our approach to new media, has gone underground, but has not disappeared. The disembodied mind is resurrected through applications such as VR – the desecration of the body has entered a new phase. The proof of the impact of such technologies (which have stretched and twisted our understanding of time and space as well as the limitations of our vulnerable, physical, human bodies) may be measured by the paranoia which they have inspired. Cyberspace has become a fertile breeding ground for multiple personalities, flaming, electronic stalking and gender-bending at the very least.

The body, in virtual space, is no mere user-interface; VR offers the chance to trade-in, remodel, or even leave behind the physical nature with which we are, in reality, burdened. Outside forces which act upon us, impose restrictions, are gone. Gravity, and the laws of physics, gone. Entropy and the passage of time become meaningless concepts. Women have always, by virtue or necessity, been adept at free fall, grounding themselves in personal physical experience. This skill will serve well as we venture into other dimensions and back home again. However skilled we become at navigating these spaces and temporarily leaving our bodies behind, it is doubtful that we will ever achieve immortality. Virtuality is patriarchy's blind spot.

Paris Is Burning, Jennie Livingstone's film about gender, identity and style, documents what was surely (before the introduction of technology-based VR into pop culture), the ultimate virtual experience – walk down a runway, through Harlem, or down Wall Street for that matter, in drag. Transsexual and cross-dressing 'walkers,' competing in the categories of 'executive,' 'college boy,' and 'fashion model,' recognize that the successful embodiment or representation of stereotypes is measured by both appearance and attitude. 'Realness' has always been the unspoken criteria for 'passing,' and women (those who have avoided being institutionalized for not 'fitting in') have become experts at that.

Through Virtual Reality, deconstruction of gender is entering the realm of pop culture, and this link with new electronic technology has implications for the philosophy of cyberfeminism. Technological convergence describes the unification of computers, television and communications technologies. However, convergence describes much more than the evolution towards an environment in which electronic technologies are pervasive. Convergence is happening on more than a technological level - it is happening on a metaphysical level as well. Cultural convergence may be described as the meeting or merging of art and technology. Cyberfeminism is entering an arena in which much more than gender is up for grabs.

Multimedia, interactive video, virtual reality; for women these new technologies present opportunities to break out of prescribed roles and away from scripted dialogues. A rabbit hole through which we may tumble. Our real experiences, when not denied, have been acknowledged only in their immediacy. Our individual histories and the attempt to isolate or remove ourselves from a patriarchal context, have always been undervalued and undermined. We have learned to live from hand to mouth. Transgressing order and linear organization of information, cyberfeminists recognize the opportunity to redefine 'reality,' on our terms and in our interest and realize that the electronic communications infrastructure or 'matrix' may be the ideal instrument for a new breed of feminists to pick up and play with.

notes

1 William Gibson. (1984). *Neuromancer.* New York, NY: Ace Books. p. 25

2 Stewart Brand (Ed.) (1987). *The Media Lab: Inventing the Future at MIT.* New York, NY: Viking. p. 9

3 Gibson, p. 51

4 Cheris Kramarae. (Ed.). (1988) *Techology & Women's Voices: Keeping in Touch,* London: Routledge, P. 15

curly, larry & PoMo nancy paterson

On February 20, 1998, in a kind of a replay of H.G. Wells' 'War of the Worlds' broadcast, satellite transmissions from CBS to numerous television stations across the U.S. carried 'practice' stories about the bombing of Iraq. For 20 minutes, Dan Rather described the first attacks, in full make-up, complete with theme music and 3D graphics of cruise missile routes, targets and 'actual' video footage of bombed out buildings in Bagdad. In addition to being viewed by several stunned television technicians who had picked up the feed, the broadcast was also viewed by individuals monitoring the G4 satellite.

As we approach the millennium the popularity of fatalistic language is reaching hysterical proportions. Cultural critics and theoreticians are suffering from the same kind of Y2K problems (Year 2000) that they are experiencing in computer programming; they can't seem to turn the year over into the millennium. There are hundreds of books which begin with the phrase 'The End of. . .' or 'The Death of. . .' So many that I began compiling a list: *The End of Art Theory* by Victor Burgin, *The End of History and the Last Man* by Francis Fukuyama, *The End of Education* by Neil Postman, *The End of Science* by John Horgan, *The End of Work* by Jeremy Rifkin, *The Death of Desire, The End of Liberalism, The Death of Ethics.* Everything, apparently, is over.

In 1984, a California state law was passed which declared that the name or likeness of a deceased person is a property right that can pass on to heirs. This law, more affectionately known as the 'Dracula' law because it was fought for and won by Bela Lugosi's son, was also used as a precedent in a more recent case which also took place in L.A.: the heirs of Curly and Larry vs. the heirs of Moe. The case was won and damages were awarded, but most interesting was the irony of the fact that the prosecuting attorney had obtained the Judge's permission to screen, at intervals during the trial, some of the Stooges' funniest clips. In the words of one reporter, When jurors began yawning – having had their fill of bookkeeping entries, accounting charts and licensing agreements – pies would start to fly, noggins would get cracked, and cries of Knucklehead would fill the air.

Postmodern culture thrives on irony – in courtrooms, in politics, in science, in art. Irony is a means for addressing the tensions created by rapidly increasing diversity and the blurring of distinctions based on both sex and gender. Irony delineates an expression of technological realism, an epistemological grounding of oneself and a way of responding to the accelerating pace of communications. Through irony we represent what is otherwise unstated or unstateable – what is meant or implicated, but never quite articulated. Irony is a key component of millennial theory. Both symptom and remedy for postmodern culture, irony represents a possible path up and out of a pessimistic quagmire of simulacra and meaninglessness.

Cultural cannibalism. In the late stages of capitalism, in the latter half of the final decade of this millennium, perversity characterizes entertainment. We can't watch enough sex, death and automobile accidents. And if the actors are having sex with dead people, or during car crashes or with dead people during car crashes – even better. In the fall-out shelters of our nuclear families we have become so estranged from authentic experience that reality has ceased to exist. In our media-saturated world, vicarious experiences are the standard against which 'reality' is judged. Picking up the telephone, as you know, is no longer 'the next best thing to being there.' It is being there. As much consciousness is manifested there as through physical presence. We are moving into a period which may be described as post-postmodern. What is that? Or, as Northrop Frye used to say, 'Where is here?' This period may be best described as Millennialism.

Both democracy and totalitarianism recognize individualism and public opinion as sources of power. Both are strategies for coping in a relativistic world. Fascism and democracy become interchangeable in this convergence of technological control. The control of information is the real discourse of power. A new ideology emerges in which terrorism and manipulation are focused more obliquely on areas such as medical research, education, advertising and telecommunications. Creativity, the processing and distribution of ideas, are also subject to the effects of convergence, which is happening in society on more than the level of communications technology. Convergence is happening on a deeper philosophical level as well. As power shifts from the political-economic realm to the technological-economic world, the real power no longer lies with elected or appointed heads of states, but is in the hands of those who control and perpetuate an economy based on electronic technologies. Microsoft world domination is one tenable example. The encounter between Bill Gates and the pie-wielding anarchist group L'Entarteur in Brussels in January 1998 might best be described as 'just deserts.'

It is time to move beyond postmodernism, which has become a comfortable philosophy for privileged, white, and mostly male theorists – a sort of sociological/aesthetic 'laissez faire.' Misogyny has found a willing host in postmodern theory. Women's link to the physical world (ie. nature) is emphasized and this entitles postmodern theorists to dismiss women as anti-intellectual. Women have also suffered from the backlash – feminist philosophers who attempt to describe themselves as postmodernists are dismissed as being in denial of their physical nature (sex). Only men, apparently, can have it both ways and be good postmodernists.

Postmodernism has outlived its usefulness, and pragmatic feminism has been one near-casualty. In our recognition and analysis of the association which has been manufactured between discourse and power it is essential, as feminists such as Irigaray, Cixous and Kristeva have pointed out, that we understand language as a patriarchal construction. We do not all bestow significance on what we name and recognize, this is a privilege reserved for a select elite who attempt to define: politics, science, art, etc. The effectiveness of irony relies on what is not spoken and it is the irony inherent in postmodernism which may halt this treacherous slide across the thin surface of our collective unconscious and compulsion for 'naming.' Words have the power you give them; language cannot explain everything.

We must also be wary of postmodernism's obsession with the 'image' and the confusion of artistic technique with creation. In fact, creativity supersedes technique, and there is nothing to be gained, but much to be lost in proclaiming the 'end' or 'death' of art.

Within millennial theory, cyberfeminism must be defined from the perspective of North American pragmatism – not a utopian vision. I am looking for a feminism that works – right here, right now. A feminism which is inclusive of all cultures, of all genders. Anyone can play. Cyberfeminism is a starting point.

As control of information has become the new measure of power, de-industrialization of first world cultures and economies are throwing the democratic 'foundational' myths of progress and growth into a tailspin. The encouragement and protection of creative work will become increasingly problematic. And there is the potential for the feminist movement to outgrow its emergence as a North American phenomenon, and take a leading role on the world stage – by addressing issues such as diversity, the ubiquity of electronic technologies and transgender politics.

How does cyberfeminism fit into contemporary culture? What is it about de-industrialization and new media that has given rise to cyberfeminism? The answers I am able to propose address the persistence and future of art – electronic media art – as we approach the millennium. The transition from postmodernism to millennialism can be examined through the fields of evolutionary biology, philosophy and feminism. The processes of communication, simulation and sex are addressed through Richard Dawkins, Jean Baudrillard and Camille Paglia – Curly, Larry & PoMo.

Richard Dawkins, one of the leading thinkers in modern evolutionary biology, introduced the concept of the 'meme' over 20 years ago in order to point out how Darwinism and natural selection are not necessarily tied to genes, but can work wherever self-replicating code exists. The meme, therefore, was intended to explore the similarities between cultural and genetic evolution – in particular, how ideas, trends and other cultural representations develop and are spread through imitation, by word-of-mouth, and through mass media. The survival of the fittest ideas, transmitted through postmodern culture like disease – is a metaphor which tells us nothing new about biology, intelligence or communication – but a great deal about postmodern culture. Millennial Anxiety, the Jerusalem Syndrome, Intellectual Copyright, the persistence of Charismatic and Apocalyptic Religions, the Human Genome Project, the obligations of the Paparazzi – these describe the state of ethics in postmodern culture – wholesale desperation and chaos. In North America, Instrumentalist theory has replaced phenomenological thinking. The cycle of 'production – distribution – consumption' no longer merely describes our economic/political system, but is emerging as our new philosophy and psychology. 'Reductionist' accounts of human behavior diminish individual responsibility in acts of horrific violence by relying on a variety of genetic, chemical or nature-and-nurture explanations. Prozac. Twinkies. Multiple intelligences. The memes are flowing thick and fast. Significantly, Dawkins' theory of 'memes' does not deal adequately with creativity - how ideas originate, how they are developed and improved through processes which are dynamic and unquantifiable. He does not deal at all with the dissemination of ideas through means of complex pattern recognition – intuition, insight and telepathy. If Artificial Intelligence research ever breaks this particular code, there will be no looking back. However, Dawkins is a biologist. He is treading in dangerous, murky waters when his theories attempt to deal with creativity and the communication of ideas.

The patriarchal basis of postmodernism – whether 'reality' or simulation – remains virtually unchallenged. It is, in fact reinforced by Baudrillard in his theory of seduction which is proposed as a way of undermining systems and meaning, and promoting the process and role of simulation. Baudrillard envisions the feminine as an uncertainty principle, and seduction as its main strength. Manipulation, sedition – a woman's charms.

In Baudrillard's theory of seduction, he proposes the deliberate and provocative manipulation of signs as an alternative to production and communicative interaction. In essentializing the differences between the 'masculine' and the 'feminine,' Baudrillard's debt to Freud emerges. He is clearly not interested in any specific issues of women's social condition or feminist theory. In fact, in a paper titled 'Plastic Surgery for the Other'[1] he dismisses feminism as 'an example of hystericization of the masculine by women, a hysterical projection of their masculinity which follows exactly the hysterical projection by men of their femininity in the mythic image of a woman.' So, women project their masculinity in order to try to define themselves, men project their femininity in order to try to define – women. Presumably it is not necessary for men to try to define themselves – as there is one sexuality, one libido for Baudrillard as for Freud, and it is masculine.

There are women who agree with Baudrillard's attacks on feminism – and some of these women, by some perverse logic of appropriation, describe themselves as feminists. Camille Paglia, for example, is quoted as saying with apparent amazement 'They're calling anti-woman a woman who has spent hundreds of hours with her head between other women's legs. And who loves it!'[2] Imagine that.

In polite circles Paglia's position is described as a naturalistic celebration of sexuality. However, in her obsession with figures such as Madonna, we see the ultimate commodification of gender. Victimization as a play for power. Very close, in fact, to Baudrillard's description of seduction. And quite in keeping with Richard Dawkins' description of how ideas become embedded in the cultural fabric. Paglia describes the development of the position which she supports as originating in the earliest mother-cults, through the book of Genesis, to Freud with more to come, presumably, in her sequel to *Sexual Personae*.[3] Paglia's star may very well be fading, and she has not achieved the same international notoriety which she has enjoyed in North America. However, she is representative of the extreme interpretations to which postmodernism lends itself and the possible perversion of this philosophy in the service of an essentialism which attempts and often succeeds in describing itself as feminist. In postmodern culture, according to Baudrillard, we must doubt more than the value of our subjective experience but also the very existence of our subjectivity. The 'subject' (we are told) has disappeared into a whirling void of spectacular and philosophical dimensions. Feminists are dismissed, told to pay homage to technological determinism, seduction, and the inevitability of the feminine ideal. Individual experience is meaningless. Our power, we are told, is not to be had through any mastery of technology – but through an acceptance of our ability to exploit (ourselves) and to manipulate (men).

Repeating a predictable analogy between sexual physiology and culture, Paglia explains that men dominate art, science and politics because of their ability to 'project.' Women are valued (and doomed) solely through their relationship with nature. Freud asserted that women lack even the capacity for pleasurable spectatorship because they lack the masculine ability to fetishize and thereby separate themselves from an object. And now that the 'object' has been replaced by a simulation, Baudrillard would say we are twice removed.

Cyberfeminism recognizes that it is precisely due to our culturally enforced distance from technology, that women are in a position to explore the three tenets of feminism after post-modernism, through artistic practice: diversity, the ubiquity of technology and transgender politics. If we lack the capacity for spectatorship, we have the capacity for action. If we lack the masculine 'ability' to fetishize technology, then we are able to understand that culture is not what you live in, but what you live through.

The individualization of feminist politics by postmodernists has demobilized women. Theorists such as Baudrillard reject Europe as a model for postmodernism because of a continental pre-occupation with difference. Disregard for difference is what he sees as America's strength. However, postmodern feminism has been largely defined by European feminists and encour-ages the idea of difference, in some sense precluding solidarity. The first written reference to 'individualism' was made by Alexis de Tocqueville, in his investigation of American democra-cy. And yet, it is North American feminists who have the history and background to support a claim that it is as a mass movement and philosophy that feminism has real power for change.

Pluralism is one postmodern concept which feminism finds no argument with, due to its widely divergent approaches within specific cultures as well as throughout the world. The usefulness of connections and dislocations, the integrity and relevance of different perspec-tives becomes particularly apparent when the site of intersection is artistic practice. There is considerably more to cultural diversity than knowing where to find the best of various 'ethnic' restaurants — and knowing what to order when you get there. Appropriation is a strategy to be avoided. And there is more to an awareness of technological ubiquity than having an email account and knowing how to use it. Being a woman and using new technologies, does not (automatically) mean you are liberated. This is what I describe as separating the cyber-femmes from the cyberfeminists. Furthermore, the promotion of transgender politics involves support for authentic expression of individual sex/gender, not the license to 'seduce' and fuck anything that moves. Diversity, technological ubiquity, transgender politics — these are all related. For example, it was through the debate surrounding the supposed 'disappearance' of the body in cyberspace and through VR technologies, that transgender politics emerged as an issue which cyberfeminism must address. Transgender politics is the most fascinating aspect of cyberfeminism — faking gender, trying on gender, multiple genders. When we moved past religion it was feared that we would believe in nothing. In fact, we have gained the ability to believe in anything. With transgender politics it is not so much that we lose definitions of gender but that anything goes. Coming soon to Hollywood (Brandon Lee, [4]Kyoko Date[5]) — identity as fleeting as the flicker of pixels.

Cyberfeminism is an opportunity for us to see the cracks in postmodernism - and the theories of Baudrillard, Dawkins and Paglia. Women are not destined to be victims, seductresses or mothers by virtue of sex or gender. We are not doomed to reiterate currently or historically popular 'memes' of femininity. Cyberfeminism is active, subversive and inclusive – of all cultures, of all genders and of technologies regardless (but not with disregard) of their origins. Creativity is not a scientific theory and it is not a sociological, psychological or philosophical phenomenon. Part mystical, part spiritual – combining insight, intuition and telepathy – advanced pattern recognition systems. The ability to simultaneously create metaphors and mythologies without precursors.

notes

1 Jean Baudrillard, "Plastic Surgery for the Other" Figures de L'altérité, Jean Baudrillard, Marc Guillaume (Paris: Descartes, 1994).

2 "Hurricane Camille reaks Havoc!" Imagine Magazine. *San Francisco Chronicle* 27, Sept 1992.

3 Camille Paglia, *Sexual Personae: Art and Decadence from Nefertiti to Emily Dickenson* (new Haven: Yale University Press, 1990).

4 *Kyoto Date*, computer software. Visual Science Laboratory, 1996. Kyoko Date is the teen singing sensation created by the Japanese modelling agency HoriPro and the engineers at Visual Science Laboratory. She was built from scratch and constructed with 40,000 polygons.

5 *The Crow*, Director Alex Proyas. 1994. This adaptation of the underground comic classic in which the superhero has returned from beyond the grave, starred Brandon Lee, who was killed during its filming.

technology ≠ art nancy paterson

One consequence of the recent proliferation of new electronic technologies is the erosion of philosophical distinctions between the body and the brain that dominated scientific and philosophical thought for most of the nineteenth and twentieth centuries. As the Cartesian body/mind split between physical/biological and rational/intellectual processes is challenged, the debate which distinguishes between chemical processes in the brain and more abstract mental operations such as metacognition and creativity is also in a state of flux. New electronic media compel us to re-think the body's relationship to technology.

The body is far from absent in the discussion of the political, economic and cultural impact of interactive media such as virtual reality technologies and their application. But whose (generic) body are we talking about? Issues of representation, access and diversity of cultural experience are undermined attributes of our bodies in these debates.

The experience of interaction in a computer-generated environment, a definitive paradigm of VR, was inaugurated in the early 1960s when Ivan Sutherland, working out of the University of Utah, developed a head-mounted display that allowed the user to look around a virtual landscape. Two small cathode ray tubes driven by vector graphics generators provided the appropriate stereo view for each eye. In the early 1970s, Fred Brooks at the University of North Carolina created a system for handling graphic objects using a mechanical manipulator. Around the same time, Myron Krueger began experimenting with interactive environments for unencumbered, full body, multi-sensory participation in computer-generated events. The intense (although not widespread) excitement inspired by such experiments was accompanied by confusion and a sense of unease. Not since the Industrial Revolution had new technologies so directly challenged our sense of physical being as well as consciousness.

"What is new about cyberspace is not so much the underlying technologies, but the way they are packaged and applied to a new way of thinking about computers and their relationship to human experience. Under the old way of looking at things, computers were regarded as tools for the mind, where the mind was regarded as a disembodied intellect. Under the new paradigm, computers are regarded as engines for new worlds of experience, and the body is regarded as inseparable from the mind." [1]

Head-mounted displays, data gloves, body suits — these systems oversee the user's spatial position and orientation with devices that track eye movement, heart rate, depth and rate of each breath taken. In VR, the body becomes an essential component of the cybernetic cycle of data input, analysis and feedback in what has been described as a systemic relationship of surveillance and control. The presence and significance of the body is indisputable. The early designers and proponents of virtual reality expressed an interest in utilizing these new tools and systems to break down barriers between class, race and gender. The disappearance of the body, however, was not an original intention. Although

Hollywood seems determined to sell us a vision of VR as a means for escaping from the body, it is increasingly apparent that the body itself has never been more present. Our physical attendance and participation has become the interface itself.

Perhaps the discussion around the "disappearance" of the body have taken our attention when we should be thinking about the disappearance or nonexistence of critical and aesthetic discourse in the field of new media art itself. An appropriate question is whether artists have missed the critical moment in the development of these new media when these issues might have been raised. Have we missed the boat entirely? For many years, the economics and politics of technological research and design have dictated the type of work being done in these fields. Aesthetic considerations and questions about content have taken a back seat to concentration on performance improvements in personal computers and the development of low cost yet powerful 3-D rendering engines. The need for support (primarily funding) has meant that the applications chosen for development reflect the influence of the US military, which invested heavily in the potential of these media for battlefield simulations and training.

As a case in point, the Architecture Machine Group at the Massachusetts Institute of Technology produced the revolutionary "Aspen Movie Map" in 1978-79, funded by the US military's "Defense Advanced Research Projects Agency" (DARPA). Numerous artists participated in this and related projects — their justification being that they could not otherwise afford or gain access to the expensive, high-end tools of the trade. Many individuals who benefited from the military funding for such projects went on to become permanent fixtures of the new media art scene, receiving sponsorships at media arts organizations in the US, Germany and Canada for projects showcasing the latest in VR and other new electronic technologies.

Drawing on her background in theater, Brenda Laurel describes the central controversy in VR as "the questions of whether virtual worlds and the experiences people may have in them are or are not designed."[2] If we forgo involvement in system design, allowing our experience of virtual worlds to be limited to systems designed for us, what responsibility are we willing or able to undertake for the types of experiences triggered by these systems?

It is no coincidence that the first Canadian "Playdium" opened by Sega is in a suburban mega-mall, thirty minutes by car outside of Toronto. Anyone looking for a quick, cheap (video) thrill can find satisfaction on the Yonge Street strip in downtown Toronto. But for those who can afford a more substantial investment of both time and money, more intense (virtual) pleasures await at the "Playdium." It offers an opportunity to experience the twenty-first century body — hard wired and in an intimate relationship with technology — in a context designed by and for a very specific sector of the population. The bodies it speaks to and about are white, Western and mostly male, reinforcing the debt owed by the designers of VR to capitalist and military mentors.

Notable as exceptions are the VR artworks of Char Davies and Brenda Laurel. Although these women are working from positions of privilege within the software industry, they must be credited with having taken the first tentative steps toward addressing an aesthetic that has been otherwise dominated by consumerism and militarism.

Char Davies, a principle at Softimage (Montreal) prior to its purchase by Microsoft created *Osmose* which she proposes as representing an alternative aesthetic for VR — one that encourages reflection and contemplation as well as a profound awareness of the body. This work is experienced in solitude. The immersant can explore several interconnected worlds, but cannot touch or change them. Translucency, subtlety of texture and spatial ambiguity describe the objects and environments that are encountered. There is no goal or mission in *Osmose*. Wearing a head-mounted display and a vest that monitors breathing, the immersant navigates through lush and abstract landscapes,utilizing the underwater breathing and learning techniques of scuba diving.Encouraged to let go of habitual percep-tions of space, the immersant must re-experience the body and its relationship to the world.

Brenda Laurel of Interval Research recently started a company called Purple Moon[3] that designs software specifically for girls and young women. It is one of a handful of companies that are considering women's needs, as compared to the many hundreds that are designing software for an adolescent male audience. Laurel's work at Interval Corp. and Purple Moon has placed her, like Davies, in a position to challenge (at least) the gender bias that has dominated VR design and development. In residence at the Banff Centre in 1993, Laurel designed a VR work with Rachel Strickland titled *Placeholder*. In this work, unlike *Osmose*, multiple users interact with each other as they explore, separately and together, several "worlds" that are connected by portals. Each participant is originally assigned a pictographic representation of an animal, for example, "snake," "crow,"and "spider." This is how they are seen by the other participants. These "costumes" lend certain powers to the wearer, but also certain limitations that quickly become apparent. "Costumes" may be exchanged or discard-ed, and so the participants are empowered to choose the body in which they are most com-fortable. The interaction between people (and animals), the places that they choose to inhabit, and the way that this relationship is described and manifested ("the places here are marked with many voices") is the focus of this work.

Both *Osmose* and *Placeholder* are exceptional media works that attempt to contribute to the development of a critical aesthetic in this field. Artists experience the same challenge as the rest of the population in gaining access to new technologies and maintaining a com-petitive level of media literacy. However, simply putting new electronic technologies in the reach and hands of artists does not equal art. Whatever our class, race or gender, we all take our bodies with us as we approach the millennium. We can only buy so much techno-logical confidence. The rest must comes from art and artist like Davies and Laurel who crit-ically envision a creative future in which we all take part.

notes

1 Randal Walser, "Elements of a Cyberspace Playhouse" in *Virtual Reality: Theory, Practice and Promise*, ed. Sandra K. Helsel and Judith Paris Roth (Westport, Connecticut: Meckler,1991), p. 53.

2 Brenda Laurel, "Virtual Reality Design: A Personal View" in *Virtual Reality: Theory, Practice and Promise*, op. cit., p. 95.

3 Purple Moon has since been purchased by Mattel.

bio nancy paterson

exhibitions

2000 *The Library*[2], Seneca@York, School of
Communication Arts. Toronto, ON
Faculty Exhibition, ON College of Art &
Design, Toronto, ON
Siggraph 2000, New Orleans Convention
Centre, New Orleans, Louisiana
3D/VRML2000, Monterey Conference
Centre, Monterey, California
Second Nature, Surrey Art Gallery, Surrey, BC

1999 *SEAFair 99: e-FUSION*, Museum of the City
of Skopje, Skopje, Macedonia
Game Girls, InterAccess Gallery, Toronto, ON
War Zones: Present Tense, ArtSpeak
Gallery, Vancouver, BC

1998 *Interface*, Canadian Museum of Contemporary
Photography/National Gallery, Ottawa, ON
Women Beyond Borders, Dufferin Mall &
tour, Toronto, ON
Stock Market Skirt: Burn-In Test, Bell
Centre for Creative Communications,
Toronto, ON
The Medusa Project (Autobiography),
Thames Art Gallery, Chatham, ON

1997 *The Medusa Project (Autobiography)*,
Thunder Bay Art Gallery, Thunder Bay, ON
The Machine in the Garden, Canadian
Cultural Centre, Paris, France
Language Games, Walter Phillips Gallery,
Banff, AB
How the Rest Was Won, McLaughlin
Gallery, Oshawa, ON
CyberLisbon, Centro Cultural de Belem,
Lisbon, Portugal
Myths from Cyberspace, Koffler Gallery,
Toronto, ON

1996 *How the Rest Was Won*, McIntosh Gallery.
London, ON
InterAktiv, Ars Electronica, Landesmuseum,
Linz, Austria

1996 *The Bridge*, Siggraph 96, New Orleans
Convention Centre, New Orleans, Louisiana
Technology as Art II, The New Gallery,
Calgary, AB

1995 *Net@Works*, Centro Nacional de las Artes,
Mexico City, Mexico
The Machine in the Garden, Art Gallery of
St. Thomas, St. Thomas, ON
Sixth International Symposium on
Electronic Art, Montreal, QC
Welcome to the Electric Skin, Gallery 401,
Toronto, ON
Mediaworks by Nancy Paterson, Art Gallery
of Peterborough, Peterborough, ON
The Processing of Perception, Ohio State,
ACCAD, Columbus, Ohio

1994 *Nancy Paterson: Cyberfeminism*, Lynnwood
Art Centre, Simcoe, ON
TechnoArt, ON Science Centre, Toronto, ON
Dreaming of You, Garnet Press Gallery,
Toronto, ON
The Machine in the Garden, Woodstock
Public Art Gallery, Woodstock, ON

1993 *Machine Culture*, SIGGRAPH 93, Anaheim
Convention Centre, Anaheim, California
Perspectives, Proximities, Perceptions,
Montage 93, Strong Museum, Rochester,
New York
Claiming Machines, SAW Gallery, Ottawa, ON

1992 *Third International Symposium on Electronic
Art*, Museum of Contemporary Art,
Sydney, Australia
InterActiva, Koln, Germany
EXPO 92, Canada Pavilion, Seville, Spain
Out of the Drawer, WARC Exhibition, A
Space, Toronto, ON

1991 *TeleVisions*, PRIM, Montreal, QC

1990 *Second International Symposium on
Electronic Art*, Groningen, The Netherlands

1990 *A Thick Book of Ideas*, Museum Fodor,
      Amsterdam, The Netherlands
      European Media Arts Festival, Osnabruk,
      Germany
      Recent Works, White Water Gallery, North
      Bay, ON
      Machinations, Galerie UQAM, Montreal, QC
      Fault Line, Art Gallery of Northumberland,
      Cobourg, ON
      Interactive Works, Gairloch Art Gallery,
      Oakville, ON
1989 *Machinations*, Centre Culturel, Trois
      Rivieres, QC
      Artware: Artists' Bookworks, A Space,
      Toronto, ON
      Hair Salon TV, Centre for Art Tapes,
      Halifax, NS
1988 *Guerilla Tactics*, MacDonald Stewart Art
      Centre, Guelph, ON
      Robert McLaughlin Gallery, Oshawa, ON
      Siting Technology, Norman MacKenzie
      Gallery, Regina, SK
      The Lunatic of One Idea, Public Access
      Videowall Project, Mississauga, ON
1987 *Siting Technology*, Walter Phillips Gallery,
      Banff, AB
      Guerilla Tactics, A Space, Toronto, ON
1983 Digicon 83, Robson Square Media Centre,
      Vancouver, BC
      Women and Architecture, Artculture
      Resource Centre. Toronto, ON
1982 *Signal Breakdown: Ear to the World*,
      Artculture Resource Centre/ARS ELEC-
      TRONICA. Toronto, ON/Linz, AUS

lectures

1999 *Ethics & Aesthetics: New Media Art*,
      University of Victoria, Fine Art Dept.
      Victoria, BC
      The $9.95 Project, Video Verite. Saskatoon,
      SK
      Serving Up New Media Art, Dunlop Art
      Gallery. Regina, SK
      *Electronics & Spiritualism: A Scientific
      Alliance*, Subtle Technologies Conference,
      Toronto, ON
      Visionary Speakers Series: *6DOS: THE
      LIBRARY*, Interactive Multimedia Arts &
      Technology Association (IMAT), Toronto, ON
1998 *Curly, Larry & PoMo*, ASTARTI Conference,
      Paris, France
      Stock Market Skirt, Carnegie Mellon
      University, Art & Robotics Group,
      Pittsburgh, Pennsylvania
      Curly, Larry & PoMo, College Art
      Association Conference, Toronto, ON
1997 *New Media Focus: Interactive Television*,
      Web TV, Banff Television Festival, Banff,
      AB (panel)
      Cyberfeminism, Vancouver Electronic Art
      Festival, Vancouver, Canada
      Cyberfeminism, Frauen Film Festival,
      Dortmund, Germany
      Lust & Wanderlust, Seminole Community
      College. Sanford, Florida
      Cyberfeminism, Kunst und Ausstellungshalle
      der Bundesrepublik Deutschland, Bonn,
      Germany
1996 *Technology as Environment and Technology
      Interventions on the Body*, University of
      Calgary, Calgary, AB (panel)
      True Lies/Digital Decentre, Media Forum
      96, Toronto, ON (panel)
1995 *Cyberfeminism*, Centro Nacional de las
      Artes, Mexico City, Mexico
      Cyberfeminism, Sixth International
      Symposium on Electronic Art, Montreal,
      QC (panel)

1995 *Rituals for Future Bodies*, Images: Festival of Independent Film & Video, Toronto, ON (panel)

Understanding Multimedia, Daytona Beach Community College, Daytona Beach, Florida

Colonialism, Tourism & Virtual Voyeurism, Fotobase Gallery, Vancouver, BC (panel), (The Spectacular State)

Lust & Wanderlust-Sex & Tourism in a Virtual World, Video In, Vancouver, BC, 1995

Cyberfeminism, University of BC, Vancouver, BC

1994 *The Virtual Museum: Electronic Ghetto or Interactive Future*, InterAccess, Toronto, ON (panel)

Creative Applications of New Technology, University of Western ON, London, ON

Cyberspace, Virtual Systems and Interactive Media, Images: Festival of Independent Film & Video, Toronto, ON (panel)

The Surprise Party: A Festival of Art, Theory & Electronic Desire, University of Florida, Gainesville, Florida (series of lectures and workshops)

1993 *Siggraph '93: Machine Culture*, Information Technology Design Centre, Toronto, ON

Art in Electronic Media: Machine Culture, Siggraph ACM Toronto, Toronto, ON

Creative Potential of Optical Discs, SAW Gallery, Ottawa, ON

Cyberspace, Virtual Reality and the Body, InterAccess, Toronto, ON (panel)

1992 *Lust & Wanderlust-Sex & Tourism in a Virtual World*, Third International Symposium on Electronic Art, Sydney, Australia

education

1986 Brock University (MEd)

1985 University of Toronto, Victoria College (BA Hons)

1983 ON College of Art (A.O.C.A.)

professional activities

2000 Visiting Artist, Seneca @ York

1996 Artist in Residence, Bell Centre for Creative Communications

1990 Instructor, ON College of Art & Design

1985 Charles Street Video, Facilities Manager

published articles/papers

"Curly, Larry & PoMo: Cyberfeminismus und Millenialismus." *Vision Ruhr,*. Westfalisches Industriemuseum Zeche Zollern II/IV und Meseum am Ostwall, Dortmund. Hatje Cantz Verlag, 2000.

"Cyberfeminizam." *Cyberfeminizam*, Centar za zenske studije, Zagreb, 1999.

"Cyberfeminismus." Der Sinn Der Sinne, *Steidl* (Germany), 1998.

"Technology (does not equal) Art." *Fuse*, Fall 1997.

"Cyberfeminism." *Fireweed*, Summer 1996.

"Towards Cyberfeminism." *Matriart*, August 1994.

"Lust & Wanderlust-Sex & Tourism in a Virtual World." *Media Information Australia*, Fall 1993.

"Feministiche Asthetik im Zeitalter des Technischen Utopismus." Feministiche Streifzuge Durch's Punkte Universum, *Femme Totale* (Germany), March 1993.

"BCTV: EXPO 92 Installation." *Leonardo*, Vol. 25 #2, 1992.

"Bicycle TV: Some Interactive Exercise." *Leonardo*, Vol 24 #4, 1991.

"Wringer/Washer TV." *Leonardo*, Vol. 24 #1, 1991.

"Hair Salon TV." *Leonardo*, Vol. 24 #1, 1991.

"Art, Technology & Public Policy, Part II." *Parallelogramme*, Summer 1990.

"Focus on Oliver Kelhammer and Janice Bowley." *Canadian Art*, Spring 1990.

"Misplaced Affection." *Leonardo*, Vol. 20 #3, 1987.

"Curating Video." *Cinema Canada*, March 1987.

"Contemporary Art and Technology: The New Ecological Era." *Art Is Communication*, Exhibition catalogue, November 1985.

"Art, Technology & Public Policy." *Parallelogramme*, Summer 1984.

"Rock Video/Video Art: An Historical Survey of Video Art and Contemporary Music." *Videoguide*, Summer 1983.

"Women and Architecture." *Fifth Column*, April 1983.

"Taboo Subjects: Rachel Rosenthal and Guiditta Tornetta." *Arts Canada*, November 1982.

catalogues

The Medusa Project, Thames Art Gallery, 1998.

How The Rest Was Won, London, ON, 1996.

Ars Electronica - Memesis, Linz, Austria, 1996.

Siggraph 96 Visual Proceedings, New Orleans, Louisiana, 1996.

Net@Works, Centro Nacional de las Artes, Mexico City, 1995.

S.I.S.E.A. Exhibition Catalogue, Montreal, QC, 1995. (CD-ROM/text)

Cyberfeminism, Peterborough, ON, 1995.

The Processing Of Perception, Columbus, Ohio, 1995. (CD-ROM/text)

Technoart, Toronto, ON, 1994.

Siggraph 93: Machine Culture, Anaheim, California, 1993.

T.I.S.E.A. Exhibition Catalogue, Sydney, Australia, 1992.

Onatrio Arts Council Annual Report, Toronto, ON, 1992.

Televisions, PRIM, Montreal, QC, 1991.

A Thick Book Of Ideas, Museum Fodor, Amsterdam, The Netherlands, 1990.

S.I.S.E.A. Exhibition Cataloque, Groningen, The Netherlands, 1990.

European Media Arts Festival, Osnabruk, West Germany, 1990.

Machinations, Louis Poissant, (Canadian tour), 1990.

Interactive Works, Dale Barrett, Oakville, ON, 1989.

Siting Technology, Daina Augaitis, Banff, AB, 1987.

selected press reviews

Rickwood. "Virtually As Easy as 1, 2, 3." *New Media Pro*, October 2000

Sherrin & Bell. "War Zones." *Blackflash* Vol. 17, #2

Perra, Daniele. "Navigando In Rete Con Gli Artisti." *Tema Celeste* (Milan). Maggio-Giugno, 1999.

Rickwood, Lee "Virtual Library Project: Waiting for the Future" *New Media Pro*, May 1999.

Pescovitz, David. "Be There Now." *Flash Art*, March/April 1999.

Silva, Horacio. "Style Bytes." *Harper's Bazaar & Mode*, September 1998.

Wawzonek, Donna "Close Encounters of the Technological Kind." *The Ottawa Citizen*, June 8, 1998.

Silva, Horacio. "Stock Frock." *Dutch*, #165, 1998.

Deepwell, Katy. "Women Artists Online." *N.Paradoxa*. Vol. 2, 1998.

Rickwood, Lee. "Electronic Media Artist Meets Her (Dress) Maker." *New Media.Pro*, May 1998.

Mirapaul, Matt. "Watching the Hemline and the Bottom Line, On Line." *New York Times*, *Cybertimes*, Feb. 5, 1998.

Hume, Chris. "Of Stocks and Bodices." *Toronto Star*, Feb. 5, 1998.

Cossette, Angie."Art Display at BCCC Melds Fashion and Technology." *The Courier*. Feb. 5, 1998.

Hansen, Sue. "Clothes-Minded Artist Plays the Stock Market." *East York Observer*, Jan. 30, 1998.

Mintz, Fredrica. "WE Focus: Nancy Paterson." *WE Magazine*, Fall/Winter 1997/98.

Miller, Earl. "Myths from Cyberspace." *Parachute*, Summer 1997.

Hoover, Michael & Stokes, Lisa. "Nancy Paterson: Live Wire." *Orlando Weekly*, Feb. 13-19, 1997.

"Electronics Artist to Give Lecture on Virtual Reality." *Orlando Sentinel*, Feb. 18, 1997.

Orzessek, Arno. "Seid nett zu den Maschinen!" *Suddeutsche Zeitung*, Munchen. Feb. 7, 1997.

Rickwood, Lee. "No Need for Weatherman..." *VPM*

Magazine. October 1996.

"Envisioning our Machine Future." *Sculpture*, July/August 1996.

Palmer, Rodney. "Multimedia Survival Kit: Who to Know -The Digerati." *Shift Magazine*, November 1995.

Rickwood, Noel. "New Media Artists Use Video Technology to Challenge Status Quo." *VPM Magazine*, March 1995.

Gustafson, Paula. "The Spectacular State Warns of Fascism's Contemporary Forms." *The Georgia Straight* (Vancouver, BC), February 10-17, 1995.

O'Donnell, Susan. "In Search of the Arts Lane of the Information Highway." *Proscenium*, March/April 1994.

"Nancy Paterson." *Intercommunication #7* (Japan), Winter 1994.

"Lynnwood Snags Successful Computer/Electronic Artist." *The Simcoe Times*, October 11, 1994.

Meads, Mickey & Curtis, Holly. "Art World: Woodstock Art Gallery." *Scene Magazine*, #143

Boucher, Mario. "Gamblers Will Love New Art Show." *Woodstock Daily Sentinel Review*, January 13, 1994.

Liebner, Judy. "Video Won't Threaten Older Forms, Artist Says." *London Free Press*, January 10, 1994.

"Jurrasic Park met z'n dinosaurussen beheerst Siggraph" *Wim van der Plas*, Av Prof #10 (The Netherlands), 1993.

Farah, Mary Ann. "Machines in the Garden." *Parallelogramme*, Spring 1993.

"Women in Science and Technology" *Canadian Woman Studies Journal*, Winter 1993.

Marchessault, Janine. "Incorporating the Gaze." *Parachute*, Winter 1992.

Lapage, Jocelyn. "Le Printemps de PRIM: Les Arcades Culturelle de L'Avenir." *La Presse*, May 25, 1991.

Carriere, Daniel. "Quand Les Machines Revent." *Le Devoir*, May 18, 1991.

Siberok, Martin. "Switch Or." *Montreal Mirror*, May 16, 1991.

Zimner, Wendlin. "Anregend, Aber Nicht Aufregend." *Neu Oz* (Osnabruk, Germany), September 13, 1990.

LePages, Jocelyn. "Les Machinations Diaboliques." *La Presse*, January 1990.

Cron, Marie Michele. "Science Friction." *Voir*, January 1990.

Vander Vennen, Mark. "Matter of Scale." *Cobourg Times*, January 1990.

Wood, William. "By the Lake: The Lunatic of One Idea." *Public*, November 1989.

Proulx, Louis Serge. "A Plein Dans L'Art Gadget." *Journal De Trois Rivieres*, May 1989.

Hubbard, Jackie. "Interactive Works." *Oakville Today*, July 27, 1989.

Werner, Hans. "This Time the Medium is Really the Message." *Toronto Star*, July 22, 1989.

Rochon, Lisa. "High Tech Works Take Their Cue From Computers." *Globe & Mail*, June 25, 1987.

Hume, Chris. "Art Exhibit Gets a Laugh Out of Technology." *Toronto Star*, June 19, 1987.

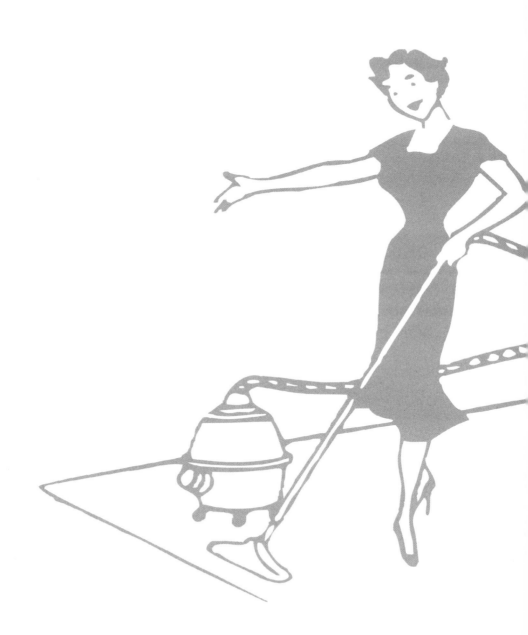